HUMAN BEHAVIOR, LEARNING,
AND THE DEVELOPING BRAIN

Human Behavior, Learning, and the Developing Brain

ATYPICAL DEVELOPMENT

EDITED BY

Donna Coch
Geraldine Dawson
Kurt W. Fischer

THE GUILFORD PRESS
New York   London

© 2007 The Guilford Press
A Division of Guilford Publications, Inc.
72 Spring Street, New York, NY 10012
www.guilford.com

Paperback edition 2010

Printed in the United States of America

This book is printed on acid-free paper.

Last digit is print number: 9 8 7 6 5 4 3 2

Library of Congress Cataloging-in-Publication Data

Human behavior, learning, and the developing brain : atypical development / edited by Donna Coch, Geraldine Dawson, Kurt W. Fischer.

   p. cm.
  Includes bibliographical references and index.
  ISBN 978-1-59385-137-8 (hardcover: alk. paper)
  ISBN 978-1-60623-966-7 (paperback: alk. paper)
  1. Developmental disabilities. 2. Developmental psychobiology.
3. Cognitive neuroscience. I. Coch, Donna. II. Dawson, Geraldine.
III. Fischer, Kurt W.
  [DNLM: 1. Developmental Disabilities. 2. Child Development Disorders, Pervasive. 3. Learning Disorders. 4. Neurobehavioral
Manifestations. 5. Brain—growth & development. 6. Child. 7. Infant.
WS 350.6 H9178 2007]
  RJ506.D47H86 2007
  618.92′8—dc22

                                             2006029878

About the Editors

Donna Coch, EdD, is Assistant Professor in the Department of Education at Dartmouth College. She earned a doctoral degree from the Harvard University Graduate School of Education and conducted postdoctoral research at the University of Oregon. Using a noninvasive brain wave recording technique, Dr. Coch's research focuses on what happens in the brain as children learn how to read, particularly in terms of phonological and orthographic processing. A goal of both her research and teaching is to make meaningful connections between the fields of developmental cognitive neuroscience and education.

Geraldine Dawson, PhD, is Professor of Psychology at the University of Washington, where she is also Director of the Autism Center. She has had an active career as a scientist and clinician specializing in autism and the effects of experience on early brain development, and is internationally recognized for her pioneering research on early diagnosis and brain function in autism and early biological risk factors for psychopathology. Dr. Dawson has published over 125 scientific articles and chapters on these topics, and edited or authored a number of books, including *Autism: Nature, Diagnosis, and Treatment* (1989), *Human Behavior and the Developing Brain* (1994), and *A Parent's Guide to Asperger Syndrome and High-Functioning Autism: How to Meet the Challenges and Help Your Child Thrive* (2002), all published by The Guilford Press. She has been the recipient of continuous research funding from the National Institutes of Health for her studies on autism and child psychopathology.

Kurt W. Fischer, PhD, is Charles Bigelow Professor of Education and Human Development at the Harvard University Graduate School of Education and founder and director of the program in Mind, Brain, and Education. He studies cognitive and emotional development from birth through adulthood, combining analysis of the commonalities across people with the diversity of pathways of learning and development. Dr. Fischer's studies concern students' learning and problem solving, brain development, concepts of self in relationships, cultural contributions to social-cognitive development, reading skills, emotions, and child abuse. One product of Dr. Fischer's research is a single scale for measuring learning, teaching, and curriculum across domains, which is being used to assess and coordinate key aspects of pedagogy and assessment in schools. He is the author of several books as well as over 200 scientific articles. Leading an international movement to connect biology and cognitive science to education, Dr. Fischer is founding president of the International Mind, Brain, and Education Society and the new journal *Mind, Brain, and Education.*

Contributors

Emma K. Adam, PhD, School of Education and Social Policy, Program in Human Development and Social Policy, Northwestern University, Evanston, Illinois. Her research focuses on how everyday life factors such as work, school, and family relationships influence levels of stress, health, and well-being in parents and their children, and how stress affects children's behavioral, cognitive, and emotional development.

Catherine C. Ayoub, EdD, Risk and Prevention Program, Harvard Graduate School of Education, Cambridge, Massachusetts, and Department of Psychiatry, Harvard Medical School, Boston, Massachusetts. She is a counseling psychologist and nurse with interests in the impact of childhood trauma and the development and evaluation of prevention and intervention systems in the educational, mental health, and legal arenas.

Theodore P. Beauchaine, PhD, Department of Psychology, University of Washington, Seattle, Washington. His research interests include the autonomic and central nervous system substrates of psychopathology; biobehavioral models of inhibition, disinhibition, and emotion dysregulation; advanced research methods; and taxometrics.

Francine M. Benes, MD, PhD, Program in Structural and Molecular Neuroscience, McLean Hospital, Belmont, Massachusetts, and Program in Neuroscience and Department of Psychiatry, Harvard Medical School, Boston, Massachusetts. Her research program uses a combination of neuroanatomical, electrophysiological, molecular, and cellular approaches to investigate limbic lobe circuitry, particularly the GABA and glutamate systems, in relation to normal and abnormal development.

Raphael Bernier, MA, Child Clinical Psychology Program, University of Washington, Seattle, Washington. His current research interests concern the neuroscience of social impairments in autism.

Elizabeth J. Carter, MA, Department of Psychological and Brain Sciences, Duke University, Durham, North Carolina. She is interested in using neuroimaging techniques to detect changes throughout development in the neural substrates underlying social perception abilities, particularly in individuals with autism.

Geraldine Dawson, PhD (see "About the Editors").

Stanislas Dehaene, PhD, INSERM, Cognitive Neuroimaging Unit, Service Hospitalier Frédéric Joliot of the Atomic Energy Commission, Orsay, France. His research investigates the neural bases of human cognitive functions such as reading, calculation, and language, with a particular interest in the differences between conscious and nonconscious processing.

Lisa M. Gatzke-Kopp, PhD, Department of Psychology, University of Washington, Seattle, Washington. Her research focuses on the neurobiological substrates of externalizing disorders and influences on central nervous system development leading to psychopathology.

Usha Goswami, PhD, Centre for Neuroscience in Education, Faculty of Education, University of Cambridge, Cambridge, England. Her research interests include the relation between phonology and reading across languages, with special reference to auditory temporal processing, rhyme and analogy in reading acquisition, and rhyme processing in dyslexic and deaf children's reading.

Elena L. Grigorenko, PhD, Child Study Center and PACE Center, Yale University, New Haven, Connecticut, and Department of Psychology, Moscow State University, Moscow, Russia. Her primary research interest is in understanding the contributions of genetic and environmental risk factors to developmental and learning disabilities in children, with specific interest in the risk factors for language and mathematical disabilities, autism, and violent criminal behaviors in young children.

Megan R. Gunnar, PhD, College of Education and Human Development, Institute of Child Development, University of Minnesota, Minneapolis, Minnesota. Her research focuses on the emotional and social processes that regulate physiological responses to stressful events in early childhood.

Bonnie Klimes-Dougan, PhD, Department of Psychiatry, University of Minnesota, Minneapolis, Minnesota. Her research with youth at risk for depression and those experiencing depressive and suicidal symptoms focuses on understanding how disruptions in the stress reactivity system may place individuals at risk for depression.

Frederique Liegeois, PhD, Developmental Cognitive Neuroscience Unit, Institute of Child Health, University College London, and Great Ormond Street Hospital for Children, London, England. Her research and clinical work are focused on the diagnosis and neurorehabilitation of language and motor–speech disorders in young people with acute brain injury or disease.

Dennis L. Molfese, PhD, Psychological and Brain Sciences, University of Louisville, Louisville, Kentucky. His research interests include developmental changes in brain, language, and cognitive processes; predicting cognitive and linguistic skills from infancy; electrophysiological measures of learning and intervention strategies in infancy and early childhood; cognitive functions in adults with head injuries; and factors underlying lateralization of language and cognitive functions.

Peter J. Molfese, BS, Psychological and Brain Sciences, University of Louisville, Louisville, Kentucky. His research interests include language, learning, human–computer interactions, neuroanalysis, and source localization.

Victoria J. Molfese, PhD, Center for Research in Early Childhood, University of Louisville, Louisville, Kentucky. Her research interests include factors affecting intelligence and achievement test performance in preschool- and school-age children, prediction of developmental delay, and the identification and prediction of early reading skills in preschool children.

Angela Morgan, PhD, Developmental Cognitive Neuroscience Unit, Institute of Child Health, University College London, and Great Ormond Street Hospital for Children, London, England. Her research and clinical work focus on the use of objective techniques to improve the diagnosis of motor–speech impairment in pediatric populations with developmental and acquired impairments.

Charles A. Nelson, PhD, Developmental Medicine Center, Laboratory of Cognitive Neuroscience, Harvard Medical School and Boston Children's Hospital, Boston, Massachusetts. His research interests are broadly concerned with the effects of early experience on the brain and behavioral development; his specific interests are concerned with memory development and the development of face and object recognition.

Kevin A. Pelphrey, PhD, Department of Psychological and Brain Sciences, Duke University, Durham, North Carolina. His research focuses on the development and neural basis of social, cognitive, and affective information processing in children with and without autism, with a specific interest in the development of the functional organization of the human brain for social perception.

Gabrielle Rappolt-Schlichtmann, EdM, Human Development and Psychology, Harvard University Graduate School of Education, Cambridge, Massachusetts. Her research focuses on the relationships among stress, brain development, and social systems.

Daniela Plesa Skwerer, PhD, Lab of Developmental Cognitive Neuroscience, Department of Anatomy and Neurobiology, Boston University School of Medicine, Boston, Massachusetts. Her work focuses on social understanding in people with developmental disorders.

Helen Tager-Flusberg, PhD, Lab of Developmental Cognitive Neuroscience, Department of Anatomy and Neurobiology, Boston University School of Medicine, Boston, Massachusetts. Her research focuses on children with developmental disorders, including Williams syndrome, specific language impairment, Down syndrome, and autism, and the connections between genes, brain pathology, and cognitive and language impairments in these populations.

Faraneh Vargha-Khadem, PhD, Developmental Cognitive Neuroscience Unit, Institute of Child Health, University College London, and Great Ormond Street Hospital for Children, London, England. Her research and clinical work are focused on understanding the cognitive and behavioral deficits of children with brain injuries in relation to the underlying neuropathology, with the goal of developing new knowledge about the ontogeny of specific neural systems.

Anna J. Wilson, PhD, INSERM, U562, Orsay, France. Her research interests include dyscalculia, numerical cognition, and educational applications of research in cognitive psychology; she is currently working on a project to implement and test rehabilitation software for dyscalculia.

Preface

The relatively new fields of developmental cognitive neuroscience and developmental psychopathology are located at the junction of brain science, cognitive science, and behavioral science in human development. These interdisciplinary fields are focused on the scientific investigation of brain–behavior relations in typical and atypical populations. In turn, this investigation is characterized by multiple levels of analysis, ranging from molecular and genetic bases to neural structure and function to behavioral manifestation to sociocultural influences and context. By necessity, then, these investigations are also marked by the use of a wide range of research methods and tools, from genetic markers to brain imaging, such as functional magnetic resonance imaging (fMRI) scans, to performance on classroom evaluations.

Each of the chapters in this volume (see also the companion volume, *Human Behavior, Learning, and the Developing Brain: Typical Development*) deftly illustrates this transdisciplinary approach to the study of atypical development. The themes of multiple levels of analysis and multiple tools for analysis are revisited in each chapter, emphasizing the intellectual importance and scientific benefit of a converging evidence approach to understanding atypical development. Summarizing across the chapters, it is abundantly clear that specific pathways of atypical development will only come to be fully understood, in terms of both strengths and weaknesses, by using this sort of multifaceted approach.

Across the chapters, the reader will also gain a sense of the dynamic nature of atypical human development, as well as an understanding of the complex etiologies of atypical developmental pathways that necessitate interdisciplinary approaches to diagnosis and remediation. This sort of understanding based on multiple perspectives has not only scientific implications but also real-world educational implications. With greater knowledge comes the prospect of prediction, accompanied by the possibility of early identification and more appropriately targeted interventions. For children and teachers in the context of the classroom, greater knowledge leads to the potential for both improved teaching and better learning.

Another theme touched upon in many chapters is the dynamic nature of our scientific and educational understanding of atypical development: Although further research is required to elucidate the intricacies of many of the atypical pathways presented in these chapters, current data and theory reveal an impressive, rich knowledge of development in various populations. Each of the chapters, introduced below, illustrates the scientific, clinical, educational, and theoretical promise of using findings from atypically developing populations to inform an understanding of human development at multiple, interactive levels.

THE CHAPTERS: A PREVIEW

Charles A. Nelson opens with a model for a developmental cognitive neuroscience approach to researching and understanding atypical development. Using infants of mothers with diabetes as an illustrative study, he demonstrates the uses of cross-sectional and longitudinal data; comparisons of typically and atypically developing populations on multiple, targeted measures; integration of biological and behavioral approaches; and the critical importance of converging evidence and interdisciplinarily informed, theory- and data-driven investigations for shedding light on the mechanisms involved in atypical development. Nelson reviews ongoing studies of memory development in infants and children of mothers with diabetes, reporting event-related potential (ERP) data that suggest that children of diabetic mothers show deficits in recognition and delayed recall memory (for voices, faces, objects, and event sequences) that are likely related to prenatal hippocampal development. Interestingly, standardized behavioral testing revealed no differences between infants of mothers with diabetes and control infants, implying that neural measures may access subtle differences to which behavioral tests are not sensitive. The research program described clearly illustrates the promise of using neuroimaging techniques to investigate the development of circuitry related to specific cognitive functions and behaviors.

Following, a pair of chapters address perhaps one of the most complex developmental disorders: autism. Geraldine Dawson and Raphael Bernier provide a developmental perspective on the social impairments that characterize this disorder. They review and connect data within five domains of social functioning often deficient in young children with autism: social orienting, attention to emotional cues, joint attention, imitation, and face processing. They then discuss how normal development of social brain networks might be compromised in autism, according to the social-motivation hypothesis. Central to this hypothesis are the roles of oxytocin and vasopressin within the dopamine reward system, particularly with regard to the emotional tagging of social stimuli and interactions. This hypothesis leads to an important discussion about research-based early intervention strategies. The authors close with a review of evidence for a genetic basis for autism, once again linking the evidence to early intervention strategies.

The second chapter of the pair explores deeply the brain bases of the social deficits observed in autism. Kevin A. Pelphrey and Elizabeth J. Carter summarize exciting recent research that is beginning to provide clues about the functioning of the neural systems that underlie the pervasive social deficits characteristic of autism spectrum disorders. Integrating findings across studies with animals, typically developing children and adults, and persons with autism, the authors identify the amygdala, the superior temporal sulcus region, and the fusiform gyrus as the structures most implicated in the social deficits observed in autism. Given the interconnectivity of these brain regions and the heterogeneity of autistic symptoms, it seems likely that the marked social deficits in autism spectrum disorders have a complex etiology that might best be differentiated by a combined behavioral and functional neuroimaging approach that takes into account developmental change over time.

Helen Tager-Flusberg and Daniela Plesa Skwerer next offer a chapter that reviews experimental, developmental, and brain imaging findings related to visual–spatial cognition and social cognition in Williams syndrome, a rare, genetically based neurodevelopmental disorder. Despite early claims of extreme impairment in visual–spatial cognition and relative sparing in social cognition in Williams syndrome, the authors report a much more complex pattern of strengths and weaknesses that rests on clever experimental design and more accurate conceptualization of the neurocognitive systems involved. Indeed, they claim that the clearly defined genetic basis of Williams syndrome makes it "a model syndrome for exploring a fine-grained analysis of the development and organization of neurocognitive architecture." This chapter clearly illustrates the promise of using findings from atypically developing populations to inform a scientific understanding of human development at multiple levels.

The chapter that follows begins a series of four chapters exploring different aspects of atypical language and reading development. In this outstanding chapter, Elena L. Grigorenko offers a clear definition of developmental dyslexia and an extensive discussion about both the genetic bases of developmental dyslexia and the environmental factors that interact with biological factors leading to reading disability. Four models presented in the chapter capture the dynamic complexity and interplay of genetic deficiencies, brain networks, and cognitive processes in developmental dyslexia—and these are just a few of many possible models. The chapter closes with a thoughtful discussion about the educational implications of the genetic research on dyslexia; because of the interactive nature of biological and environmental factors, it is concluded that the protective environmental factor of good teaching is currently the best intervention for atypical reading development.

Usha Goswami further expands the discussion about language and reading development in a chapter on developmental dyslexia across cultures. She reviews evidence indicating that poor phonological awareness—an insensitivity to phonological structure or the sounds of language—is associated with developmental dyslexia across orthographies. According to the psycholinguistic grain-size framework, phonological development is essentially universal but the ways in which orthographic units are mapped to sounds are language specific. In inconsistent orthographies, such as English, developmental dyslexia can be diagnosed on the basis of reduced accuracy on phonological awareness tasks, whereas in languages with more consistent orthographies, such as Italian, developmental dyslexia is usually diagnosed on the basis of reduced speed and poor spelling. Goswami argues that, given the universal phonological deficit behavioral marker of developmental dyslexia, it follows that "biological unity" could be expected in terms of the brain bases of this disorder, motivating the need for appropriate cross-cultural data.

Frederique Liegeois, Angela Morgan, and Faraneh Vargha-Khadem continue the discussion about language and reading development in a chapter that focuses on members of the KE family who have a severe speech and language disorder that is characterized as chronic developmental verbal and orofacial dyspraxia (DVOFD) and encoded by the FOXP2 gene. Many of the behaviors of the affected KE family members are similar to behaviors observed in children with developmental verbal dyspraxia (DVD) or specific language impairment; indeed, the authors conclude that current evidence is insufficient to provide a differential diagnosis between DVOFD and DVD. In the second part of the chapter, the authors attempt to connect both the behavioral phenotype and the genotype observed in affected members of the KE family to neural processes. They review the results of functional neuroimaging studies that suggest atypical processing in both motor and language regions. Liegeois and colleagues conclude that fluent, intelligible speech is the product of multiple sensory and cognitive systems in complex and dynamic interaction, and that meaningfully teasing apart both the contributin̦ ponents and the interactions is an area ripe for future research.

In the final chapter on atypical language and reading, Denni Molfese, Victoria J. Molfese, and Peter J. Molfese look more specifically at early language development and review persuasive evidence indicating that recordings of ERPs in infancy and early childhood can be used to predict later language and reading outcomes. They provide a historical review of their own pioneering work as well as others' longitudinal studies showing that ERP responses to speech sounds in infants are related to standardized behavioral measures of language and reading in the same children when they have reached preschool and school age. These results highlight the critical role of speech perception abilities in language and reading development and offer the real possibility of combined brain–behavior approaches to early identification, intervention, and remediation for language-related disorders and disabilities. In their conclusion, the authors speculate that such a combined approach might be powerful enough not only to mitigate later emerging cognitive disabilities, but possibly to eliminate them.

Moving on from discussions of language and reading, Anna J. Wilson and Stanislas Dehaene review behavioral and biological evidence related to developmental dyscalculia. They convincingly build their arguments for a core deficit in number sense and the possibility of subtypes of developmental dyscalculia by connecting evidence about the localization of numerical cognition functions in typical adults, the causes of acalculia, and the typical development of numerical cognition to what is known about developmental dyscalculia. Emphasizing brain–behavior relations and the preliminary nature of much of the data, they encourage further research in this area and demonstrate with an example of their own remediation software the importance of an interdisciplinary scientific and educational understanding of mathematical difficulties.

Once again shifting focus, in the next chapter Lisa M. Gatzke-Kopp and Theodore P. Beauchaine review the evidence for a frontostriatal, dopaminergic deficit in developmental disorders of impulsivity. In particular, they review findings indicating nigrostriatal, mesocortical (cognitive), and mesolimbic (motivational) system deficits in attention-deficit/hyperactivity disorder (ADHD) and conduct disorder (CD). Although the precise mechanism—in terms of hyperactivity or hypoactivity of the dopaminergic system—remains unknown, it appears that each of these functionally integrated systems may contribute to different symptoms observed in the ADHD syndrome. The authors suggest that this complex etiology may result in different patterns of symptoms across individuals diagnosable with ADHD and may necessitate a combined behavioral and neurobiological approach to diagnosis.

In the chapter that follows, Emma K. Adam, Bonnie Klimes-Dougan, and Megan R. Gunnar provide a broad review of studies investigating social effects on the regulation of the hypothalamic–pituitary–adrenal (HPA) system involved in the human response to stress. They present developmental findings indicating regulation of the HPA axis in infants, children, and adolescents by varied social experiences, including institutional rearing, maternal depression, abuse and neglect, and everyday interpersonal interactions and relationships. Furthermore, they highlight a convincing connection among exposure to social stress, HPA axis functioning, and the development of both internalizing and externalizing psychopathologies. In closing, they contextualize these links among brain, behavior, and environment by thoughtfully considering the implications of the research they have reviewed for education.

In the next chapter, Catherine C. Ayoub and Gabrielle Rappolt-Schlichtmann provide a review of findings relating brain and behavior development in the case of child maltreatment. The authors argue that the behaviors of maltreated children are highly complex and adaptive in context, but can be maladaptive outside the context of the mistreatment; maltreated children are not simply delayed in development but grow along an alternative, trauma-induced developmental pathway. The authors contend that understanding the plasticity of neurobiological systems affected by abuse and neglect can clarify the immediate and long-term vulnerabilities of maltreated children and guide the design of intervention plans. They conclude that both behavior and biology are both adaptive and maladaptive in cases of child maltreatment and that only by investigating the relations among different components of the developing system in context can an understanding of the whole child be established.

To close the volume and reiterate many of the themes introduced in previous chapters, Francine M. Benes provides a fascinating tour of the phylogenetic and ontogenetic development of brain systems involved in the integration of emotion and thought processes: the corticolimbic system. Focusing on structures within the hippocampal formation and the neocortex, this chapter provides integrated reviews of evolution and maturation that allow for an exploration of the bases of the complex emotional and cognitive behaviors found in humans. This extensive developmental framework provides the background for a discussion of the hypothesis that maturational changes in adolescence may serve as a "trigger" for the appearance of a mental illness phenotype; schizophrenia is used as an illustrative example. Interestingly, it seems that maturational changes in the corticolimbic system during the teenage years can be related to either typical or atypical behavioral development, demarcating a fine line between normal and abnormal maturation.

Contents

A Developmental Cognitive Neuroscience Approach to the Study of Atypical Development

A MODEL SYSTEM INVOLVING INFANTS OF DIABETIC MOTHERS

Charles A. Nelson

In an earlier publication (Dawson & Fischer, 1994) I focused on the utility of recording the brain's electrical activity—specifically, the recording of event-related potentials (ERPs)—in the context of studying the neural correlates of memory development. Over the ensuing decade my colleagues and I have continued this work with typically developing infants and children, and have expanded our research focus to include infants and children at risk for developing disorders of memory. We have focused our efforts on such populations for two reasons. First, the study of atypical development can inform the study of typical development. In this context, our hope was to shed light on the neural systems involved in typical memory development by studying infants who had experienced perturbations in the development of such systems. Second, we felt that our work had matured to the point at which it was appropriate to extend our armamentarium of tools to various clinical populations. The value of doing so is hopefully obvious: Improved diagnostic imaging with greater neural specificity should lead to earlier and better diagnosis, which in turn should lead to better treatment.

This chapter takes the following form. I begin with a brief tutorial on ERPs in general and on the recording of ERPs in developmental populations. I then talk about the virtues and limitations of studying atypical populations and draw an analogy to the classic lesion approach used for over 100 years in neuropsychology. In the last section of the chapter I review a research program, in which my colleagues and I have been engaged for nearly a decade, that focuses on one specific population of children at risk for developing a memory disorder: infants born to mothers with diabetes.

WHAT IS AN ERP?

Because our group has extensively discussed the utility of ERPs in the study of cognitive development (see DeBoer, Scott, & Nelson, 2004; Nelson & Monk, 2001), my review of the ERP here is relatively brief. ERPs represent the summation of electrical activity generated by large populations of neurons that volume conduct to the scalp surface. This activity can then be recorded by means of electrodes placed on the scalp surface. Figure 1.1 illustrates several of the ways in which we have recorded ERPs over the years.

It is generally believed that ERPs represent the activity of pyramidal cell neurons whose orientation is configured in such a way so as to permit their recording at the scalp surface (if oriented in the "wrong" direction, the currents generated by such neurons would not be detectable). The implications of this constraint are worth mentioning. First, in theory, neural structures or circuits that do not contain pyramidal cells (e.g., amygdala) should not give rise to electrical currents that take the form of ERPs. Second, because the electrical currents that give rise to ERPs are created by the simultaneous activity of large populations of neurons that volume conduct to the surface of the scalp, the spatial resolution of ERPs is limited; even with dense-array sampling (see far right image of Figure 1.1), it has been hypothesized that the spatial resolution is approximately 1 centimeter (cm; far less than is obtained with fMRI). Of course, with low-density array sampling, the resolution is likely less than 1 cm.

Despite the relatively poor spatial resolution of ERPs, their many advantages over other neuroimaging tools are noteworthy. First, ERPs have exquisite temporal resolution, on the order of milliseconds, comparable to magnetoencephalography (MEG) and far superior to fMRI (which reflects neural activity on the order of seconds). Second, ERPs are entirely non-invasive, there are no safety issues that can concern institutional review boards (IRBs), they do not depend on motor or verbal responses, and they can be used across the entire lifespan without a change in methods. Finally,

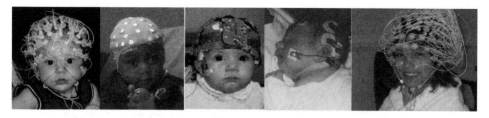

FIGURE 1.1. *From left to right*: an infant wearing a 64-channel sensor net, an infant wearing a 32-channel electrode cap, an infant on whose head has been placed 12 electrodes held in place with adhesive foam and headbands, a newborn infant in the intensive care nursery wearing disposable electrodes, and a 10-year-old wearing a 128-channel sensor net.

although fMRI has yielded profound insights into the functional neuro-anatomy of a number of cognitive functions, fMRI cannot be used (easily) before the age of 5–7 years. Moreover, fMRI is expensive; for example, at most institutions a single subject's scan costs at least $500, and the equipment itself costs approximately $3 million. In contrast, even a high-end dense-array ERP system costs approximately $100,000, and there are minimal costs per subject once electrodes and electrode supplies have been purchased.

HOW HAVE ERPs BEEN USED TO STUDY COGNITIVE DEVELOPMENT?

The ways in which ERPs have been used to study cognitive development have received considerable attention from our lab, and again, the reader is encouraged to consult recent reviews (e.g., DeBoer et al., 2004; Nelson & Monk, 2001). In brief, functions that have received most attention include memory, face/object processing, attention, working memory, and speech and language processing. The vast majority of this work has focused on typically developing infants and children, although a number of labs have increasingly focused their attention on various atypical populations, such as children with autism (e.g., Dawson, Webb, Carver, Panagiotides, & McPartland, 2004), children with language learning impairments (e.g., Kraus, 2001), neonatal intensive care unit (NICU) "graduates" (e.g., deRegnier, Georgieff, & Nelson, 1997), children with attention-deficit disorder (Klorman et al., 2002), children with histories of neglect/abuse (e.g., Pollak, Klorman, Thatcher, & Cicchetti, 2001), and children who experienced institutional rearing early in life (Parker, Nelson, Bucharest Early

Intervention Project Core Group, 2005a, 2005b). Virtually all of these studies have been performed with infants or school-age children; very few have been done with adolescent-age children, although such work is now under way in several laboratories (e.g., Davies, Segalowitz, & Gavin, 2004).

In a typical cognitive paradigm, participants are presented with punctuated trains of visual or auditory stimuli while ERPs are recorded. A behavioral measure (e.g., reaction time) may or may not be recorded simultaneously. Depending on the age of the participant, as few as 40–50 trials to several hundred trials might be presented. A typical experimental session generally lasts 5–15 minutes. If data have been collected continuously (e.g., to record EEG), they are then down-sampled to create epochs or trials; in many cases, however, data are not recorded continuously and instead trials are constructed at the outset. After rigorously rejecting and/or correcting artifactual data (e.g., eye movements), individual trials are typically averaged and these averages are then averaged across participants in order to examine components that exist in the full group of participants.

Conventional data analysis tools historically have been confined to examining the amplitude, latency, and scalp topography of individual components. With higher-density arrays of electrodes, more sophisticated analyses can be run, such as independent components analysis and source analysis (see Johnson et al., 2001, for discussion in the context of development).

WHAT ARE THE VIRTUES AND LIMITATIONS OF STUDYING ATYPICAL POPULATIONS?

As I elaborate below, there are two broad reasons for considering the advantages and disadvantages of studying atypical developmental populations: to provide insight into clinical phenomena, per se, and to use the study of atypical development to inform the study of typical development.

The Study of Clinical Populations for Their Own Sake

The primary driving force in the study of clinical populations is to use ERPs to shed light on the pathophysiology of atypical development. A case in point might be work by Dawson and colleagues in the field of autism. For example, this group has reported that ERPs elicited by face stimuli in children with autism differ considerably from ERPs in response to the same stimuli in control children, whereas the ERPs to objects are remarkably similar (Dawson et al., 2002). This observation provides critical information as to the neural correlates of face-processing deficits, something that has not been possible by studying overt behavior alone. Similarly, Pollak and colleagues have reported that the ERPs generated in response to discrete facial expressions (e.g., anger) differ in children with histories of neglect/abuse from those who are reared in typical environments (e.g., Pollak et al., 2001). And, we (Parker et al., 2005a, 2005b) have reported that the ERPs elicited by facial emotion differ in toddlers with a history of institutionalization relative to a community sample. In all cases the motivation underlying this work was to illuminate the neuropathophysiology of a specific cognitive function.

The Study of Clinical Populations as a Means of Shedding Light on Typical Development

The work I present below in some detail is a case in point. Specifically, because of my interest in the neural architecture that underlies typical memory development, I have been drawn to the study of populations of children with damage to the structures/circuits of the brain that underlie memory. In so doing I provide a form of converging operations on the study of memory. Thus, for example, if I hypothesize that the hippocampus is critically involved in some forms of recognition memory, and that a particular component of the ERP reflects such memory, then children with hippocampal damage should show perturbations in that particular component. In the following section I focus my attention on one particular population, the study of which is designed to shed light on typically developing children while, at the same time, adding to what is known about the neuropathophysiology of this particular condition.

A MODEL SYSTEM: THE INFANT OF THE DIABETIC MOTHER

Here I begin by laying out the rationale for studying infants of diabetic mothers (IDMs). I then proceed to review our ERP findings to date.

Background

The fetal metabolic milieu of the diabetic pregnancy is characterized by significant risk factors to the developing brain, including chronic hypoxia and iron deficiency, with intermittent metabolic acidosis and hyper/hypoglycemia (Georgieff et al., 1990; Petry et al., 1992; Widness, 1989). All of these risk factors are a function of lack of maternal glycemic control during the third trimester of pregnancy (Georgieff et al., 1990). Maternal hyperglycemia (i.e., too much sugar in the blood) results in fetal hyperglycemia and reactive fetal hyperinsulinemia (i.e., too much insulin in the fetus's blood). The latter two factors independently (Milley, Papacostas, & Tabata, 1986; Stonestreet, Golstein, Oh, & Widness, 1989) and collectively (Widness et al., 1981) increase the fetal rate of oxygen consumption beyond the placental capacity to transport oxygen. The resultant fetal hypoxemia (i.e., lack of oxygen—see Milley et al., 1986; Stonestreet et al., 1989; Widness et al., 1981) is pervasive and chronic, as evidenced by an elevated serum erythropoietin concentration and a compensatory rise in fetal hemoglobin concentration (Georgieff et al., 1990; Widness et al., 1981). Chronic hypoxia constitutes a significant risk factor to the developing brain, with some circuitry (e.g., the hippocampus) more vulnerable than other circuitry (Nelson & Silverstein, 1994). The differential regional vulnerability may relate to areas that have high metabolic rates during late fetal and early postnatal life. The theme of regional brain vulnerability (Burdo & Connor, 2002; de Ungria et al., 2000) is consistently seen with metabolic insults during the perinatal period and is important in our targeting of hippocampal function in our studies.

Fetal hyperinsulinemia secondary to chronic maternal hyperglyemia leads to stimulation of pancreatic islet cells and increases the fetal risk of intermittent hypoglycemia. When the glucose flow from the mother vacilates abruptly, the fetus is at particular risk. For example, when the mother is hyperglycemic, the fetus will respond to the surge of maternally derived glucose by secreting an appropriately large amount of insulin. As the mother treats her diabetes with exogenous insulin, her blood glucose falls rapidly, cutting off the supply to the fetus, lowering the fetal glucose concentration, and leaving the fetus unprotected from its own hyperinsulinemia. The resultant fetal hypoglycemia constitutes a significant risk to the developing hippocampus (Barks, Sun, Malinak, & Silverstein, 1995).

Further neurological risk is conferred by a state of chronic brain iron deficiency in the fetus. Early iron deficiency affects multiple developing brain functions, including myelination (Connor & Menzies, 1996; Roncagliolo, Garrdio, Walter, Peirano, & Lozoff, 1998), monoamine neurotransmitter metabolism (Nelson, Erikson, Piner, & Beard, 1997), and oxidative metabolism (de Ungria et al., 2000; Rao et al., 1999). The fetal brain shows regional variability with these effects, with the energy metabolism effects being most striking in the hippocampus (de Ungria et al., 2000), whereas dopaminergic effects are found primarily in the striatum (Georgieff, Petry, Mills, McKay, & Wobken, 1997).

The 40% decrease in hippocampal neuronal metabolism results in striking dendritic truncation and alteration in the ontogeny of NMDA subunit appearance in area hippocampal CA1 in the perinatal rat. These structural changes persist beyond the period of iron repletion. Furthermore, studies using high-field (9.4 Tesla) magnetic resonance (MR) spectroscopy in the developing rat demonstrate significant increases in glutamate concentrations in the hippocampus in the resting state. More alarming, these changes are enhanced following exposure to hypoxia, a condition prevalent in the diabetic fetus. The etiology of iron deficiency in the diabetic fetus is due to the inability of the diabetic placenta to up-regulate iron transport due to hyperglycosylation of the transferrin receptor (Georgieff et al., 1997). The inability to meet the increased iron demands for augmented fetal hemoglobin synthesis results in a shunting of available fetal iron into the red blood cells at the expense of the developing human brain (Petry et al., 1992). The result is a reduction in hippocampal volume.

Multiple risk factors are associated with the diabetic pregnancy, and a plethora of animal models have been used to elucidate the pathophysiology associated with these risk factors. In addition, several studies have demonstrated that neurobehavioral outcomes in human children who were born to diabetic mothers are correlated with the quality of metabolic regulation during pregnancy (e.g., Ornoy et al., 2001; Rizzo, Metzger, Burns, & Burns, 1991; Rizzo, Metzger, Dooley, & Cho, 1997; Silverman et al., 1991). However, these investigations have typically examined global cognitive development in children well downstream from the proposed insult. Although important from an educational perspective, the disadvantage of using global measures is their inability to reveal (1) specific domains of dysfunction that may be responsible for the global deficits and (2) the specific neural circuitry that underlies deficits in behavior. Moreover, most measures of global functioning cannot easily (or meaningfully) be performed during the early infancy period, thereby placing limits on early detection and prediction of subsequent developmental course. Because of the infant's limited behavioral repertoire, we have placed a premium in our studies on employing noninvasive electrophysiological imaging during the first few years of life (starting at birth).

The logic of our work is as follows. First, as reviewed in an earlier publication (Nelson, 1994) as well as in more recent writings (e.g., Nelson & Webb, 2002; Nelson, Thomas, & de Haan, 2006), we know that ERPs can be used to evaluate different forms of memory, including recognition memory. Second, we know that the forms of memory in which we are most interested are subserved, in large part, by structures that reside in the medial temporal lobe—the hippocampus, in particular. Third, if the adverse fetal milieu experienced by IDMs is, in fact, "toxic" to the developing hippocampus, then such infants should show impairments in memory, and ERPs should, in turn, provide an index of such impairments.

Our study is longitudinal in nature; here, however, I focus most on our cross-sectional findings. We have employed a battery of tasks, including conventional developmental testing, elicited imitation, neuropsychological testing, and, now that our children are school-age, structural and functional MRI. However, for purposes of this chapter I confine myself to a discussion of our ERP findings.

All infants (both IDMs and controls) were screened for various confounds (e.g., maternal drug use, neurological history) and then enrolled prenatally. At the delivery we obtained cord blood and placental tissue so we could ascertain the degree of iron deficiency (and attempt to infer information about hypoxemia). We began our investigation within 2 days of birth, then continued to see our study subjects throughout the next few years.

Newborn Infants' Recognition of the Mother's Voice

We examined the 1- to 2-day-old infant's ability to discriminate the mother's voice from a stranger's voice, based on the assumption that the former would be familiar to the infant after being exposed to that voice prenatally. ERPs were recorded as infants were presented with sound clips (via ear insert) of their mother's voice or a stranger's voice (random 50% probabilities) pronouncing the word *baby*. The grand means displayed in Figure 1.2 show electrophysiological responses by group to the mother's voice (thick line) and stranger's voice (thin line). Within this sample, we examined two components of interest, the P2 and the negative slow wave (NSW) that follows the P2. We have associated the P2 with early perceptual processing of the content of the stimuli, and the NSW with the ability to detect a novel stimulus set against a background of familiar stimuli. Our results reveal P2 amplitudes to be greater to the mother's versus a stranger's voice among controls but not the IDM group. In terms of the NSW (our metric of memory), our controls display significantly greater NSW area to a stranger's than to the mother's voice (particularly at leads Fz and T4), whereas no such differences are observed among IDMs (for details, see deRegnier, Nelson, Thomas, Wewerka, & Georgieff, 2000).

Brain Iron Deficiency versus Sufficiency

We have recently had the opportunity to reclassify some of our newborn data based on the degree of iron deficiency experienced, focusing specifically on those infants we presume to be truly brain iron deficient (BID) (see Siddappa et al., 2004). Ten BID infants were compared to 22 IDMs who were presumably brain iron sufficient (BIS) (concentration > 30 µg/L < 60

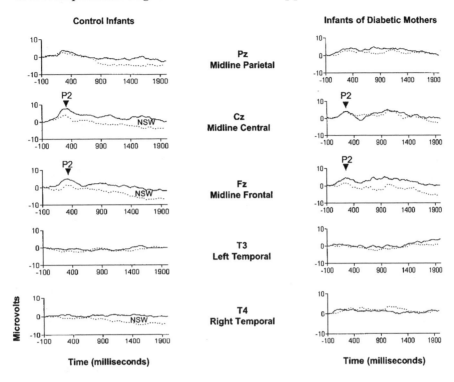

FIGURE 1.2. ERPs recorded from newborn IDMs (right side) and controls (left side) to brief auditory clips of the infant's mother's voice and the voice of a stranger. Note differences between groups for the P2 and NSW components at lead Cz. Reproduced with permission from Elsevier from deRegnier, R.-A., Nelson, C.A., Thomas, K., Wewerka, S., & Georgieff, M.K. (2000). Neurophysiologic evaluation of auditory recognition memory in healthy newborn infants and infants of diabetic mothers. *Journal of Pediatrics, 137,* 777–784.

µg/L). Two manipulations were performed: a simple auditory discrimination task (speech vs. nonspeech) and the mother-versus-stranger voice task (both with ERPs). There were no differences between groups on the former task, suggesting no differences in sensory processing. On the latter, only the BIS infants manifested a slow wave to a stranger's voice that was significantly more negative than that to the mother's voice, indicating discrimination; the BID group showed no such difference (see Figure 1.3).

On the whole, we interpreted our newborn ERP findings to support our contention that IDMs will show impairments in recognition memory that are likely of prenatal origin (when exposure to the mother's voice occurred). These effects are particularly pronounced if the infant's brain is

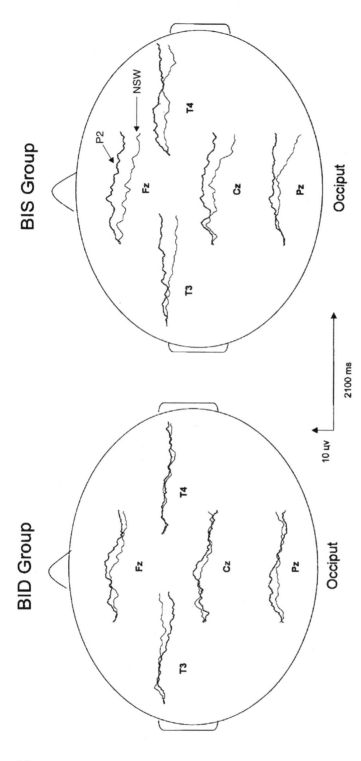

FIGURE 1.3. Data collected as described in Figure 1.2, with IDMs sorted into those with suspected brain iron deficiency (BID—left side of figure) and brain iron sufficiency (BIS—right side of figure). Note the lack of difference between mother versus stranger voice among BID versus BIS infants. Adapted with permission from Lippincott Williams & Willkins from Siddappa, A. M., Georgieff, M. K., Wewerka, S., Worwa, C., Nelson, C. A. & deRegnier, R.-A. (2004). Iron deficiency alters auditory recognition memory in newborn infants of diabetic mothers. *Pediatric Research, 55,* 1034–1041.

iron deficient (which is more likely to occur if the mother's diabetes is poorly controlled, leading to an even more adverse fetal environment).

Six-Month-Old Infants' Recognition of Mother's Face

To examine memory for material that should be well encoded from prior experience, at 6 months we studied the electrophysiological correlates of the infant's ability to recognize his or her mother's face (Nelson et al., 2000). The ERP paradigm consists of presenting infants with alternating digitized images of their mother's face and a stranger's face. We focused our examination on the negative central component (NC) and the positive slow wave (PSW; see Nelson & Monk, 2001, for review and discussion). As seen from the grand means in Figure 1.4 (see lead C4 in particular), group differences in the amplitude of the NC to the mother's face (thick line) as well as group differences in the PSW to the stranger's face (thin line) are prominent for the control group over the right hemisphere. The IDM group did not demonstrate any differences in condition for either component.

Eight-Month-Old Infants' Cross-Model Recognition Memory

At 8 months we evaluated cross-modal recognition memory. Here cross-modal (tactile to vision) recognition memory was evaluated using ERPs. Infants palpated an object without seeing it and were then presented with a series of ERP test trials, in which they viewed pictures of the object they had palpated juxtaposed with pictures of a novel object. As seen in Figure 1.5, our control infants showed a significantly greater NC to the novel stimulus (thin line) as compared to the familiar, palpated stimulus (thick line), particularly over the left hemisphere (see lead C3). In addition, control infants displayed a greater PSW to the novel stimulus, again over the left hemisphere (see lead T3), indicating their ability to encode and update their memory of the novel stimulus. IDMs failed to show ERP evidence of distinguishing novel from familiar stimuli for any component.

Infants with Iron Deficiency at Birth Are Iron Sufficient at 8 Months of Age

We obtained follow-up ferritin levels at 8 months of age on infants at risk for perinatal iron deficiency. Ten infants with birth serum ferritin concentrations of < 70 ng/ml (iron deficient) were compared to 12 infants with birth serum ferritin concentrations of > 80 ng/ml. The birth iron deficient

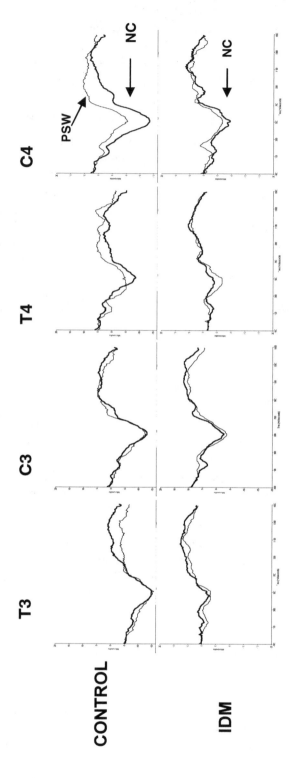

FIGURE 1.4. ERPs recorded from 6-month-old IDMs and controls presented with brief images of their mother's faces and the face of a stranger. Note difference in the NC and PSW at lead C4 for control versus IDM infants. Adapted with permission from the American Psychological Association from Nelson, C. A., Wewerka, S., Thomas, K.M., Tribby-Walbridge, S., deRegnier, R.-A., & Georgieff, M. (2000). Neurocognitive sequelae of infants of diabetic mothers. *Behavioral Neuroscience, 114,* 950–956.

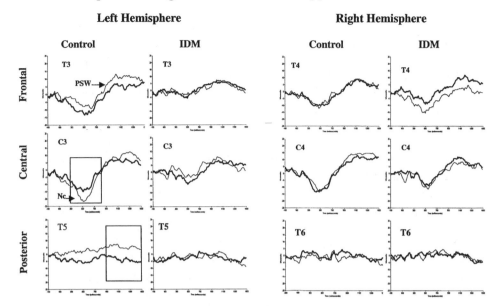

FIGURE 1.5. ERPs recorded from 8-month-old IDMs and controls familiarized haptically to one object and then tested visually with familiar and novel objects. Note differences in the PSW at lead T3 for control versus IDMs. Reproduced with permission from Elsevier from Nelson, C. A., Wewerka, S., Borscheid, A. J., deRegnier, R.-A., & Georgieff, M.K. (2003). Electrophysiologic evidence of impaired cross-modal recognition memory in 8-month-old infants of diabetic mothers. *Journal of Pediatrics, 142,* 575–582.

group had statistically lower mean ferritin levels at 8 months (30 ± 17 vs. 57 ± 33 µg/dl), but no infant had iron deficiency (serum ferritin < 10 ng/ml) or iron deficiency anemia (hemoglobin < 11.5 g/dl). Thus, at the time of 8-month testing on cross-modal recognition memory (and possibly even earlier), the infants were iron sufficient and the abnormal ERPs recorded at that time (see above) were not due to ongoing iron deficiency. Based on our perinatal rat model (see earlier discussion), we speculate that important structural changes in CA1 during the period of perinatal iron deficiency continue to exist at follow-up.

Twelve-, 18-, and 24-Month-Old Infants' Explicit Memory for Event Sequences

This portion of our project is still in progress and is being overseen by Tracy DeBoer. Here the goal is to employ a task designed to evaluate memory in 1- to 2-year-old infants—elicited imitation. Elicited imitation typically involves showing an infant a series of objects, which, when assembled in a particular order, create an event sequence (e.g., putting the baby doll in the bathtub, washing the baby, drying the baby; for review, see Bauer, 2006). The age of the infant, in part, determines (1) how many steps in the sequence to present, and (2) the length of the delay between initial presentation and retest. In the current study, we evaluated infants at 12, 18, and 24 months of age on an elicited imitation task in which two types of recall were assessed: immediate and after a 10-minute delay. After an experimenter modeled the action sequences, infants' behavioral memory performance was assessed based on the number of target actions infants correctly reproduced and the order of those actions. Each participant's response score was an average over two trials. In addition, for both the 12- and 24-month age groups, recognition memory was assessed via ERP measures 1 week after the behavioral session. ERPs were recorded from 32 electrodes while infants watched pictures of a familiar event sequence (seen in the immediate imitation task) and pictures of a novel sequence. To date, we have tested forty-six 12-month-old infants (31 controls, 15 IDMs), forty-one 18-month-old infants (28 controls, 13 IDMs), and seventy 24-month-old infants (52 controls, 18 IDMs—for discussion, see DeBoer, Wewerka, Bauer, Georgieff, & Nelson, 2005; DeBoer, Georgieff, & Nelson, in press).

Behavioral Results

Thus far, there are no group differences in immediate test performance at any age, indicating that all infants were able to imitate the sequences when allowed to do so immediately following modeling by the experimenter. However, under delay conditions, 12-month-old control infants recalled significantly more pairs of target actions than 12-month-old IDMs (DeBoer et al., 2005). This effect was marginally significant at 24 months of age, with IDMs producing slightly fewer target actions after a delay than control infants.

ERP Results

As with our previous studies, we analyzed the electrophysiological data focusing on the NC and PSW. Preliminary results indicate that at both 12 (Figure 1.6) and 24 months of age (Figure 1.7), the control infants' NC amplitude (see lead Fz at 12 months and P4 at 24 months) and PSW (see lead Cz at 12 and 24 months) differentiated between the novel sequence (thin line) and the familiar sequence (thick line), whereas the IDMs' did not.

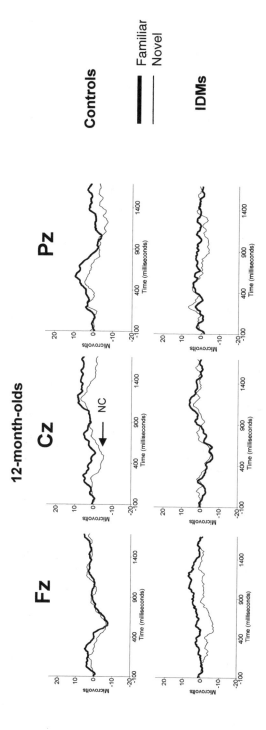

FIGURE 1.6. ERPs recorded from 12-month-old infants tested in an elicited imitation paradigm. Here infants are first presented with various props in a particular sequence. One week after initial exposure, infants are presented with visual images of a familiar prop and a novel prop while ERPs are recorded. Note differences between responses to familiar versus novel stimuli among controls only, at leads Cz and Pz, in particular, and the lack of such differences among IDMs.

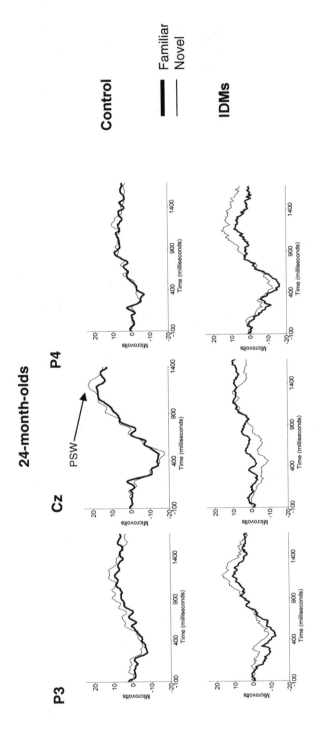

FIGURE 1.7. ERPs recorded from 24-month-old infants tested in an elicited imitation paradigm (see Figure 1.6 for details). Analysis of the data indicated that the PSW was greater to novel versus familiar stimuli at lead Cz for control infants only. (Although there appears to be a difference for both the NC and PSW among IDMs, these differences were, in fact, not statistically significant.)

Relations between Behavioral Recall and ERPs

At both 12 and 24 months, immediate imitation of target actions also correlated with PSW activity to the familiar stimulus at Cz after a 1-week delay. Specifically, the number of target actions produced at Session 1 was associated with greater positive slow wave activity at Session 2. Because we interpret the PSW to reflect memory, we were not surprised to see that the amplitude of this component correlated with the number of target actions produced.

Summary

The observation that the 12-month-old control infants recalled more than IDMs on the delayed imitation task but not the immediate imitation task (and the trend in this same direction at 24 months of age) suggests that IDMs show evidence of forgetting over delays as short as 10 minutes. Furthermore, at 12 months, newborn ferritin levels were marginally related to performance on the delayed recall task (DeBoer et al., 2005). The electrophysiological data, collected after a 1-week delay for both the 12- and 24-month-old infants, also suggest that there are group differences in long-term memory storage. Specifically, although the infants did not show differences in behavioral recall of the sequences immediately, they did show differential brain activity to pictures of these same sequences after a delay, and correlations between immediate recall performance and positive slow wave activity indicate that ERPs may allow for detection of subtler differences in the processing of the information related to recall performance.

A Follow-Up on Explicit Memory for Event Sequences in 36- and 48-Month-Old Children

In order to characterize more accurately differences in behavioral recall between controls and IDMs, we recently added a follow-up investigation at 36 and 48 months. Specifically, at these follow-up assessments children are given three nine-step sequences of different degrees of difficulty (one easy, one medium, and one difficult, with difficulty level determined by the number of causal relations in the sequence) and tested for recall of target actions and the order of those actions both immediately and after a 1-week delay. As at 12 and 24 months, an electrophysiological assessment is obtained after the 1-week delay to allow for direct comparison with previous ages; in addition, a 1-year delay ERP to familiar and novel stimuli from 36 months of age is also collected at 48 months. To date we have tested twenty-two 36-month-olds (14 controls, 8 IDMs) and nineteen 48-month-olds (13 controls, 6 IDMs).

Behavioral Results

Preliminary analyses indicate that, as was the case at 12 and 24 months, there do not appear to be group differences in *immediate* test performance on the medium and easy sequences at 36 months or any of the sequences at 48 months. However, there were marginal group differences in immediate performance on the difficult imitation task at 36 months. Thus, on the whole, both groups were able to imitate these sequences when allowed to do so immediately. However, when a 1-week delay was imposed, 36-month-old control infants recalled significantly more target actions than IDMs on both the medium and difficult sequences.

ERP Results

Although the current sample size at 36 and 48 months prohibits statistical tests regarding group differences in ERP responses, visual inspection of the grand mean at 36 months (see Figure 1.8) suggests possible differences in Nc amplitude and PSW to familiar and novel stimuli. Specifically, Nc amplitude in controls appears larger to the familiar stimulus, whereas Nc amplitude in the IDM group appears larger to the novel stimulus, especially at the frontal midline lead (Fz). Although this differential pattern of results suggests differences by group, interpretation of these findings relative to elicited imitation data collected from younger infants awaits additional data collection from both the 36- and 48-month age groups, which is ongoing.

Summary

It is important to stress that on developmental testing our IDMs are performing equivalently to our controls. Specifically, we performed the Bayley Scales of Infant Development II at 12 and 30 months, and the Wechsler Preschool and Primary Scales of Intelligence, Revised, at older ages. On both measures our groups are quite comparable in their performance, falling well within the normal range.

In contrast, delayed recall appears to remain deficient in the IDM group compared to the control group when a targeted memory task is somewhat challenging (i.e., on medium and difficult sequences). However, when the task is simple (easy sequences), there appear to be no differences between the two groups after a delay. Thus, the IDM group does recall

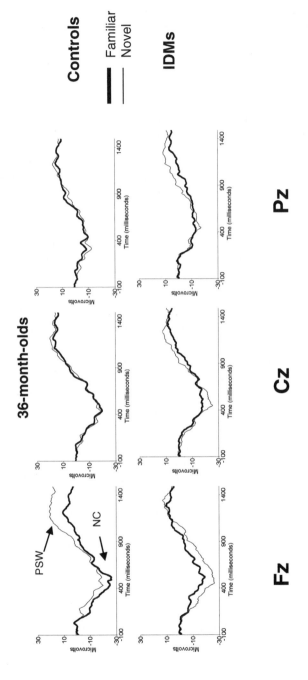

FIGURE 1.8. ERPs recorded from 36-month-old infants tested in an elicited imitation paradigm (see Figure 1.6 for details). Differences in the PSW (greater to novel vs. familiar) can be seen at lead Fz in controls, whereas no such differences are seen among IDMs.

19

some information over a delay, especially when the to-be-remembered materials support such recall. However, when the task is more challenging, deficits in recall remain apparent. Whether this difference decreases with age remains to be seen, as data collection with these older age groups continues.

Electrophysiological Measures of Continuous Recognition Memory

Many in our sample are now approaching 7 years of age, and we have embarked on an ambitious follow-up program that involves high-density ERP recordings and fMRI (being overseen by Kathleen Thomas). Below I report our preliminary ERP data with control children and adults only; thus far only three IDMs have been tested.

Eighteen adults (M = 24 years; nine males and nine females) and 12 children (M = 8 years, 3 months; five males and seven females) are participating in electrophysiological investigation of recognition memory, using a 128-channel high-density electrode array (see far right image of Figure 1.1). Stimuli consist of color photos or three-dimensional drawings of everyday objects (concrete) and unnamable objects (abstract). Stimuli are presented on a black background for a duration of 500 milliseconds (ms), followed by a 3,500-ms interstimulus interval (ISI). These parameters were selected specifically to duplicate those necessary for the fMRI paradigm.

On each trial, participants indicate whether the presented image is new (never seen previously) or old (seen previously), using the index and middle fingers of the right hand, respectively. Behavioral and electrophysiological data are collected in three runs of 72 trials. Electrophysiological and behavioral responses are compared for the first occurrence of a stimulus compared to a repeat occurrence following either 2 or 5 intervening trials. New stimuli are presented in each run, resulting in a total of 120 *new* trials, 42 trials of *lag 2*, and 42 trials of *lag 5*. Foil trials, which consist of stimuli that never repeated or stimuli repeating after a nonstandard lag (1 or 3 intervening trials), are interspersed to prevent anticipatory recognition responses. Factors for analysis included lag condition (new, lag 2, or lag 5 trials) and stimulus category (concrete or abstract).

As we have now reported at several conferences (see Hunt, Couperus, Nelson, & Thomas, 2004a, 2004b; Hunt, Couperus, et al., 2005a; Hunt, Townsend, et al., 2005b; Thomas et al., 2004a, 2004b), behavioral data indicate that adults perform the task more accurately and more quickly than children (93% vs. 88%, 746 ms vs. 1,325 ms). Response accuracy decreased with memory load for adults (94%, 93%, 92%) but not for children. Both adults and children performed more poorly for abstract items than for concrete items. For adults, this effect did not differ by memory lag; however, for children, this effect was not apparent for long memory delays (lag 5). Reaction time differences were observed by age group but not by condition.

Electrophysiologically, effects of memory lag were observed for the parietal P3b component for adults (~500 ms). The P3b to old items was faster than that to new items, with items at lag 2 peaking prior to items at lag 5. Both adults and children showed evidence of an old/new effect for the P3a (~350 ms), with greater amplitude for old items compared to new items. This P3 difference was accompanied by a slower return to baseline for old items than for new items in both adults and children (negative component at 1,000 ms). Adults evidenced a very prominent difference in P3 amplitude for concrete compared to abstract objects, despite comparable behavioral performance across stimulus types. These P300 data suggest peak latency differences for old compared to new concrete objects, whereas no such difference is apparent for abstract objects. Children did not demonstrate significant P300 differences by stimulus type, although some leads showed a trend in this direction.

Source analysis techniques were used to estimate the number and location of neural generators of the recorded scalp activity. Eye-movement artifacts were modeled first using regional dipoles with three orthogonal directions. Scalp data were then modeled with single dipoles based on a principal components analysis (PCA) of the scalp-recorded data. The location and orientation of the dipoles were unconstrained. Data were modeled separately for adults and children. Residual variance of each model was less than 5%. Both models produced dipole generators in temporal, parietal, and cingulate cortices, as well as sources in medial temporal lobe regions near the hippocampus or parahippocampal gyrus. Both models showed good fit with the opposite age group (<5% residual variance), suggesting that the two groups showed essentially the same dipole generators. Current source density (CSD) plots (not shown) in adults showed differential activity for old and new items at temporal lobe dipoles around 960 ms (old > new). A similar effect was observed for children around 1,040 ms (lag 5 > lag 2 > new).

The current data support the feasibility of using these methods, both high-density ERPs and the continuous recognition memory task, in this age range. Seven- to 8-year-old children as well as adults showed differential scalp-recorded brain activity as a function of memory load and, in some cases, by stimulus type. Dipole source modeling techniques suggest that at least some of these memory effects stem from dipole sources in medial temporal lobe brain regions hypothesized to be affected in IDMs.

CONCLUSIONS

Data drawn from our longitudinal study of IDMs reveal a reliable pattern of electrophysiological findings consistent with our hypothesis that the diabetic pregnancy places the fetus at risk for developing memory problems postnatally, due to underlying perturbations in hippocampal development. Over and above the clinical implications of such work (e.g., to alert pediatricians who care for such infants to monitor the children later in life for learning and memory problems), these data also serve as a model system for how we can use ERPs to examine the neural circuitry involved in the development of a specific cognitive function—in our case, various types of explicit memory. Thus, we should think of this research as an example of the value of converging operations: Specifically, studying this particular population has permitted us to examine more directly our hypothesis that the hippocampus is involved in recognition memory.

Although our source modeling efforts are providing invaluable information about the neural sources responsible for various ERP components, the spatial resolution of ERPs will always be limited. For this reason we believe that coregistering ERP data with MRI and fMRI data will prove extremely useful. Specifically, the superior spatial resolution of MRI-based measures, coupled with the superior temporal resolution of ERP measures, will provide investigators with temporal–spatial information that cannot be provided by either measure alone. Unfortunately, MRI-based measures lack feasibility for children younger than approximately 6 years. For this reason it is important for those recording from high-density electrode arrays to continue developing source modeling algorithms that have increased precision, thereby affording investigators a tool that permits reasonable inferences to be drawn about the neural sources that underlie ERP components. This effort will be aided by conducting research with atypical populations in whom there is a suspicion of discrete neural injury (as we have done in our IDM population). For example, if we demonstrate among typically developing children that a particular ERP component is localized to the hippocampus, then when the same experimental manipulation is performed with children who have experienced hippocampal damage, source modeling should reveal the *lack* of (normal) hippocampal activation. This method of converging operations will go a long way toward providing a fuller understanding of the development of function–structure relations among both typically developing and atypically developing children.

One additional area worthy of new investigation unique to early development concerns the ability to time-lock overt behavior with ERPs. Currently most ERP investigations do not record behavior coincident with

ERPs, for the very simple reason that most ERP designs do not permit the simultaneous recording of behavior (e.g., when stimuli are presented for 500 ms, there is no infant behavior that can be measured). We and others have devoted considerable attention to this problem over the past few years, thus far with little to show for our effort. Still, we are optimistic that new eye-tracking technology may permit us to record some visual behaviors simultaneously with ERPs, furthering our efforts to investigate brain–behavior links.

In conclusion, the field of developmental cognitive neuroscience has made tremendous advances in the last decade. This is particularly true in the domain of ERPs, where the number of laboratories employing this method has increased exponentially. It is my hope that when in another decade hence, the field will have advanced even further.

ACKNOWLEDGMENTS

The writing of this chapter was made possible, in part, by support from the National Institutes of Health (Grant No. NS32755). I gratefully acknowledge the many contributions of the developmental cognitive neuroscience laboratory and my collaborators Drs. Michael Georgieff and Raye-ann deRegnier.

REFERENCES

Barks, J. D., Sun, R., Malinak, C., & Silverstein, F. S. (1995). Gp120, an HIV-1 protein, increases susceptibility to hypoglycemic and ischemic brain injury in perinatal rats. *Experimental Neurology, 132,* 123–133.

Bauer, P. J. (2006). Event memory. In W. Damon, R. Lerner, D. Kuhn, & R. Siegler (Eds.), *Handbook of child psychology* (6th ed.): *Vol. 2. Cognition, perception and language* (pp. 373–425). Hoboken, NJ: Wiley.

Burdo, J. R., & Connor, J. R. (2002). Iron transport in the central nervous system. In D. Templeton (Ed.), *Molecular and cellular iron transport* (pp. 487–505). New York: Dekker.

Connor, J. R., & Menzies, S. L. (1996). Relationship of iron to oligodendrocytes and myelination. *Glia, 17,* 83–93.

Davies, P. L., Segalowitz, S. J., & Gavin, W. J. (2004). Development of error-monitoring event-related potentials in adolescents. *Annals of the New York Academy of Sciences, 1021,* 324–328.

Dawson, G., Carver, L., Meltzoff, A. N., Panagiotides, H., McPartland, J., & Webb, S. J. (2002). Neural correlates of face and object recognition in young children with autism spectrum disorder, developmental delay, and typical development. *Child Development, 73,* 700–717.

Dawson, G., & Fischer, K. W. (Eds.). (1994). *Human behavior and the developing brain*. New York: Guilford Press.

Dawson, G., Webb, S. J., Carver, L., Panagiotides, H., & McPartland, J. (2004). Young children with autism show atypical brain responses to fearful versus neutral facial expressions of emotion. *Developmental Science, 7,* 340–359.

DeBoer, T., Georgieff, M. K., & Nelson, C. A. (in press). Declarative memory performance in infants of diabetic mothers. In P. J. Bauer (Ed.), *Varieties of early experience: Influences on declarative memory development*. Mahwah, NJ: Erlbaum.

DeBoer, T., Scott, L., & Nelson, C. A. (2004). Event-related potentials in developmental populations. In T. Handy (Ed.), *Event-related potentials: A methods handbook* (pp. 263–297). Cambridge, MA: MIT Press.

DeBoer, T., Wewerka, S., Bauer, P. J., Georgieff, M. K., & Nelson, C. A. (2005). Explicit memory performance in infants of diabetic mothers at 1 year of age. *Developmental Medicine and Child Neurology, 47,* 525–531.

deRegnier, R.-A., Georgieff, M. K., & Nelson, C. A. (1997). Visual event-related brain potentials in 4–month-old infants at risk for neurodevelopmental impairments. *Developmental Psychobiology, 30,* 11–28.

deRegnier, R.-A., Nelson, C. A., Thomas, K., Wewerka, S., & Georgieff, M. K. (2000). Neurophysiologic evaluation of auditory recognition memory in healthy newborn infants and infants of diabetic mothers. *Journal of Pediatrics, 137,* 777–784.

De Ungria, M., Rao, R., Wobken, J. D., Luciana, M., Nelson, C. A., & Georgieff, M. K. (2000). Perinatal iron deficiency decreases cytochrome$_c$oxidase (CytOx) activity in selective regions of neonatal rat brain. *Pediatric Research, 48,* 169–176.

Georgieff, M. K., Landon, M. B., Mills, M. M., Hedlund, B. E., Faassen, A. E., Schmidt, R. L., et al. (1990). Abnormal iron distribution in infants of diabetic mothers: Spectrum and maternal antecedents. *Journal of Pediatrics, 117,* 455–461.

Georgieff, M. K., Petry, C. D., Mills, M. M., McKay, H., & Wobken, J. D. (1997). Increased N-glycosylation and reduced transferrin-binding capacity of transferrin receptor isolated from placentae of diabetic women. *Placenta, 18,* 563–568.

Hunt, R. H., Couperus, J. W., Nelson, C. A., & Thomas, K. M. (2004a, June). *Continuous recognition memory in adults and children: An ERP study of parametric memory load manipulation*. Poster presented at the annual meeting of the Organization for Human Brain Mapping, Budapest, Hungary.

Hunt, R. H., Couperus, J. W., Nelson, C. A., & Thomas, K. M. (2004b, April). *Electophysiological correlates of continuous recognition memory in adults and children: A parametric manipulation of memory load*. Poster presented at the annual meeting of the Cognitive Neuroscience Society, San Francisco.

Hunt, R. H., Couperus, J. W., Townsend, E. L., Nelson, C. A., & Thomas, K. M. (2005, April). *Developmental differences in continuous recognition memory: An fMRI and ERP study of parametrically manipulated memory load*. Paper presented at the annual meeting of the Society for Research in Child Development, Atlanta, GA.

Hunt, R. H., Townsend, E. L., Couperus, J. W., Nelson, C. A., & Thomas, K. M. (2005, April). *A developmental fMRI study of medial temporal lobe function: Differences in continuous recognition memory.* Poster presented at the annual meeting of the Society for Research in Child Development, Atlanta, GA.

Johnson, M. H., de Haan, M., Oliver, A., Smith, W., Hatzakis, H., Tucker, L. A., et al. (2001). Recording and analyzing high-density event-related potentials with infants: Using the Geodesic sensor net. *Developmental Neuropsychology, 19,* 295–323.

Klorman, R., Thatcher, J. E., Shaywitz, S. E., Fletcher, J. M., Marchione, K. E., Holahan, J. M., et al. (2002). Effects of event probability and sequence on children with attention-deficit/hyperactivity, reading, and math disorder. *Biological Psychiatry, 52,* 795–804.

Kraus, N. (2001). Auditory pathway encoding and neural plasticity in children with learning problems. *Audiology Neurootolaryngology, 6,* 221–227.

Milley, J. R., Papacostas, J. S., & Tabata, B. K. (1986). Effect of insulin on uptake of metabolic substrates by the fetus. *American Journal of Physiology—Endocrinology and Metabolism, 251,* E349–E359.

Nelson, C. A. (1994). Neural correlates of recognition memory in the first postnatal year of life. In G. Dawson & K. W. Fischer (Eds.), *Human behavior and the developing brain* (pp. 269–313). New York: Guilford Press.

Nelson, C., Erikson, K., Pinero, D. J., & Beard, J. L. (1997). In vivo DA metabolism is altered in iron deficient anemic rats. *Journal of Nutrition. 127,* 2282–2288.

Nelson, C. A., & Monk, C. (2001). The use of event-related potentials in the study of cognitive development. In C. A. Nelson & M. Luciana (Eds.), *Handbook of developmental cognitive neuroscience* (pp. 125–136). Cambridge, MA: MIT Press.

Nelson, C., & Silverstein, F. S. (1994). Acute disruption of cytochrome oxidase activity in brain in a perinatal rat stroke model. *Pediatric Research, 36,* 12–19.

Nelson, C. A., Thomas, K. M., & de Haan, M. (2006). Neural bases of cognitive development. In W. Damon, R. Lerner, D. Kuhn, & R. Siegler (Eds.), *Handbook of child psychology* (6th ed.): *Vol. 2. Cognition, perception and language* (pp. 3–57). Hoboken, NJ: Wiley.

Nelson, C. A., & Webb, S. J. (2002). A cognitive neuroscience perspective on early memory development. In M. de Haan & M. H. Johnson (Eds.), *The cognitive neuroscience of development* (pp. 99–125). London: Psychology Press.

Nelson, C. A., Wewerka, S., Borscheid, A. J., deRegnier, R.-A., & Georgieff, M. K. (2003). Electrophysiologic evidence of impaired cross-modal recognition memory in 8–month-old infants of diabetic mothers. *Journal of Pediatrics, 142,* 575–582.

Nelson, C. A., Wewerka, S., Thomas, K. M., Tribby-Walbridge, S., deRegnier, R.-A., & Georgieff, M. (2000). Neurocognitive sequelae of infants of diabetic mothers. *Behavioral Neuroscience, 114,* 950–956.

Ornoy, A., Ratson, N., Greenbaum, C., Wolf, A., & Dulitzky, M. (2001). School-age children born to diabetic mothers and to mothers with gestational diabetes exhibit a high rate of inattention and fine and gross motor impairment. *Journal of Pediatric Endocrinology and Metabolism, 14,* 681–689.

Parker, S. W., Nelson, C. A., & Bucharest Early Intervention Project Core Group. (2005a). An event-related potential study of the impact of institutional rearing on face recognition. *Development and Psychopathology, 17,* 621–639.

Parker, S. W., Nelson, C. A., & Bucharest Early Intervention Project Core Group. (2005b). The impact of deprivation on the ability to discriminate facial expressions of emotion: An event-related potential study. *Child Development, 76,* 54–72.

Petry, C. D., Eaton, M. D., Wobken, J. D., Mills, M. M., Johnson, D. E., & Georgieff, M. K. (1992). Iron deficiency of liver, heart and brain in infants of diabetic mothers. *Journal of Pediatrics, 121,* 109–114.

Pollak, S. D., Klorman, R., Thatcher, J. E., & Cicchetti, D. (2001). P3b reflects maltreated children's reactions to facial displays of emotion. *Psychophysiology, 38,* 267–274.

Rao, R., De Ungria, M., Sullivan, D., Wu, P., Wobken, J. D., Nelson, C. A., et al. (1999). Perinatal iron deficiency increases the vulnerability of rat hippocampus to hypoxic ischemic insult. *Journal of Nutrition, 129,* 199–206.

Rizzo, T., Metzger, B. E., Burns, W. J., & Burns, K. (1991). Correlations between antepartum maternal metabolism and intelligence of offspring. *New England Journal of Medicine, 325,* 911–916.

Rizzo, T. A., Metzger, B. E., Dooley, S. L., & Cho, N. H. (1997). Early malnutrition and child neurobehavioral development: Insights from the study of children of diabetic mothers. *Child Development, 68,* 26–38.

Roncagliolo, M., Garrdio, M., Walter, T., Peirano, P., & Lozoff, B. (1998). Evidence of altered central nervous system development in infants with iron deficiency anemia at 6 months: Delayed maturation of auditory brainstem responses. *American Journal of Clinical Nutrition 68,* 683–690.

Siddappa, A. M., Georgieff, M. K., Wewerka, S., Worwa, C., Nelson, C. A., & deRegnier, R.-A. (2004). Iron deficiency alters auditory recognition memory in newborn infants of diabetic mothers. *Pediatric Research, 55,* 1034–1041.

Silverman, B. L., Rizzo, T., Green, O. C., Cho, N. H., Winter, R. J., Ogata, E. S., et al. (1991). Long-term prospective evaluation of offspring of diabetic mothers. *Diabetes, 40,*121–125.

Stonestreet, B. S., Golstein, M., Oh, W., & Widness, J. A. (1989). Effect of prolonged hyperinsulinemia on erythropoiesis in fetal sheep. *American Journal of Physiology, 257,* R1199–R1204.

Thomas, K. M., Hunt, R. H., Townsend, E. L., Couperus, J. W., Nelson, C. A., & Mueller, B. A. (2004a, June). *Developmental differences in continuous recognition memory: An fMRI study of medial temporal lobe function.* Poster presented at the annual meeting of the Organization for Human Brain Mapping, Budapest, Hungary.

Thomas, K. M., Hunt, R. H., Townsend, E. L., Couperus, J. W., Nelson, C. A., & Mueller, B. A. (2004b, April). *Developmental differences in hippocampal function: An fMRI study of continuous recognition memory*. Poster presented at the annual meeting of the Cognitive Neuroscience Society, San Francisco.

Widness, J. A. (1989). Fetal risks and neonatal complications of diabetes mellitus. In S. A. Brody & K. Ueland (Eds.), *Endocrine disorders in pregnancy* (pp. 273–297). Norwalk, CT: Appleton & Lange.

Widness, J. A., Susa, J. B., Garcia, J. F., Singer, O. B., Sehgal, O., Oh, W., et al. (1981). Increased erythropoiesis and elevated erythropoietin in infants born to diabetic mothers and in hyperinsulinemic rhesus fetuses. *Journal of Clinical Investigation, 67*, 637–642.

CHAPTER 2

Development of Social Brain Circuitry in Autism

Geraldine Dawson
Raphael Bernier

The past two decades have witnessed a tremendous expansion in our knowledge of the neural basis of social behavior. Improved neuroimaging techniques have allowed us to study the brain in action in young children, offering insights into the brain basis of early social behavior. This knowledge has provided new understanding of brain-based disorders that affect social development. In turn, studies of such disorders have provided unique perspectives on the normal development of the social brain.

Autism, most fundamentally, is a disorder of social communication. Young children with autism fail to show early preferences for the social environment; higher-order social behaviors, such as shared attention and theory of mind, are core impairments found in the disorder. As we learn more about the neural basis of autism, we come to understand the biological underpinnings of fundamental aspects of social behavior. Which neural substrates are critical to an ability to imitate others, to share emotional states, and to engage in coordinated, reciprocal interactions with others? When do such neural substrates come on line and how do they influence the child's ability to engage with the social environment, thereby providing the basis and mechanism for further development? These are the types of questions that the disorder of autism poses.

In this chapter, we begin by describing some of the early impairments in social behavior found in autism. Next, a developmental model for the normal emergence of social brain circuitry during early infancy is described, along with a theory of how this development might be disrupted in autism. Finally, we discuss research on the genetic basis of aspects of social behavior and the potential role of this research in understanding the etiology of autism.

EARLY SOCIAL IMPAIRMENTS IN AUTISM

Five domains of social behavior that typically emerge during the first year of life have been found to be affected in autism. As reviewed below, these domains are social orienting, joint attention, attention to others' emotions, motor imitation, and face processing.

Social Orienting

Dawson and her coworkers coined the term "social orienting impairment" to refer to the failure of young children with autism to spontaneously orient to naturally occurring social stimuli in their environment (Dawson, Meltzoff, Osterling, Rinaldi, & Brown, 1998). Mundy and Neal (2001) proposed that the developmental pathway of young children with autism is altered by this social orienting impairment because the children are deprived of appropriate social stimulation. Very early in life, typical infants show remarkable sensitivity to social stimuli (Rochat, 1999). Neonates are naturally attracted to people, including human sounds, human movements, and features of the human face (Maurer & Salapatek, 1976; Morton & Johnson, 1991). For example, infants as young as 5 months observe even very small deviations in eye gaze during social interactions with adults and stop smiling and look away when the adult partner's eyes are averted (Symons, Hains, & Muir, 1998). This early emerging sensitivity and attention to the social world is reflexive rather than voluntary. Very likely, the acquisition of subsequent social behaviors depends on this very early propensity to devote particular attention to people (Rochat & Striano, 1999). Active volitional orienting to a social stimulus, such as head turning when one's name is called, typically emerges by 5–7 months of age. Around this age early joint attention skills also may begin to develop: Typically developing infants between the ages of 6 and 12 months have been shown to match the direction of mother's head turn toward a target (Brooks & Meltzoff, 2002; Morales, Mundy, & Rojas, 1998).

One of the earliest and most basic social impairments in autism is a failure to orient to social stimuli, and this failure almost certainly contributes to the later social and communicative impairments observed in the disorder (Dawson, Meltzoff, Osterling, & Rinaldi, 1998; Mundy & Neal, 2001). Retrospective studies of home videotapes of first birthdays have shown that, in comparison to typically developing 12-month-olds, 1-year-old infants later diagnosed with autism fail to orient to their names, attend less to people, and show impairments in joint attention (Osterling & Dawson, 1994; Osterling, Dawson, & Munson, 2002). A home videotape study examining behaviors in even younger infants demonstrated that 8- to 10-month-old infants later diagnosed with autism were much less likely to orient when their names were called, compared to typically developing infants of the same age (Werner, Dawson, Osterling, & Dinno, 2000). These behaviors are also seen in toddlers with autism. Swettenham and colleagues observed attentional patterns in 20-month-old toddlers with autism, typical development, and developmental delay and found that the toddlers with autism spent less time overall looking at people, looked more briefly at people, and looked longer at objects (Swettenham et al., 1998). Dawson and colleagues demonstrated in two experimental studies that, compared to children with mental retardation without autism and typically developing children, children with autism more frequently failed to orient to both social and nonsocial stimuli, but this failure was much more extreme for social stimuli (Dawson, Meltzoff, Osterling, Rinaldi, & Brown, 1998; Dawson, Toth, et al., 2004). These studies also indicated that children with autism were more impaired in their joint attention ability; furthermore, severity of their joint attention ability was strongly correlated with social orienting ability but not with nonsocial orienting ability.

Joint Attention

Joint attention is the ability to coordinate attention between interactive social partners with respect to objects or events in order to share an awareness of the objects or events (Mundy, Sigman, Ungerer, & Sherman, 1986). There is a range of joint attention behaviors that includes sharing attention (e.g., through the use of alternating eye gaze), following the attention of another (e.g., following eye gaze or a point), and directing the attention of another. Typically developing infants generally demonstrate all of these skills by 12 months of age (Carpenter, Nagell, & Tomasello, 1998), but some infants as young as 6 months display aspects of joint attention (e.g., matching direction of mother's head turn to a visible target; Morales et al., 1998).

The absence of joint attention ability has been unequivocally established as an early emerging and fundamental impairment in autism, present by 1 year of age in children wiht early-onset autism and incorporated into the diagnostic criteria for the disorder (American Psychiatric Association, 1994; Mundy et al., 1986). Through numerous studies, joint attention ability has been shown to distinguish preschool-age children with autism from those with developmental delays and typical development (Bacon, Fein, Morris, Waterhouse, & Allen, 1998; Charman et al., 1998; Dawson, Meltzoff, Osterling, & Rinaldi, 1998; Mundy et al., 1986; Sigman, Kasari, Kwon, & Yirmiya, 1992). Joint attention skills have also been found to be a good predictor of both concurrent and future language skills in children with autism. In a longitudinal study of social competence and language skills in children with autism and Down syndrome, Sigman and Ruskin (1999) found that joint attention skills were concurrently associated with language ability for both groups and for the children with autism were predictive of long-term gains in expressive language skills. Using path analysis in a sample of 72 young children with autism, Dawson and colleagues found that social orienting ability was *indirectly* related to language ability through its contribution to joint attention skills. The authors hypothesized that a child's ability to attend to social information contributes critically to the acquisition of joint attention skills because such skills require the child to attend actively to social cues, particularly those expressed on the face (e.g., direction of eye gaze; Dawson, Meltzoff, Osterling, Rinaldi, & Brown, 1998). Other perspectives posit that it is a lack of a "shared attention mechanism" that is fundamentally responsible for the joint attention impairments seen in autism, rather than an impairment in attention to social stimuli (Baron-Cohen, 1995).

Attention to Others' Emotions

Another early emerging social behavior is noticing and responding to others' emotions. Infants within the first 6 months of life show great sensitivity to the emotions displayed by others (Trevarthen, 1979) and differentially respond to faces showing different emotions (e.g., neutral, happy, sad). Infants will attend longer and smile more frequently to a happy face as compared to a neutral or sad face (Rochat & Striano, 1999; Tronick, Als, Adamson, Wise, & Brazelton, 1978). Social referencing, whereby children seek emotional information from an adult's face when presented with a stimulus of uncertain valence, is established by 9–12 months of age (Feinman, 1982; Moore & Corkum, 1994). By 2 years of age, children begin to respond to another person's distress affectively and prosocially by helping, comforting, and sharing (Rheingold, Hay, & West, 1976; Zahn-Waxler & Radke-Yarrow, 1990).

   Many, but not all, children with autism demonstrate a lack of sensitivity to the emotional states of others. Studies have shown that, when adults displayed facial expressions of distress, children with autism looked less at the adult and showed less concern compared to children with mental retardation and typical development (Bacon et al., 1998; Charman et al., 1998; Dawson, Meltzoff, Osterling, & Rinaldi, 1998; Dawson, Toth, et al., 2004; Sigman et al., 1992). Further examination of these behaviors has shown that when a neutral affect condition was included, children with autism could distinguish between negative and neutral affect displays. Children with autism looked more at the examiner's face and showed more concern when the examiner showed a distressed expression than a neutral expression. However, they looked for shorter durations and showed less interest and concern in both conditions than did children with mental retardation (Corona, Dissanayake, Arbelle, Wellington, & Sigman, 1998).

   Dawson and colleagues used event-related electrical brain potentials (ERPs) to examine whether young children with autism responded differentially to distinct emotional expressions. Differential ERPs to different facial expressions of emotion have been shown in adults (Eimer & Holmes, 2002), in typically developing children (de Haan, Nelson, Gunnar, & Tout, 1998), and even in infants as young as 7 months (Nelson & de Haan, 1996). To assess emotion perception skills in young children with autism, Dawson and colleagues showed 3- to 4-year-old children pictures of two facial expressions. In one picture the model's face depicted a neutral expression; in the other her face depicted a prototypic expression of fear (Dawson, Webb, et al., 2004). Compared to typically developing children, the children with autism exhibited significantly slower early (N300) brain responses to the facial expression of fear. Children with autism also failed to show a larger amplitude negative slow-wave response to the fearful face that characterized the ERPs of typically developing children. Moreover, the children with autism displayed aberrant ERP scalp topography in response to the fearful face. The delayed response to the fearful face suggests that information-processing speed is compromised, and the abnormal topography suggests a failure of cortical specialization or atypical recruitment of cortical areas in autism. Additionally, individual differences in N300 latency to the fearful face were associated with performance on behavioral tasks requiring social attention (tasks that were administered on a different day from ERP testing). The children with better joint attention skills, fewer social orienting errors, and who spent more time looking at an experimenter expressing distress displayed a faster N300 latency to the fearful face. In contrast, there was no association between N300 latency and performance on nonsocial tasks. These findings suggest that slower information-processing speed for emotional face stimuli is associated with more severe social attention impairments in children with autism.

Motor Imitation

The ability to imitate is a very early emerging and pivotal aspect of social development. Even newborns are capable of imitating facial expressions (Meltzoff & Moore, 1977, 1979, 1983), and imitation ability develops rapidly such that, by 1 year of age, infants are able to imitate actions on objects and gestures, such as waving. The imitation of observed actions later in new contexts, termed *deferred imitation*, emerges between the first and second year, although some researchers suggest that it develops much earlier (Meltzoff & Moore, 1994).

The importance of imitation in social development has long been recognized. Imitation has been proposed to serve as a basis for social connectedness with others as well as a basis for the child's ability to differentiate self from others (Eckerman, Davis, & Didow, 1989; Meltzoff & Gopnick, 1993; Nadel, Guerini, Peze, & Rivet, 1999; Trevarthen, Kokkinaki, & Fiamenghi, 1999; Užgiris, 1981). Imitation also promotes learning and understanding about the intentions and goals of others (Kugiumutzakis, 1999; Užgiris, 1999) and likely serves as a precursor for the development of a theory of mind (Meltzoff & Gopnick, 1993; Rogers & Pennington, 1991). Imitation also plays a role in symbolic play (Piaget, 1962), peer relationships (Trevarthen al., 1999), language (Avikainen, Wohlschlager, Liuhanen, Hanninen, & Hari, 2003; Charman et al., 2003), and emotional sharing (Hatfield, Cacioppo, & Rapson, 1994).

A failure to spontaneously imitate others, especially in social play contexts, appears to be a core early impairment in autism (Dawson & Adams, 1984; Dawson & Lewy, 1989; Rogers, Bennetto, McEvoy, & Pennington, 1996; Rogers & Pennington, 1991; Williams, Whiten, Suddendorf, & Perrett, 2001). Imitation ability discriminates toddlers with autism from those with mental retardation or a communication disorder (Stone, Lemanek, Fishel, Fernandez, & Altemeier, 1990; Stone, Ousley, & Littleford, 1997). Numerous studies have demonstrated that individuals with autism perform poorly in virtually all aspects of imitation (Rogers, Hepburn, Stackhouse, & Wehner, 2003), including imitating motor movements (Hertzig, Snow, & Sherman, 1989), facial expressions (Loveland et al., 1994), the style of tasks (Hobson & Lee, 1999), actions involving imaginary objects (Rogers et al., 1996), and vocalizations (Dawson & Adams, 1984).

Williams and colleagues (2001) hypothesize that the imitation deficits observed in autism are the result of a deficit in self–other mapping. That is, imitation deficits reflect an impairment in the ability to map the complex actions of others onto a reference for the self. Meltzoff and colleagues (Meltzoff & Decety, 2003; Meltzoff & Gopnick, 1993) have proposed a similar concept in the "Like Me" hypothesis.

Face Processing

Faces have special significance and provide nonverbal information important for communication for typically developing infants (Darwin, 1872/ 1965). Face recognition ability is present very early in life. Indeed, at birth, neonates show the capacity for very rapid face recognition (Walton & Bower, 1993) and a visual preference for faces (Goren, Sarty, & Wu, 1975). By 4 months, infants recognize upright faces better than upside down faces (Fagan, 1972) and by 6 months, infants show differential ERPs to familiar versus unfamiliar faces (de Haan & Nelson, 1997, 1999). By the end of the first year of life, infants are capable of differentiating facial gestures, determining the direction of eye gaze, and attending to expressions of emotion. These early developing abilities, particularly attention and response to the face and gaze, are essential to successful joint attention and social orienting interactions. Face processing has also been suggested to be important in the development of social relationships and theory of mind (Baron-Cohen, 1995; Brothers, Ring, & Kling, 1990; Perrett, Harries, Mistlin, & Hietanen, 1990; Perrett, Hietanen, Oram, & Benson, 1992; Williams et al., 2001).

Face processing abilities in individuals with autism have consistently been shown to be impaired. In a retrospective study using videotapes of first birthday parties, the failure to look at others was the single best discriminator between infants who were later diagnosed with an autism spectrum disorder and those with typical development (Osterling & Dawson, 1994; see also Adrien et al., 1991). In a case study published by Dawson and colleagues (Dawson, Osterling, Meltzoff, & Kuhl, 2000), a young infant who was diagnosed with autism at 1 year of age and rediagnosed at 2 years of age was reported to show atypical eye contact. In early medical records chronicling his first 6 months, he reportedly demonstrated "generally good eye contact, although at times he averted his eyes" and smiled responsively. However, on four different evaluations from 9 to 13 months, his eye contact was reported as "a transfixed stare," "poor," and "within normal limits." Thus, the infant's use of eye gaze appeared to develop normally at first, becoming variable and typical only during the second half of the first year of postnatal life. Reportedly, during this same period, the infant showed reduced social responsiveness, and social interactions were described as "aversive" to the infant.

Using ERPs Dawson, Carver, and colleagues (2002) examined face recognition abilities in 3- to 4-year-old children with autism, developmental delay, and typical development. In this study, high-density ERPs were recorded from the children while they watched images of familiar (mother) and unfamiliar (another female) faces and familiar (favorite toy) and unfamiliar (novel toy) objects. The typical children demonstrated increased amplitude to the novel faces and objects for two ERP components. The children with autism showed the same differential ERP response for the objects, but did not show the differential response for the faces. These findings indicate that children with autism demonstrate selective face recognition impairments as early as 3 years of age.

Studies of face memory in autism have shown that by middle childhood, children with autism perform worse than mental-age- and chronological-age-matched peers on a number of face processing tasks. These tasks include tests of both face recognition (Boucher & Lewis, 1992; Boucher, Lewis, & Collis, 1998; Gepner, de Gelder, & de Schonen, 1996; Klin et al., 1999) and face discrimination (Tantam, Monoghan, Nicholson, & Stirling, 1989). Whereas typically developing children show better memory performance for faces than non-face visual stimuli, children with autism perform comparably on face and non-face tasks (Serra et al., 2003) or show better performance on non-face tasks (e.g., memory for buildings) than on face tasks (Boucher & Lewis, 1992). Studies also suggest that individuals with autism process faces using abnormal strategies. By middle childhood, typically developing children (1) are better at recognizing parts of a face when the parts are presented in the context of a whole face, (2) perform better when recognition involves the eyes versus the mouth (Joseph & Tanaka, 2003), (3) show a greater decrement in memory for inverted versus upright faces as compared with non-face visual stimuli, and (4) attend to upright faces for longer lengths of time than inverted faces (van der Geest, Kemner, Verbatem, & van Engeland, 2002). In contrast, children with autism are better at recognizing isolated facial features and partially obscured faces than typical children (Hobson, Ouston, & Lee, 1988; Tantam et al., 1989) and show better memory performance for the lower half of the face than the upper half during childhood (Langdell, 1978). Other studies of visual attention to faces indicate that individuals with autism exhibit reduced attention to the core features of the face, such as the eyes and nose, relative to typical individuals (Klin, Jones, Schultz, Volkmar, & Cohen, 2002; Pelphrey et al., 2002; Trepagnier, Sebrechts, & Peterson, 2002).

HYPOTHESES REGARDING THE NEURAL BASIS OF EARLY SOCIAL IMPAIRMENTS IN AUTISM

As reviewed above, autism is associated with a wide range of early impairments in social behavior. We now address the question of what the neurodevelopmental basis of such impairments in autism might be. We describe a general model of the emergence of social brain circuitry in the first year of life and discuss how the trajectory of normal development of social brain circuitry is altered in autism.

At least two alternatives can be offered to explain the early social impairments found in autism. The first is that there might exist basic perceptual–cognitive impairments. For example, these might be deficits in general abilities that are important for face processing, such as the ability to perceptually bind features of a stimulus (Dawson, Webb, et al., 2002) or to form prototypes (Klinger & Dawson, 2001), or deficits in specific neural mechanisms that are specialized for processing social information, such as the fusiform gyrus for faces (Haxby et al., 1994, 1999; Hoffman & Haxby, 2000; Kanwisher, McDermott, & Chun, 1997) or the superior temporal sulcus for eye movements (Perrett et al., 1985, 1992; see also Pelphrey & Carter, Chapter 3, this volume). A primary perceptual deficit would impact other aspects of social brain circuitry, especially those aspects that rely on social perception, such as joint attention, interpretation of emotional expression, and even speech perception.

The second hypothesis, referred to as the *social motivation hypothesis*, posits a primary impairment in social motivation—that is, the affective tagging of socially relevant stimuli (Dawson, Webb, & McPartland, 2005; Dawson, Carver, et al., 2002; Grelotti, Gauthier, & Schultz, 2002; Waterhouse, Fein, & Modahl, 1996). The evidence for a social motivation impairment in autism comes from both clinical observations and research findings. Clinically, diagnostic criteria for autism include "a lack of spontaneous seeking to share enjoyment, interests, or achievements with other people" and "lack of social or emotional reciprocity" (American Psychiatric Association, 1994). Dawson, Hill, Galpert, Spencer, and Watson (1990) found that preschool-age children with autism were less likely to smile when looking at their mothers during social interaction, and young children with autism have been found to be less likely to express positive emotion during joint attention episodes (Kasari, Sigman, Mundy, & Yirmiya, 1990).

According to this hypothesis, reduced social motivation results in less time spent paying attention to faces as well as to all other social stimuli, such as the human voice, hand gestures, and so forth. Previously, Dawson hypothesized that social motivational impairments in autism are related to a difficulty in forming representations of the reward value of social stimuli (Dawson, Carver, et al., 2002). One of the primary neural systems involved in processing reward information is the dopamine system (Schultz, 1998). Dopaminergic projections to the striatum and frontal cortex, particularly the orbitofrontal cortex, are critical in mediating the effects of reward on approach behavior. The orbitofrontal cortex, which is dependent on input from the basolateral amygdala, is implicated in the formation of representations of reward value (Schoenbaum, Setlow, Saddoris, & Gallagher,

2003). The dopamine reward system is activated in response to social rewards, including eye contact (Kampe, Frith, Dolan, & Frith, 2001). Gingrich, Liu, Cascio, Wang, and Insel (2000) showed that dopamine D2 receptors in the nucleus accumbens are important for social attachment in voles. Dawson, Munson, and colleagues (2002) reported that performance on neurocognitive tasks that tap the medial temporal lobe–orbitofrontal circuit (e.g., object discrimination reversal) is strongly correlated with the severity of joint attention impairments in young children with autism. We hypothesize that dysfunction of the dopamine reward system, especially its functioning in social contexts, might account for impairments in social motivation found in autism.

Oxytocin and Its Relation to the Dopamine Reward System

Waterhouse and colleagues (1996) hypothesized that impaired functioning of the oxytocin system in autism reduces social bonding and affiliation. Insel (1997) has discussed the role of peptides, specifically oxytocin and vasopressin, in the modulation of the dopamine reward circuit in social contexts. These peptides play an important role in linking social input to the reinforcement system (Pedersen et al., 1994). Several animal studies have shown that vasopressin and oxytocin are critical in facilitating "social memory." For example, oxytocin knockout mice show a profound and specific deficit in social memory (Ferguson, Young, Hearn, Insel, & Winslow, 2000; Ferguson, Young, & Insel, 2002; Nishimori et al., 1996). These knockout mice studies provide support for the notion that social memory has a neural basis distinct from other forms of memory. Interestingly, during the initial exposure to a familiar conspecific, oxytocin acts in the medial amygdala to facilitate social recognition. Indeed, both oxytocin and vasopressin appear to play a role in a variety of social behaviors, including social affiliation (Witt, Winslow, & Insel, 1992), maternal behavior (Pedersen et al., 1994), and social attachment (Insel & Hulihan, 1995; Winslow, Hastings, Carter, Harbaugh, & Insel, 1993). Insel and Fernald (2004) suggest that these peptides may operate on social behavior through their influence on the mesocorticolimbic dopamine circuit that links the anterior hypothalamus to the ventral tegmental area and the nucleus accumbens. This circuit may be especially important for mediating sensitivity to social reward in the context of social interaction.

We hypothesize that reduced reward value ("emotional tagging") of social stimuli may result in the profound social impairments found in individuals in autism as well as contribute to the language processing impairments characteristic of the disorder. Like Insel, O'Brien, and Leckman

(1999), we speculate that this factor might be related to abnormalities in peptides such as oxytocin and/or vasopressin, which modulate the dopamine reward pathway, specifically in the context of social interactions. In fact, there is some evidence of abnormalities in oxytocin and vasopressin in autism. In one study, reduced plasma concentrations of oxytocin were found in children with autism (Modahl et al., 1998). In another, Kim and colleagues (2002) found a nominally significant transmission disequilibrium between autism and an AVPR1A microsatellite, a V_{1a} receptor in the brain that has been shown to mediate the action of vasopressin. Clearly, this is an interesting area for future research in autism.

Emergence of Social Brain Circuitry in the First Year of Life

Dawson, Webb, and colleagues (2005) have described a developmental model for the normal emergence of social brain circuitry during early infancy, stressing the key role of the reward system in the development of the social brain (see Figure 2.1). In the model, drawing upon the work of Insel and colleagues (1999), modulation of the dopamine reward circuit by oxytocin is important for shaping the infant's early preference for social stimuli and attention to such stimuli. As mentioned above, in normal development, neonates display a particular attraction to people, especially to the sounds, movements, and features of the human face (Maurer & Salapatek, 1976; Morton & Johnson, 1991). Spontaneous orienting to a social stimulus, such as head turning when one's name is called, can be seen in infants by about 6–7 months of age.

We hypothesize that volitional orienting occurs, in part, because the infant anticipates pleasure (reward) to be associated with such stimuli. This type of interaction involves activation of the reward circuit, including parts of the prefrontal regions, such as the orbital prefrontal cortex, that play a role in the formation of reward representations. With increasing experience with faces and voices, which occurs in the context of social interactions, cortical specialization for faces and linguistic stimuli develops. This specialization involves the fine-tuning of perceptual systems. Furthermore, areas specialized for the perceptual processing of social stimuli, such as the fusiform gyrus and superior temporal sulcus, become tightly integrated with regions involved in reward (e.g., amygdala) as well as regions involved in motor actions and attention (e.g., cerebellum, prefrontal/cingulate cortex). Through this integration process, increasingly complex social brain circuitry emerges. In turn, this developing circuitry supports more complex behaviors, such as disengagement of attention, joint attention, intentional communication, and delayed imitation.

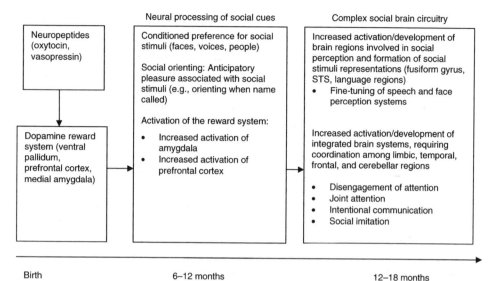

Neural processing of social cues | Complex social brain circuitry

| Neuropeptides (oxytocin, vasopressin) | Conditioned preference for social stimuli (faces, voices, people) | Increased activation/development of brain regions involved in social perception and formation of social stimuli representations (fusiform gyrus, STS, language regions) |

Social orienting: Anticipatory pleasure associated with social stimuli (e.g., orienting when name called)

• Fine-tuning of speech and face perception systems

Activation of the reward system:

Dopamine reward system (ventral pallidum, prefrontal cortex, medial amygdala)

• Increased activation of amygdala
• Increased activation of prefrontal cortex

Increased activation/development of integrated brain systems, requiring coordination among limbic, temporal, frontal, and cerebellar regions

• Disengagement of attention
• Joint attention
• Intentional communication
• Social imitation

Birth — 6–12 months — 12–18 months

FIGURE 2.1. The role of social reward in the emergence of social brain circuitry in the first years of life. Reproduced with permission from Dawson, G., et al. (2005). Neurocognitive and electrophysiological evidence of altered face processing in parents of children with autism: Implications for a model of abnormal development of social brain circuitry in autism. *Development and Psychopathology, 17,* 679–697.

Implications for Autism

One of the earliest symptoms of autism is a lack of "social orienting" (Dawson, Meltzoff, Osterling, Rinaldi, & Brown, 1998; Dawson, Toth, et al., 2004). This reduced attention to social stimuli and concomitant reduced experience with social stimuli likely results in a failure to become an expert face and language processor (Dawson et al., 2005; Grelotti et al., 2002). Because experience drives cortical specialization (Nelson, 2001), reduced attention to faces and speech would lead to a failure of specialization of brain regions that typically mediate face and language processing. This failure would be reflected in decreased cortical specialization and abnormal brain circuitry for face processing, resulting in slower information-processing speed. In two ERP studies (McPartland, Dawson, Webb, & Panagiotides, 2004; Webb, Dawson, Bernier, & Panagiotides, 2006), young children as well as adolescents and adults with autism exhibited slower ERPs to faces and failed to show the normal right lateralization of ERPs to faces relative to well-matched comparison groups. These studies suggest that autism is associated with both slower information-processing speed and atypical cortical specialization for face processing.

The abnormal trajectory for brain development in autism is not caused by a simple lack of exposure to human faces and voices. Infants with autism, like typically developing infants, are held, talked to, and fed by their parents during face-to-face interactions. However, if the infant with autism does not find such interactions inherently interesting or rewarding, then the infant might not actively attend to the face and voice or perceive the face within a larger social–affective context. Recent research suggests that simple exposure to language does not necessarily facilitate the development of brain circuitry specialized for language (Kuhl, Tsao, & Liu, 2003). Rather, for speech perception to develop, language needs to be experienced by the infant within a socially interactive context. Very early in life, infants are capable of discerning differences among the phonetic units of all languages, including both native and foreign languages. However, between 6 and 12 months of age, as the brain becomes proficient at speech perception, the ability to discriminate foreign language phonetic units declines (Kuhl et al., 1997). Kuhl and colleagues (2003) investigated the possibility of preventing this decline in foreign language phonetic perception by exposing American infants to native Mandarin Chinese speakers. They found that the decline of foreign language phonetic perception was preventable, *but only if exposure to speech occurred in the context of interpersonal interaction.* That is, an experimental condition in which infants were exposed to the same speech stimuli via audiotapes without social interaction did not avoid the narrowing of speech perception for the non-native language.

In the case of autism, if the child is not *actively attending to* faces and speech sounds as part of the social context, his or her early exposure to these social stimuli might not facilitate face and speech perception. The results of a recent study are consistent with this notion. Kuhl, Coffey-Corina, Padden, and Dawson (2004) found that listening preferences in 3- to 4-year-old children with autism differed dramatically from those of typically developing children. The children with autism preferred listening to mechanical-sounding auditory signals (computer-based signals acoustically matched to speech) rather than speech (motherese). The preference for the mechanical-sounding stimuli was associated with lower language ability, more severe autistic symptoms, and abnormal ERPs to speech sounds. The children with autism who did prefer motherese were more likely to show differential ERPs to different phonemes, whereas those who preferred the mechanical-sounding signal showed no such ERP waveform differences. We hypothesize that a failure to affectively tag social and linguistic stimuli as relevant and rewarding, and the resultant failure to attend to such stimuli, impedes the cortical specialization for brain regions typically associated with face and language processing. Therefore, perceptual fine-tuning of such social stimuli and the formation of representations of these stimuli are hampered. As a result, more complex behaviors that require the integration of social stimuli with coordinated, intentional movements and volitional attention, such as disengagement of attention and joint attention, then fail to emerge.

Potential Impact of Early Intervention

If the social motivation hypothesis is correct, it should be possible to alter children's attention to, and experience with, faces and speech through early intervention aimed at making social interactions more rewarding and meaningful. The impact of such an intervention on the development of face processing could then be assessed by examining the brain's responses to faces by using ERPs (Dawson & Zanolli, 2003). Through intervention, children can increase their use of eye contact, their use of affective exchanges, and their joint attention skills. An increase in these behavioral skills may be related to improvements such as increasing specialization in the neural face processing system. Indeed, interventions based on applied behavior analysis are designed to enhance the reward value of social stimuli through learning principles (see Figure 2.2). For example, during most early intervention programs, the therapist's face (a previously neutral stimulus) is deliberately paired with a nonsocial reinforcer (usually access to food or a toy). Via classical conditioning, the face then acquires reinforcer value. Early intervention could facilitate the development of the face processing system in two ways: first, by helping the child engage in meaningful social interactions that might lead to active attention to faces, and second, by altering the child's motivational preferences for faces so that engaging in face-to-face interaction becomes more rewarding and therefore more frequent (Dawson & Zanolli, 2003).

The timing of intervention might also have important consequences in relation to the plasticity of the face processing system. Increases in social motivation and active attention to faces might have differing results in children as compared to adults. For example, adults with autism might benefit from being trained to attend to faces and being taught explicit face processing strategies. However, although these interventions might result in better behavioral performance, it is unclear if they would result in alterations in patterns of neural activation. That is, interventions might support compensatory processes but fail to activate or develop typical processing mechanisms. Conversely, given the plasticity of the developing brain, young children who receive early intervention might demonstrate both improved behavioral performance (e.g., increases in eye contact, joint attention, and face recognition) as well as normalized brain functioning. This normalized brain functioning could be observed in differential responses to familiar versus unfamiliar faces, different phonemes, speed of neural responses, and

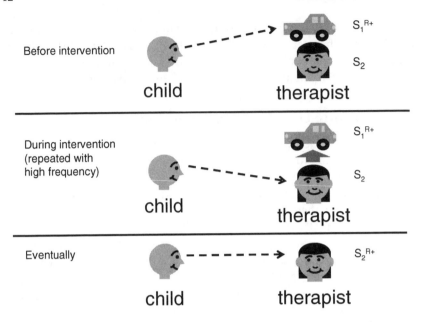

FIGURE 2.2. A model of the acquisition of social motivation in autism. Reproduced with permission from Dawson, G., & Zanolli, K. (2003). Early intervention and brain plasticity in autism. In G. Bock & J. Goode (Eds.), *Autism: Neural bases and treatment possibilities* (pp. 266–280). Chichester, UK: Wiley.

patterns of cortical specialization, as reflected in scalp topography and latency of ERP components during face and language processing tasks. Dawson is currently examining this possibility in an NIMH-funded randomized clinical trial of early intensive (25–30 hours a week for 2 years) behavioral intervention for toddlers with autism. The intervention combines both traditional applied behavior analytic strategies with more play-based approaches that emphasize the affective relationship between the child and his or her partner. We theorize that the emphasis on affective reciprocity is important for addressing the social motivational deficits found in autism, which, as argued above, theoretically affect how representations for social and language stimuli are acquired and stored.

EVIDENCE FOR A GENETIC BASIS
OF SOCIAL IMPAIRMENTS IN AUTISM

We conclude by describing recent evidence for a genetic basis for social impairments in autism. Studies of typical individuals are beginning to link specific genes to aspects of social behavior (Bertolino et al., 2005; Brown et

al., 2005; Hariri et al., 2005), but autism risk genes have yet to be identified. However, evidence for a genetic basis of autism does exist. There is
strong evidence for genetic influence in autism, with estimates of heritability ranging from 91–93% (Bailey et al., 1995). Several studies have
shown that identical twins are 60–95% concordant for autism (Bailey et
al., 1995; Folstein & Rutter, 1977; Ritvo, Freeman, Mason-Brothers, Mo,
& Ritvo, 1985; Steffenburg et al., 1989), whereas fraternal twins and siblings have a much lower concordance rate, with estimates ranging from 3–
7% (August, Stewart, & Tsai, 1981; Bailey et al., 1995; Bolton et al., 1994;
Smalley, Asarnow, & Spence, 1988). This rapid decrease in risk rates from
identical twins to siblings and differential risk rates for male versus female
siblings suggest epistatic effects involving interactions among as many as
10 or more genes (Delong & Dwyer, 1988; Jorde, Mason-Brothers,
Waldmann, & Ritvo, 1990; Pickles et al., 1995; Risch et al., 1999; Smalley
et al., 1988). Several linkage studies have reported moderate positive signals on several chromosomes; however, findings have not been strongly
consistent across these studies.

One challenging issue for genetic studies is the complex phenotype that
comprises the autism syndrome. The disorder involves at least three different symptom domains (social, communication, and restrictive behaviors/
flexibility) and its presentation is extremely heterogeneous. Furthermore,
the autism phenotype appears to extend beyond classic autism to "lesser
variant" phenotypes, referred to as the "broader autism phenotype"
(Rutter, Bailey, Bolton, & Le Couteur, 1993). Numerous studies have
shown that relatives of individuals with autism, including parents and siblings, exhibit higher than normal rates of autism-related impairments
(Bailey et al., 1995; Bailey, Phillips, & Rutter, 1996; Baker, Piven,
Schwartz, & Patil, 1994; Bolton et al., 1994; Landa, Folstein, & Isaacs,
1991; Landa et al., 1992; Narayan, Moyes, & Wolff, 1990; Wolff,
Narayan, & Moyes, 1988). For example, Piven and colleagues (Piven,
Palmer, Jacobi, Childress, & Arndt, 1997; Piven, Palmer, Landa, et al.,
1997) found that parents of two or more children with autism showed elevated rates of social and communication impairments and stereotyped
behaviors, and Bolton and colleagues (1994) reported that 10–20% of siblings of individuals with autism exhibit symptoms related to the disorder,
including language, learning, communication, and social impairments.

To date, most linkage studies have characterized the autism phenotype
in terms of qualitative discrete diagnoses. However, it is likely that autism
susceptibility genes increase the chance of developing one or more components of the syndrome rather than causing autism, per se. In theory, it
might be the case that multiple genetically related traits accumulate to cross
a threshold into the full-blown syndrome autism. If so, in order to identify
the genes related to autism it would be essential to define these genetically

related traits, or endophenotypes, and determine their association with specific genes (Dawson, Webb, et al., 2002; Holden, 2003). Such biological or behavioral markers of latent vulnerability to autism are likely not discrete, all-or-nothing characteristics, but rather continuously distributed traits.

There have been few genetic studies that have attempted to measure autism-related traits along a continuum. Constantino and colleagues (Constantino, Przybeck, Friesen, & Todd, 2000; Constantino, Davis, et al., 2003) conducted one such study by developing a questionnaire that captured autism as one continuous trait. They found evidence for a genetic basis of this trait in twin studies (Constantino, Hudziak, & Todd, 2003; Constantino & Todd, 2000, 2003). More recently, Dawson and colleagues (2006) have developed a quantitative measure of the autism broader phenotype that separately assesses several distinct domains of autism symptoms (social motivation, social expressiveness, conversation skills, and restrictive behaviors/flexibility) as well as age of language onset. The Broader Phenotype Autism Symptom Scale (BPASS) assesses autism-related traits in both parents and siblings of children with autism through interview and direct observation of behaviors. Parents are interviewed about their own functioning or the functioning of their children and observations of both parent and child are made by the interviewer through direct interactions. Nonverbal behaviors, such as eye contact, are assessed via direct observation, whereas behaviors related to restricted activities and routines are assessed via interview. A genetic investigation of these quantitative traits was conducted using BPASS data collected on a sample of 201 autism multiplex families that included 694 individuals (Sung et al., 2005). Participants included parents, probands, and nonaffected siblings from nuclear families that had at least two children on the autism spectrum. Multivariate polygenic models with ascertainment adjustment to estimate heritabilities and genetic and environmental correlations between the traits were used. Among the traits analyzed, social motivation and restricted activities/flexibility showed the highest heritability (0.19 and 0.16, respectively), indicating that these traits may be promising for gene mapping. These two traits also showed strong genetic correlation (0.92), suggesting a shared genetic basis.

Interestingly, in studies of face processing, not only children with autism but also parents of children with autism show decrements in this skill (Dawson, Webb, et al., 2005). Viewing faces typically is associated with a faster and larger negative ERP component over the right temporal region at about 170 milliseconds (ms) poststimulus presentation (this face-sensitive ERP is referred to as the N170; Bentin, Allison, Puce, Perez, & McCarthy, 1996; Kanwisher et al., 1997). As mentioned previously, it was found that the N170 was atypical in individuals with autism: They did not exhibit the expected N170 latency advantage for faces as compared to non-face stimuli, and they showed bilateral rather than right lateralized ERP responses to faces (McPartland et al., 2004). Dawson, Webb, and colleagues (2005) examined performance of parents of children with autism on standardized Wechsler cognitive tasks assessing verbal (Vocabulary, Verbal Comprehension), visual spatial (Block Design, Object Assembly), and face recognition (Immediate Memory for Faces) abilities. It was found that the parents of children with autism showed a significant deficit on the face recognition task relative to their performance on the visual spatial and verbal tasks; in fact, 29% of the sample had face recognition scores that were 1 standard deviation (SD) lower (> 3 points) than the other cognitive tasks. High-density ERPs to faces and chairs were recorded from a subset of the parents of children with autism and control adults with no familial history of autism. Control adults demonstrated the expected larger right-than-left hemisphere N170 to faces, whereas parents of children with autism demonstrated reduced right hemisphere N170 amplitude to faces, resulting in bilaterally distributed ERPs to faces. Furthermore, control adults exhibited the expected pattern of a faster N170 to upright faces than upright chairs, whereas parents of children with autism showed no significant difference in N170 latency to upright faces versus upright chairs. Based on these results, it can be hypothesized that face processing might be a functional neural trait marker of genetic susceptibility to autism.

Although these initial studies suggest that quantitative analysis of autism symptom-related traits is a promising approach for genetic studies, ultimately, a more refined measure of functional neural trait markers—one that is informed by contemporary affective and social neuroscience—will likely yield greater precision and validity. Through the discovery of autism susceptibility genes, it may someday be possible to identify newborn infants at risk for autism, allowing for very early intervention. By providing appropriate stimulation during the early years when social brain circuitry is first developing, prevention or at least meaningful amelioration of symptoms of autism might eventually be possible, especially for children without significant comorbid mental retardation. As our understanding of the development of social brain circuitry evolves, our interventions can become more targeted and focused on those aspects of social behavior that are considered fundamental and pivotal for the acquisition of more complex social and communication skills over time.

ACKNOWLEDGMENTS

The writing of this chapter was supported by Grant No. U19HD34565 from the National Institute of Child Health and Human Development (NICHD), as part of the NICHD Collaborative Program of Excellence in Autism, and Center Grant No. U54MH066399 from the National Institute of Mental Health, as part of the National Institutes of Health STAART Centers Program.

REFERENCES

Adrien, J., Faure, M., Perrot, A., Hameury, L., Garreau, B., Barthelemy, C., et al. (1991). Autism and family home movies: Preliminary findings. *Journal of Autism and Developmental Disorders, 21,* 43–49.

American Psychiatric Association. (1994). *Diagnostic and statistical manual of mental disorders* (4th ed.). Washington, DC: Author.

August, G. J., Stewart, M., & Tsai, L. (1981). The incidence of cognitive disabilities in the siblings of autistic children. *British Journal of Psychiatry, 138,* 416–422.

Avikainen, S., Wohlschlager, A., Liuhanen, S., Hanninen, R., & Hari, R. (2003). Impaired mirror-image imitation in Asperger and high-functioning autistic subjects. *Current Biology, 13*(4), 339–341.

Bacon, A. L., Fein, D., Morris, R., Waterhouse, L., & Allen, D. (1998). The responses of autistic children to the distress of others. *Journal of Autism and Developmental Disorders, 28*(2), 129–142.

Bailey, A., Le Couteur, A., Gottesman, I., Bolton, P., Simonoff, E., Yuzda, E., et al. (1995). Autism as a strongly genetic disorder: Evidence from a British twin study. *Psychological Medicine, 25,* 63–77.

Bailey, A., Phillips, W., & Rutter, M. (1996). Autism: Toward an integration of clinical, genetic, neuropsychological, and neurobiological perspectives. *Journal of Child Psychology and Psychiatry and Allied Disciplines, 37,* 89–126.

Baker, P., Piven, J., Schwartz, L., & Patil, S. (1994). Brief report: Duplication of chromosome 15q11–13 in two individuals with autistic disorder. *Journal of Autism and Developmental Disorders, 24*(4), 529–535.

Baron-Cohen, S. (1995). *Mindblindness: An essay on autism and theory of mind.* Cambridge, MA: Bradford/MIT Press.

Bentin, S., Allison, T., Puce, A., Perez, E., & McCarthy, G. (1996). Electrophysiological studies of face perception in humans. *Journal of Cognitive Neuroscience, 8,* 551–565.

Bertolino, A., Arciero, G., Rubino, V., Latorre, V., De Candia, M., Mazzola, V., et al. (2005). Variation of human amygdala response during threatening stimuli as a function of 5'httlpr genotype and personality style. *Biological Psychiatry, 57*(12), 1517–1525.

Bolton, P., MacDonald, H., Pickles, A., Pios, P., Goode, S., Crowson, M., et al. (1994). A case-control family history of autism. *Journal of Child Psychology and Psychiatry, 35,* 877–900.

Boucher, J., & Lewis, V. (1992). Unfamiliar face recognition in relatively able autistic children. *Journal of Child Psychology and Psychiatry, 33,* 843–859.

Boucher, J., Lewis, V., & Collis, G. (1998). Familiar face and voice matching and recognition in children with autism. *Journal of Child Psychology and Psychiatry, 39,* 171–181.

Brooks, R., & Meltzoff, A. N. (2002). The importance of eyes: How infants interpret adult looking behavior. *Developmental Psychology, 38*(6), 958–966.

Brothers, L., Ring, B., & Kling, A. (1990). Response of temporal lobe neurons to social stimuli in *maraca arctoides. Society of Neuroscience Abstract, 16,* 184.

Brown, S. M., Peet, E., Manuck, S. B., Williamson, D. E., Dahl, R. E., Ferrell, R. E., et al. (2005). A regulatory variant of the human tryptophan hydroxylase-2 gene biases amygdala reactivity. *Molecular Psychiatry, 10*(9), 884–888.

Carpenter, M., Nagell, K., & Tomasello, M. (1998). Social cognition, joint attention, and communicative competence from 9 to 15 months of age. *Monograph of the Society for Research in Child Development, 63*(4), 1–143.

Charman, T., Baron-Cohen, S., Swettenham, J., Baird, G., Drew A., & Cox, A. (2003). Predicting language outcome in infants with autism and pervasive developmental disorder. *International Journal of Language and Communication Disorders, 38*(3), 265–285.

Charman, T., Swettenham, J., Baron-Cohen, S., Cox, A., Baird, G., & Drew, A. (1998). An experimental investigation of social-cognitive abilities in infants with autism: Clinical implications. *Infant Mental Health Journal, 19*, 260–275.

Constantino, J., Davis, S. A., Todd, R. D., Schindler, M. K., Gross, M. M., Brophy, S. L., et al. (2003). Validation of a brief quantitative measure of autistic traits: Comparison of the social responsiveness scale with the Autism Diagnostic Interview—Revised. *Journal of Autism and Developmental Disorders, 33*, 427–433.

Constantino, J., Hudziak, J. J., & Todd, R. D. (2003). Deficits in reciprocal social behavior in male twins: Evidence for a genetically independent domain of psychopathology. *Journal of the American Academy of Child and Adolescent Psychiatry, 42*, 458–467.

Constantino, J., Przybeck, T., Friesen, D., & Todd, R. D. (2000). Reciprocal social behavior in children with and without pervasive developmental disorders. *Journal of Developmental and Behavioral Pediatrics, 21*(1), 2–11.

Constantino, J., & Todd, R. D. (2000). Genetic structure of reciprocal social behavior. *American Journal of Psychiatry, 157*, 2043–2045.

Constantino, J., & Todd, R. D. (2003). Autistic traits in the general population: A twin study. *Archives of General Psychiatry, 60*(5), 524–530.

Corona, R., Dissanayake, C., Arbelle, S., Wellington, P., & Sigman, M. (1998). Is affect aversive to young children with autism? Behavioral and cardiac responses to experimenter distress. *Child Development, 69*, 1494–1502.

Darwin, C. (1965). *The expression of the emotions in man and animals.* London: Murray. (Original work published 1872)

Dawson, G., & Adams, A. (1984). Imitation and social responsiveness in autistic children. *Journal of Abnormal Child Psychology, 12*, 209–225.

Dawson, G., Carver, L., Meltzoff, A., Panagiotides, H., McPartland, J., & Webb, S. (2002). Neural correlates of face and object recognition in young children with autism spectrum disorder, developmental delay, and typical development. *Child Development, 3*(3), 700–717.

Dawson, G., Estes, A., Munson, J., Schellenberg, G., Bernier, R., & Abbott, R. (2006). Quantitative Assessment of Autism Symptom–related traits in probands and parents: Broader Phenotype Autism Symptom Scale. *Journal of Autism and Developmental Disorders.*

Dawson, G., Hill, D., Galpert, L., Spencer, A., & Watson, L. (1990). Affective exchanges between young autistic children and their mothers. *Journal of Abnormal Child Psychology, 18*, 335–345.

Dawson, G., & Lewy, A. (1989). Arousal, attention, and the socioemotional impairments of individuals with autism. In G. Dawson (Ed.), *Autism: Nature, diagnosis, and treatment* (pp. 49–74). New York: Guilford Press.

Dawson, G., Meltzoff, A. N., Osterling, J., & Rinaldi, J. (1998). Neuropsychological correlates of early symptoms of autism. *Child Development, 69,* 1276–1285.

Dawson, G., Meltzoff, A. N., Osterling, J., Rinaldi, J., & Brown, E. (1998). Children with autism fail to orient to naturally occurring social stimuli. *Journal of Autism and Developmental Disorders, 28,* 479–485.

Dawson, G., Munson, J., Estes, A., Osterling, J., McPartland, J., Toth, K., et al. (2002). Neurocognitive function and joint attention ability in young children with autism spectrum disorder versus developmental delay. *Child Development, 73*(2), 345–358.

Dawson, G., Osterling, J., Meltzoff, A., & Kuhl, P. (2000). Case study of the development of an infant with autism from birth to two years of age. *Journal of Applied Developmental Psychology, 21*(3), 299–313.

Dawson, G., Toth, K., Abbott, R., Osterling, J., Munson, J., Estes, A., et al. (2004). Early social attention impairments in young children with autism: Social orienting, joint attention, and attention to distress. *Developmental Psychology, 40,* 271–283.

Dawson, G., Webb, S., Carver, L., Panagiotides, H., & McPartland, J. (2004). Young children with autism show atypical brain responses to fearful versus neutral facial expressions. *Developmental Science, 7,* 340–359.

Dawson, G., Webb, S., & McPartland, J. (2005).Understanding the nature of face processing impairment in autism: Insights from behavioral and electrophysiological studies. *Developmental Neuropsychology, 27*(3), 403–424.

Dawson, G., Webb, S., Schellenberg, G., Aylward, E., Richards, T., Dager, S., et al. (2002). Defining the broader phenotype of autism: Genetic, brain, and behavioral perspectives. *Development and Psychopathology, 14,* 581–611.

Dawson, G., Webb, S., Wijsman, E., Schellenberg, G., Estes, A., Munson, J., et al. (2005). Neurocognitive and electrophysiological evidence of altered face processing in parents of children with autism: Implications for a model of abnormal development of social brain circuitry in autism. *Development and Psychopathology, 17,* 679–697.

Dawson, G., & Zanolli, K. (2003). Early intervention and brain plasticity in autism. In G. Bock & J. Goode (Eds.), *Autism: Neural bases and treatment possibilities* (pp. 226–280). Chichester, UK: Wiley.

de Haan, M., & Nelson, C. (1997). Recognition of the mother's face by 6-month-old infants: A neurobehavioral study. *Child Development, 68,* 187–210.

de Haan, M., & Nelson, C. (1999). Electrocortical correlates of face and object recognition by 6-month-old infants. *Developmental Psychology, 35,* 1113–1121.

de Haan, M., Nelson, C. A., Gunnar, M. R., & Tout, K. A. (1998). Hemispheric differences in brain activity related to the recognition of emotional expressions by 5-year-old children. *Developmental Neuropsychology, 14*(4), 495–518.

Delong, G. R., & Dwyer, J. H. (1988). Correlation of family history with specific autistic subgroups: Aspergers and bipolar affective disease. *Journal of Autism and Developmental Disorders, 18,* 593–600.

Eckerman, C., Davis, C., & Didow, S. (1989). Toddlers' emerging ways of achieving social coordinations with a peer. *Child Development, 60*(2), 440–453.

Eimer, M., & Holmes, A. (2002). An ERP study on the time course of emotional face processing. *NeuroReport, 13*(4), 427–431.

Fagan, J. (1972). Infants' recognition memory for face. *Journal of Experimental Child Psychology, 14,* 453–476.

Feinman, S. (1982). Social referencing in infancy. *Merrill–Palmer Quarterly, 28,* 445–470.

Ferguson, J., Young, H., Hearn, E., Insel, T., & Winslow, J. (2000). Social amnesia in mice lacking the oxytocin gene. *Nature Genetics, 25,* 284–288.

Ferguson, J., Young, H., & Insel, T. R. (2002). The neuroendocrine basis of social recognition. *Frontiers in Neuroendocrinology, 23,* 200–224.

Folstein, S., & Rutter, M. (1977). Infantile autism: A genetic study of 21 twin pairs. *Journal of Child Psychology and Psychiatry, 18,* 297–321.

Gepner, B., de Gelder, B., & de Schonen, S. (1996). Face processing in autistics: Evidence for a generalized deficit? *Child Neuropsychology, 2*(2), 123–139.

Gingrich, B., Liu, Y., Cascio, C., Wang, Z., & Insel, T. R. (2000). Dopamine D2 receptors in the nucleus accumbens are important for social attachment in female prairie voles. *Behavioral Neuroscience, 114,* 173–183.

Goren, C., Sarty, M., & Wu, P. (1975). Visual following and pattern discrimination of face-like stimuli by newborn infants. *Pediatrics, 56,* 544–549.

Grelotti, D., Gauthier, I., & Schultz, R. (2002). Social interest and the development of cortical face specialization: What autism teaches us about face processing. *Developmental Psychobiology, 40,* 213–225.

Hariri, A. R., Drabant, E. M., Munoz, K. E., Kolachana, B. S., Mattay, V. S., Egan, M. F., et al. (2005). A susceptibility gene for affective disorders and the response of the human amygdala. *Archives of General Psychiatry, 62*(2), 146–152.

Hatfield, E., Cacioppo, H., & Rapson, R. (1994). *Emotional contagion.* New York: Cambridge University Press.

Haxby, J., Horwitz, B., Ungerleider, L., Maisog, J., Pietrini, P., & Grady, C. (1994). The functional organization of human extrastriate cortex: A PET–rCBF study of selective attention to faces and locations. *Journal of Neuroscience, 14,* 6336–6353.

Haxby, J., Ungerleider, L., Clark, A., Schouten, J., Hoffman, E., & Martin, A. (1999). The effect of face inversion on activity in human neural systems for face and object perception. *Neuron, 22,* 189–199.

Hertzig, M., Snow, M., & Sherman, T. (1989). Affect and cognition in autism. *Journal of the American Academy of Child and Adolescent Psychiatry, 28,* 195–199.

Hobson, P., Ouston, J., & Lee, A. (1988). Emotion recognition in autism: Coordinating faces and voices. *Psychological Medicine, 18,* 911–923.

Hobson, R., & Lee, A. (1999). Imitation and identification in autism. *Journal of Child Psychology and Psychiatry, 40*(4), 649–659.

Hoffman, E., & Haxby, J. (2000). Distinct representations of eye gaze and identity in the distributed human neural system for face perception. *Nature Neuroscience, 3,* 80–84.

Holden, C. (2003). Deconstructing schizophrenia. *Science, 299,* 333–335.

Insel, T. R. (1997). A neurobiological basis of social attachment. *American Journal of Psychiatry, 154*(6), 726–735.

Insel, T. R., & Fernald, R. D. (2004). How the brain processes social information: Searching for the social brain. *Annual Review of Neuroscience, 27,* 697–722.

Insel, T. R., & Hulihan, T. J. (1995). A gender-specific mechanism for pair bonding: Oxytocin and partner preference formation in monogamous voles. *Behavioral Neuroscience, 109,* 782–789.

Insel, T. R., O'Brien, D. J., & Leckman, J. F. (1999). Oxytocin, vasopressin, and autism: Is there a connection? *Biological Psychiatry, 45,* 145–157.

Jorde, L. B., Mason-Brothers, A., Waldmann, R., & Ritvo, E. (1990). The UCLA–University of Utah epidemiology survey of autism: Genealogical analysis of familial aggregation. *American Journal of Medical Genetics, 36,* 85–88.

Joseph, R., & Tanaka, J. (2003). Holistic and part-based face recognition in children with autism. *Journal of Child Psychology and Psychiatry, 44*(4), 529–542.

Kampe, K., Frith, C., Dolan, R., & Frith, U. (2001). Attraction and gaze—the reward of social stimuli. *Nature, 413,* 589.

Kanwisher, N., McDermott, J., & Chun, M. (1997). The fusiform face area: A module in human extrastriate cortex specialized for face perception. *Journal of Neuroscience, 17,* 4302–4311.

Kasari, C., Sigman, M., Mundy, P., & Yirmiya, N. (1990). Affective sharing in the context of joint attention interactions of normal, autistic, and mentally retarded children. *Journal of Autism and Developmental Disorders, 20,* 87–100.

Kim, S. J., Young, L. J., Gonen, D., Veenstra-VanderWeele, J., Courchesne, R., Courchesne, E., et al. (2002). Transmission disequilibrium testing of arginine vasopressin receptor 1A (AVPR1A) polymorphisms in autism. *Molecular Psychiatry, 7*(5), 503–507.

Klin, A., Jones, W., Schultz, R., Volkmar, F., & Cohen, D. (2002). Visual fixation patterns during viewing of naturalistic social situations as predictors of social competence in individuals with autism. *Archives of General Psychiatry, 59,* 809–816.

Klin, A., Sparrow, S., deBildt, A., Cicchetti, D., Cohen, D., & Volkmar, F. (1999). A normed study of face recognition in autism and related disorders. *Journal of Autism and Developmental Disorders, 29,* 499–508.

Klinger, L., & Dawson, G. (2001). Prototype formation in children with autism and Down syndrome. *Development and Psychopathology, 13,* 111–124.

Kugiumutzakis, G. (1999). Genesis and development of early infant mimesis to facial and vocal models. In J. Nadel & G. Butterworth (Eds.), *Imitation in infancy* (pp. 36–59). Cambridge, UK: Cambridge University Press.

Kuhl, P., Andruski, J., Chistovich, I. A., Chistovich, L. A., Kozhevnikova, E., Ryskina, V., et al. (1997). Cross-language analysis of phonetic units in language addressed to infants. *Science, 277,* 684–686.

Kuhl, P., Coffey-Corina, S., Padden, D., & Dawson, G. (2004). Links between social and linguistic processing of speech in preschool children with autism: Behavioral and electrophysiological measures. *Developmental Science, 7,* 19–30.

Kuhl, P., Tsao, F., & Liu, H. (2003). Foreign-language experience in infancy: Effects of short-term exposure and social interaction on phonetic learning. *Proceedings of the National Academy of Sciences USA, 100*(15), 9096–9101.

Landa, R., Folstein, S., & Isaacs, C. (1991). Spontaneous narrative discourse performance of parents of autistic individuals. *Journal of Speech and Hearing Research, 34,* 1339–1345.

Landa, R., Piven, J., Wzorek, M., Gayle, J., Chase, G., & Folstein, S. (1992). Social language use in parents of autistic individuals. *Psychological Medicine, 22,* 245–254.

Langdell, T. (1978). Recognition of faces: An approach to the study of autism. *Journal of Child Psychology and Psychiatry, 19,* 255–268.

Loveland, K., Tunali-Kotoski, B., Pearson, D., Bresford, K., Ortegon, J., & Chen, C. (1994). Imitation and expression of facial affect in autism. *Development and Psychopathology, 6,* 433–444.

Maurer, D., & Salapatek, P. (1976). Developmental changes in the scanning of faces by young infants. *Child Development, 47*(2), 523–527.

McPartland, J., Dawson, G., Webb, S., & Panagiotides, H. (2004). Event-related brain potentials reveal anomalies in temporal processing of faces in autism. *Journal of Child Psychiatry and Psychology, 45*(7), 1235.

Meltzoff, A., & Decety, J. (2003). What imitation tells us about social cognition: A rapprochement between developmental psychology and cognitive neuroscience. *Philosophical Transactions of the Royal Society: Biological Sciences, 358,* 491–500.

Meltzoff, A., & Gopnick, A. (1993). The role of imitation in understanding persons and developing a theory of mind. In S. Baron-Cohen, H. Tager-Flusberg, & D. J. Cohen (Eds.), *Understanding other minds: Perspectives from autism* (pp. 335–336). Oxford, UK: Oxford University Press.

Meltzoff, A., & Moore, M. (1977). Imitation of facial and manual gestures by human neonates. *Science, 198,* 75–78.

Meltzoff, A., & Moore, M. (1979). Interpreting "imitative" responses in early infancy. *Science, 205,* 217–219.

Meltzoff, A., & Moore, M. (1983). Newborn infants imitate adult facial gestures. *Child and Development, 54*(3), 702–709.

Meltzoff, A., & Moore, M. (1994). Imitation, memory, and the representation of persons. *Infant Behavior and Development, 17,* 83–99.

Modahl, C., Green, L., Fein, D., Morris, M., Waterhouse, L., Feinstein, C., et al. (1998). Plasma oxytocin levels in autistic children. *Biological Psychiatry, 43,* 270–277.

Moore, C., & Corkum, V. (1994). Social understanding at the end of the first year of life. *Developmental Review, 14,* 349–372.

Morales, M., Mundy, P., & Rojas, J. (1998). Brief report: Following the direction of gaze and language development in 6-month-olds. *Infant Behavior and Development, 21,* 373–377.

Morton, J., & Johnson, M. H. (1991). CONSPEC and CONLERN: A two-process theory of infant face recognition. *Psychological Review, 2,* 164–181.

Mundy, P., & Neal, R. (2001). *Neural plasticity, joint attention, and a transactional social-orienting model of autism.* San Diego, CA: Academic Press.

Mundy, P., Sigman, M., Ungerer, J., & Sherman, T. (1986). Defining the social deficits of autism: The contribution of nonverbal communication measure. *Journal of Child Psychology and Psychiatry, 27,* 657–669.

Nadel, J., Guerini, C., Peze, A., & Rivet, C. (1999). The evolving nature of imitation as a format for communication. In J. Nadel & G. Butterworth (Eds.), *Imitation in infancy* (pp. 209–234). Cambridge, UK: Cambridge University Press.

Narayan, S., Moyes, B., & Wolff, S. (1990). Family characteristics of autistic children: A further report. *Journal of Autism and Developmental Disorders, 20*(4), 523–535.

Nelson, C. A. (2001). The development and neural bases of face recognition. *Infant and Child Development, 10*(1–2), 3–18.

Nelson, C. A., & de Haan, M. (1996). Neural correlates of infants' visual responsiveness to facial expressions of emotion. *Developmental Psychobiology, 29,* 577–595.

Nishimori, K., Young, L., Guo, Q., Wang, Z., Insel, T. R., & Matzuk, M. M. (1996). Oxytocin is required for nursing but is not essential for parturition or reproductive behavior. *Proceedings of the National Academy of Science USA, 93,* 11699–11704.

Osterling, J., & Dawson, G. (1994). Early recognition of children with autism: A study of first birthday home videotapes. *Journal of Autism and Developmental Disorders, 24,* 247–257.

Osterling, J., Dawson, G., & Munson, J. (2002). Early recognition of one-year-old infants with autism spectrum disorder versus mental retardation: A study of first birthday party home videotapes. *Development and Psychopathology, 14,* 239–251.

Pedersen, C., Caldwell, J., Walker, C., Ayers, G., & Mason, G. (1994). Oxytocin activates the postpartum onset of rat maternal behavior in the ventral tegmental and medial preoptic areas. *Behavioral Neuroscience, 108,* 1163–1171.

Pelphrey, K., Sasson, N., Reznick, J., Paul, G., Goldman, B., & Piven, J. (2002). Visual scanning of faces in autism. *Journal of Autism and Developmental Disorders, 32*(4), 249–261.

Perrett, D., Harries, M., Mistlin, A., & Hietanen, J. (1990). Social signals analyzed at the single cell level: Someone is looking at me, something touched me, something moved. *International Journal of Comparative Psychology, 4,* 25–55.

Perrett, D., Hietanen, J., Oram, M., & Benson, P. (1992). Organization and functions of cells responsive to faces in the temporal cortex. In V. Bruce & A. Cowey (Eds.), *Processing the facial image* (pp. 23–30). New York: Clarendon Press.

Perrett, D., Smith, P., Mistlin, A., Chitty, A., Head, A., Potter, D., et al. (1985).

Visual analysis of body movements by neurons in the temporal cortex of the macaque monkey: A preliminary report. *Behavioral Brain Research, 16,* 153–170.

Piaget, J. (1962). *Play, dreams and imitation in childhood.* New York: Norton.

Pickles, A., Bolton, P., MacDonald, H., Bailey, A., Le Couteur, A., Sim, C. H., et al. (1995). Latent-class analysis of recurrence risks for complex phenotypes with selection and measurement error: A twin and family history study of autism. *American Journal of Human Genetics, 57,* 717–726.

Piven, J., Palmer, P., Jacobi, D., Childress, D., & Arndt, S. (1997). Broader autism phenotype: Evidence from a family history study of multiple-incidence autism families. *American Journal of Psychiatry, 154,* 185–190.

Piven, J., Palmer, P., Landa, R., Santangelo, S., Jacobi, D., & Childress, D. (1997). Personality and language characteristics in parents from multiple-incidence autism families. *American Journal of Medical Genetics, 74,* 398–411.

Rheingold, H. L., Hay, D. F., & West, M. J. (1976). Sharing in the second year of life. *Child Development, 47,* 1148–1158.

Risch, N., Spiker, D., Loptspeich, L., Nouri, N., Hinds, D., Hallmayer, J., et al. (1999). A genomic screen of autism: Evidence for a multilocus etiology. *American Journal of Human Genetics, 65*(2), 493–507.

Ritvo, E., Freeman, B., Mason-Brothers, A., Mo, A., & Ritvo, A. (1985). Concordance for the syndrome of autism in 40 pairs of afflicted twins. *American Journal of Psychiatry, 142,* 74–77.

Rochat, P. (1999). *Early social cognition: Understanding others in the first months of life.* Mahwah, NJ: Erlbaum.

Rochat, P., & Striano, T. (1999). Emerging self-exploration by 2-month-olds. *Developmental Science, 2,* 206–218.

Rogers, S., Bennetto, L., McEvoy, R., & Pennington, B. (1996). Imitation and pantomime in high-functioning adolescents with autism spectrum disorders. *Child Development, 67*(5), 2060–2073.

Rogers, S., Hepburn, S., Stackhouse, T., & Wehner, E. (2003). Imitation performance in toddlers with autism and those with other developmental disorders. *Journal of Child Psychology and Psychiatry, 44*(5), 763–781.

Rogers, S., & Pennington, B. (1991). A theoretical approach to the deficits in infantile autism. *Development and Psychopathology, 3,* 137–162.

Rutter, M., Bailey, A., Bolton, P., & Le Couteur, A. (1993). Autism: Syndrome definition and possible genetic mechanisms. In R. Plomin & G. E. McClearn (Eds.), *Nature, nurture, and psychology* (pp. 269–284). Washington, DC: American Psychological Association.

Schoenbaum, G., Setlow, B., Saddoris, M., & Gallagher, M. (2003). Encoding predicted outcome and acquired value in orbitofrontal cortex during cue sampling depends upon input from basolateral amygdala. *Neuron, 39*(5), 731–733.

Schultz, W. (1998). Predictive reward signal of dopamine neurons. *Journal of Neurophysiology, 80,* 1–27.

Serra, M., Althaus, M., de Sonneville, L. M., Stant, A.D., Jackson, A. E., & Minderaa, R. B. (2003). Face recognition in children with a pervasive developmental disorder not otherwise specified. *Journal of Autism and Developmental Disorders, 33*(3), 303–317.

Sigman, M., Kasari, C., Kwon, J., & Yirmiya, N. (1992). Responses to the negative emotions of others by autistic, mentally retarded, and normal children. *Child Development, 63,* 796–807.

Sigman, M., & Ruskin, E. (1999). Continuity and change in the social competence of children with autism, Down syndrome, and developmental delays. *Monographs of the Society for Research in Child Development, 64*(1), Serial No. 256.

Smalley, S. L., Asarnow, R. F., & Spence, A. (1988). Autism and genetics: A decade of research. *Archives of General Psychiatry, 45,* 953–961.

Steffenburg, S., Gillberg, C., Hellgren, L., Andresson, L., Gillberg, I., Jakobsson, G., et al. (1989). A twin study of autism in Denmark, Finland, Iceland, Norway, and Sweden. *Journal of Child Psychology and Psychiatry, 30,* 405–416.

Stone, W., Lemanek, K., Fishel, P., Fernandez, M., & Altemeier, W. (1990). Play and imitation skills in the diagnosis of autism in young children. *Pediatrics, 86,* 267–272.

Stone, W., Ousley, O., & Littleford, C. (1997). Motor imitation in young children with autism: What's the object? *Journal of Abnormal Child Psychology, 25,* 475–485.

Sung, J. U., Dawson, G., Munson, J., Estes, A., Schellenberg, J., & Wijsman, E. M. (2005). Genetic investigation of quantitative traits related to autism: Use of multivariate polygenic models with ascertainment adjustment. *American Journal of Human Genetics, 76,* 68–81.

Swettenham, J., Baron-Cohen, S., Charman, T., Cox, A., Baird, G., Drew, et al. (1998). The frequency and distribution of spontaneous attention shifts between social and nonsocial stimuli in autistic, typically developing, and nonautistic developmentally delayed infants. *Journal of Child Psychology and Psychiatry, 39*(5), 747–753.

Symons, L., Hains, S., & Muir, S. (1998). Look at me: 5-month-old infants' sensitivity to very small deviations in eye-gaze during social interactions. *Infant Behavior and Development, 21,* 531–536.

Tantam, D., Monaghan, L., Nicholson, J., & Stirling, J. (1989). Autistic children's ability to interpret faces: A research note. *Journal of Child Psychology and Psychiatry, 30,* 623–630.

Trepagnier, C., Sebrechts, M., & Peterson, R. (2002). Atypical face gaze in autism. *Cyberpsychological Behavior, 5*(3), 213–217.

Trevarthen, C. (1979). Communication and cooperation in early infancy: A description of primary intersubjectivity. In M. Bullowa (Ed.), *Before speech: The beginnings of interpersonal communication* (pp. 321–347). Cambridge, UK: Cambridge University Press.

Trevarthen, C., Kokkinaki, T., & Fiamenghi, G., Jr. (1999). What infants' imitations communicate: With mothers, with fathers, and with peers. In J. Nadel & G. Butterworth (Eds.), *Imitation in infancy* (pp. 127–185). Cambridge, UK: Cambridge University Press.

Tronick, E., Als, H., Adamson, L., Wise, S., & Brazelton, T. B. (1978). The infant's response to entrapment between contradictory messages in face-to-face interaction. *Journal of the American Academy of Child Psychiatry, 17,* 1–13.

Užgiris, E. (1981). Probing immune reactions by laser light scattering spectroscopy. *Methods in Enzymology, 74,* 177–198.

Užgiris, E. (1999). Imitation as activity: Its developmental aspect. In J. Nadel & G. Butterworth (Eds.), *Imitation in infancy* (pp. 209–234) Cambridge, UK: Cambridge University Press.

van der Geest, J., Kemner, C., Verbatem, M., & van Engeland, H. (2002). Gaze behavior of children with pervasive developmental disorder toward human faces: A fixation time study. *Journal of Child Psychiatry and Psychology, 443,* 669–678.

Walton, G., & Bower, T. (1993). Amodal representations of speech in infants. *Infant Behavior and Development, 16*(2), 233–243.

Waterhouse, L., Fein, D., & Modahl, C. (1996). Neurofunctional mechanisms in autism. *Psychological Review, 103,* 457–489.

Webb, S. J., Dawson, G., Bernier, R., & Panagiotides, H. (2006). ERP evidence of atypical face processing in young children with autism. *Journal of Autism and Developmental Disorders, 36,* 881–890.

Werner, E., Dawson, G., Osterling, J., & Dinno, J. (2000). Recognition of autism before 1 year of age: A retrospective study based on home videotapes. *Journal of Autism and Developmental Disorders, 30,* 157–162.

Williams, J., Whiten, A., Suddendorf, T., & Perrett, D. (2001). Imitation, mirror neurons and autism. *Neuroscience and Biobehavioral Review, 25*(4), 287–295.

Winslow, J., Hastings, N., Carter, C. S., Harbaugh, C. R., & Insel, T. R. (1993). A role for central vasopressin in pair bonding in monogamous prairie voles. *Nature, 365,* 545–548.

Witt, D. M., Winslow, J. T., & Insel, T. R. (1992). Enhanced social interactions in rats following chronic, centrally infused oxytocin. *Pharmacology, Biochemistry, and Behavior, 43*(3), 855–861.

Wolff, S., Narayan, S., & Moyes, B. (1988). Personality characteristics of parents of autistic children: A controlled study. *Journal of Child Psychology and Psychiatry, 29,* 143–153.

Zahn-Waxler, C., & Radke-Yarrow, M. (1990). The origins of empathic concern. *Motivation and Emotion, 14,* 107–130.

CHAPTER 3

Brain Mechanisms Underlying
Social Perception Deficits in Autism

Kevin A. Pelphrey
Elizabeth J. Carter

Autism is a severe and pervasive neurodevelopmental disorder character-ized by the presence and distinct developmental course of a triad of deficits: (1) social reciprocity and engagement deficits, (2) communication and lan-guage skills deficits, and (3) stereotyped, repetitive behaviors and limited interests (American Psychiatric Association, 1994; see also Dawson & Bernier, Chapter 2, this volume). Within these three domains, there is a great deal of variability in the extent of deficits. For example, social domain symptoms can range from a nearly complete absence of interest in interper-sonal interaction to subtler difficulties in managing complex social interac-tions, understanding social contexts, and detecting the intentions of others. Language deficits can vary from mutism to mild pragmatic language defi-cits. The restricted, repetitive, and stereotyped behaviors and interests can be anything from a preference for sameness and exhibition of simple motor stereotypies to performance of extremely elaborate, complex rituals with severe distress upon their interruption. Along with the great variability in these three behavioral domains, there is also a wide range in general intel-lect, with the majority of individuals with autism exhibiting mental retarda-tion, but others possessing intelligence quotients (IQs) that are average or superior.

Approximately two to three per 1,000 individuals meet the criteria for a diagnosis of autism (Fombonne, 1999); however, this number would be significantly higher if it included other disorders falling on the "autism spectrum," such as Asperger syndrome and pervasive developmental disorder not otherwise specified (Folstein & Rosen-Sheidley, 2001). These other developmental disorders share many of the same features of autism, such as early social and communication deficits, but do not include the full range of symptoms. The spectrum is further expanded by the inclusion of the broad autism phenotype for describing individuals who do not meet criteria for the other autism spectrum disorders but who have milder deficits in the three major domains (Folstein & Rutter, 1977; see Piven, 2001, for a review). In their twin study of autism, on the basis of finding a higher concordance rate for a broad autism phenotype, Folstein and Rutter (1977) proposed the idea that the genetic liability for autism might be expressed in nonautistic relatives in characteristics that were milder but qualitatively similar to those seen in autism. Often, these characteristics are seen in family members of individuals with autism. In parents, this may include subtle difficulties in language and communication (Landa et al., 1992; Piven, Palmer, Jacobi, Childress, & Arndt, 1997), social impairments and certain personality characteristics (e.g., aloofness and rigidity; Murphy et al., 2000; Piven et al., 1994; Wolff, Narayan, & Moyes, 1988), and higher rates of depression and social phobia (Piven & Palmer, 1997, 1999). Additionally, executive functioning deficits have been found in parents (Hughes, Leboyer, & Bouvard, 1997) and siblings (Hughes, Plumet, & Leboyer, 1999) of individuals with autism.

Higher rates of concordance in monozygotic twins and of recurrence within families than typically are seen in the general population suggest that there is a significant genetic component to autism (Cook et al., 1998; see Bailey et al., 1995, for a review), and heritability rates are estimated at 60–70% (Veenstra-VanDerWeele, Cook, & Lombroso, 2003). In addition, significantly more males than females meet criteria for the disorder, with estimates of this ratio as high as 4:1 (Wing, 1981; Yeargin-Allsopp et al., 2003). The source of this sex difference could be relatively indirect; for example, it might emerge through the effects of gonadal steroids on brain development. But it could also be more direct, vis-à-vis expression of proteins on the sex chromosomes in neurons. Approximately 10% of individuals with autism are also affected by a medical condition associated with the disorder, such as fragile X syndrome, tuberous sclerosis, or Smith–Lemli–Opitz syndrome (Bailey, Hatton, Skinner, & Mesibov, 2001; Baker, Piven, & Sato, 1998; Martin et al., 2001). In those without another medical condition (i.e., idiopathic autism), the underlying mechanism is probably the result of the interactions of a number of genes (Pickles et al., 1995; Risch et al., 1999).

Although individuals with autism differ in the extent to which they demonstrate each of these impairments, evidence suggests that social deficits are the primary feature of autism (Kanner, 1943; Wing & Gould, 1979), and only the social deficits are specific to autism and its related disorders. Indeed, early emerging problems with social engagement might initiate a developmental cascade that leads to the commonly seen communication delays and deficits. For instance, social isolation has been shown to cause stereotyped and repetitive behaviors in monkeys that are similar to those observed in autism (e.g., Cross & Harlow, 1965). Moreover, deficits in social perception, including visual joint attention, are important early indicators of autism (Baron-Cohen, 1995; Dawson, Munson, et al., 2002; Lord et al., 1997; Sigman et al., 1999). Finally, research and theory in developmental psychology support the notion that cognitive operations, including executive functions and learning strategies, are coconstructed over ontogeny in the context of social and cultural interactions (e.g., Fischer & Bidell, 1998; Rogoff, 1990; Valsiner, 1987; Vygotsky, 1978) in which children with autism do not readily participate. Here, we review the growing knowledge base concerning the neural basis of specific deficits in social functioning in autism.

Social perception refers to the initial stages of evaluating the intentions of others by analyzing gaze direction, body movement, and other types of biological motion (Allison, Puce, & McCarthy, 2000). This construct falls within a domain of cognitive skills referred to by different laboratories as social cognition, social attention, theory of mind, and mentalizing. The essence of social perception is captured by the notion of an "intentional stance," introduced by the philosopher Dennett (1987) to describe the assumptions human beings tend to make when interpreting and predicting the behavior of others:

> Here is how it works: first you decide to treat the object whose behavior is to be predicted as a rational agent; then you figure out what beliefs that agent ought to have, given its place in the world and its purpose. Then you figure out what desires it ought to have, on the same considerations, and finally you predict that this rational agent will act to further its goals in the light of its beliefs. A little practical reasoning from the chosen set of beliefs and desires will in most instances yield a decision about what the agent ought to do; that is what you predict the agent will do. (p. 17)

Here Dennett eloquently described a set of processes that occurs in a rapid, automatic fashion during social perception in typically developing individuals.

Abnormalities in social perception are a striking feature of autism. For example, children with autism fail to recognize biological motion from point-light displays (Blake, Turner, Smoski, Pozdol, & Stone, 2003; Klin, Jones, Schultz, & Volkmar, 2003). Additionally, individuals with autism do not look at faces in the same way as do typically developing individuals: In many studies, they spend significantly less time looking at the eyes and more time on a speaker's mouth or body (Klin, Jones, Schultz, Volkmar, & Cohen, 2002; Pelphrey et al., 2002). Also, people with autism find it difficult to identify emotional facial expressions (Adolphs, Sears, & Piven, 2001; Pelphrey et al., 2002), especially expressions of fear and anger. Baron-Cohen (1995) described an experiment that illustrates the nature of these social perception deficits in autism. They showed pictures of a cartoon face (Figure 3.1) named "Charlie" looking at one of four different kinds of candy and asked children to identify Charlie's preferred candy. Typically developing children and mentally retarded children readily indicated the candy toward which Charlie was gazing. This response implied that they linked the direction of gaze with its social and mental significance. They inferred that Charlie liked the candy at which his gaze was directed. In contrast, children with autism failed to select the candy at which Charlie

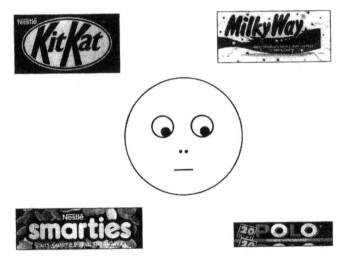

FIGURE 3.1. Sample stimulus from Baron-Cohen (1995). Children with and without autism were asked which candy "Charlie" preferred. Children without autism correctly indicated that Charlie's favorite was the one at which he was looking, but children with autism were not able to use the eye information to make accurate judgments. Adapted with permission from MIT Press from Baron-Cohen, S. (1995). *Mindblindness: An essay on autism and theory of mind.* Cambridge, MA: MIT Press.

was looking. This deficit was not due simply to an inability to perceive the direction of gaze: In a different task, children with autism scored as well as typically developing or mentally retarded children when shown faces looking toward or away from them and asked, "Which one is looking at you?" In other words, children with autism were able to perceive the direction of gaze but were unable to use such information to infer the mental state of the other person.

Whereas extensive descriptions of social perception deficits are available at the behavioral and cognitive levels of developmental analysis, much less is known about the neural basis of social perception dysfunction in autism. Cognitive neuroscientists have begun to identify a set of key brain regions involved in aspects of social perception and cognition in typically developing individuals, consistently implicating the amygdala, the superior temporal sulcus, and the fusiform gyrus (see Figure 3.2). More recently, advances in techniques for studying brain–behavior relationships have allowed researchers to link particular deficits in autism to dysfunction in specific brain structures. In this chapter we focus on two cognitive neuroscientific methods: functional magnetic resonance imaging (fMRI) and neuropsychological marker tasks. fMRI uses an endogenous property

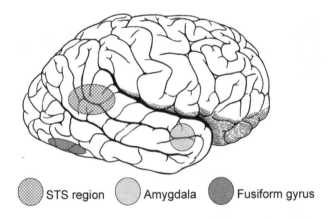

STS region   Amygdala   Fusiform gyrus

FIGURE 3.2. Brain structures thought to be important for the cognitive neuroscience of social deficits in autism. The superior temporal sulcus (STS) has been implicated in eye-gaze processing, voice perception, and attribution of intentionality deficits in autism. The amygdala (here projected to the cortical surface for illustration) has been linked to emotion recognition and theory-of-mind deficits in autism. Hypoactivation of the fusiform gyrus has been proposed as a mechanism underlying face processing deficits in autism. Reproduced with permission from John Wiley & Sons from Pelphrey, K., Adolphs, R., & Morris, J. P. (2004). Neuroanatomical substrates of social cognition dysfunction in autism. *Mental Retardation and Developmental Disabilities Research Review, 10*(4), 259–271.

of the brain called *blood oxygenation level dependent* (BOLD) contrast. By tracking relative changes in the BOLD signal in different areas of the brain, fMRI provides an indirect measure of regional brain activity. This *in vivo* imaging method can be used repeatedly in relatively large numbers of individuals because it is noninvasive and does not rely on the use of ionizing radiation. This technique can be used with marker tasks, which are developed by comparing neurologically normal individuals with individuals who have known brain lesions in order to explore the function of the lost neural structures. Researchers can combine these methods in order to further knowledge of the neural structures that appear to be dysfunctional in autism spectrum disorders. Using this information, neurophysiological models of autism are being developed along with candidate mechanisms for the expression of individual differences in behavioral and treatment outcomes.

In this chapter, we describe progress toward understanding the brain mechanisms underlying social perception and social perception deficits in autism. We begin with an analytic approach, dissecting the individual contributions of the three aforementioned social brain structures. We present basic research aimed at identifying the functional significance of each brain region in social perception. With this fundamental neuroscientific work as a backdrop, we then present translational studies that have implicated each structure in autism, comparing findings, when possible, from nonhuman primates, neurologically normal humans, and individuals with lesions to research on people with autism. After examining the contributions of each structure in isolation, we adopt a more integrative posture and discuss research that has added to our understanding of how the social brain operates at the level of neural circuitry (i.e., characterizations of normal and abnormal functional interactions among the individual structures). In presenting this work, we emphasize the potential benefits of a developmental perspective and propose several future research directions. We conclude with a discussion of the potential for the cognitive neuroscience of autism to inform educational interventions and treatment efforts.

AMYGDALA

The amygdala is a complex structure that is comprised of at least 13 different nuclei and is highly interconnected with other brain structures, including the thalamus, hippocampus, brainstem, basal forebrain, and claustrum (Amaral & Insausti, 1992; Amaral, Veazey, & Cowan, 1982). Brothers (1990) proposed that the amygdala is a key component of a neural circuit that forms the neurobiological basis of social perception and social cogni-

tion, along with the superior temporal sulcus and gyrus and the orbitofrontal cortices. Some of the most compelling data for the function of the
amygdala in a variety of socially relevant behaviors come from animal
research. For example, in studies of mice, LeDoux (1996) discovered that
the amygdala is critical for fear conditioning, which is the acquisition of
fear-related responses to a stimulus via its association with a different,
strongly aversive stimulus. Additionally, in nonhuman primates, neurons in
the amygdalae of monkeys respond both to the basic motivational significance of stimuli and their complex social significance (Brothers, Ring, &
Kling, 1990; Rolls, 1992). Studies in macaques with bilateral lesions of the
amygdala illuminate the importance of a developmental perspective. Specifically, adult macaques with lesions of the amygdala and surrounding
medial temporal structures have been described as tamer and as possessing
abnormal food preferences and sexual behaviors (Brown & Schafer, 1888;
Kluver & Bucy, 1938, 1939). Macaques with amygdala lesions at 2 weeks
of age demonstrate an absence of fear in response to typically fear-inducing
stimuli, but more screams and fear grimaces during conspecific social interactions (Prather et al., 2001). Macaques with neonatal lesions of bilateral
medial temporal lobes, including the amygdala, appear more severely
affected, displaying autistic-like behaviors such as decreased eye contact,
locomotor stereotypies, and increased social avoidance (Bachevalier, 1994,
1996; Bachevalier & Mishkin, 1994).

The abovementioned work was limited by a lack of precision regarding the extent and specificity of the lesions. A more precise tool for
lesioning brain regions is the use of ibotenic acid, which destroys the cell
bodies in the area but leaves the axons passing through it intact. Researchers used this technique to create bilateral amygdala lesions in adult
rhesus monkeys, which were later observed to make more approaches and
be less inhibited during dyadic social interactions with unlesioned control conspecifics and also to lack normal fear behaviors to novel, fear-
provoking stimuli (Emery et al., 2001; Prather et al., 2001). Such findings
led to the proposal that the primary role of the amygdala is the assessment
of threat and danger in the environment (Emery et al., 2001).

In humans, lesion and functional neuroimaging studies have also
pointed to the amygdala's role in social perception and social behavior. For
example, humans with lesions of the amygdala show social information-
processing deficits, including problems in recognizing and judging emotions, particularly fear (Adolphs, Tranel, Damasio, & Damasio, 1994;
Anderson & Phelps, 2000; Broks et al., 1998; Sprengelmeyer et al., 1999).
In neuroimaging studies, amygdala activation is consistently detected in
response to viewing facial expressions of fear, even when participants are
not asked to judge the emotions portrayed in the stimuli (Breiter et al.,

1996; Morris et al., 1996). Whalen and others (1998) found that when fearful faces were briefly presented and then backward-masked so as to be subliminal, amygdala activation was still seen, suggesting that rapid, automatic processing takes place in this structure. A recent study by Whalen and colleagues (2004) demonstrated that the amygdala responds to fearful eye sclera presented alone, suggesting that emotional eye information alone is sufficient to evoke activity in the amygdala.

The performance of patients with amygdala lesions is also compromised in social judgments. When asked to determine certain characteristics of photographed people, these individuals consider the people in the images to be more trustworthy and approachable than do nonlesioned controls (Adolphs, Tranel, & Damasio, 1998). Neurologically normal individuals show activation in the amygdala, superior temporal sulcus, orbitofrontal cortex, and insular cortex during this task (Winston, Strange, O'Doherty, & Dolan, 2002). This finding further supports the hypothesis derived from animal research that the amygdala is involved in danger and threat assessment (Adolphs et al., 1999; Adolphs, Damasio, Tranel, Cooper, & Damasio, 2000).

The role of the amygdala in autism has been explored in several functional neuroimaging studies (see summary in Table 3.1). The first, performed by Baron-Cohen and colleagues (1999), explored the ability of the participants to judge the mental or emotional state of a person in a photograph that only showed the eyes. Previously, high-functioning individuals with autism had been found to perform poorly in a behavioral version of this task outside of the scanner (Baron-Cohen, Jolliffe, Mortimore, & Robertson, 1997). In typically developing subjects, the left amygdala, superior temporal gyri, and insula were activated. However, in the high-functioning subjects with autism, there was less frontal cortical and amygdala activation.

Critchley and others (2000) compared neurologically normal individuals to those with autism on two versions of a task with emotional faces, one requiring judgments of the expressions (an explicit emotion-processing task) and the other requiring gender identification (an implicit task). Unlike the other participants, those with autism showed no fusiform gyrus activation in the explicit task and no left amygdala activation in the implicit task. A later study explored the modulation of amygdala activation in children and adolescents with and without autism when viewing faces in two different tasks: labeling the emotions and matching the expressions (Wang, Dapretto, Hariri, Sigman, & Bookheimer, 2004). There were no significant group differences in the labeling task, but the subjects with autism showed lower fusiform gyrus and higher precuneus activation in the matching task. In the control subjects, the amygdala was modulated by task demands;

TABLE 3.1. Summaries of Functional Neuroimaging Studies Implicating the Social Brain Structures in Autism

Study	Stimuli	Key finding
Amygdala		
Baron-Cohen et al. (1999)	Inferring mental states from the eye region	Decreased activity in the amygdala
Critchley et al. (2000)	Implicit and explicit processing of emotional facial expressions	Failed to activate amygdala in the implicit task and the fusiform gyrus in the explicit task
Wang et al. (2004)	Face labeling versus matching by emotional expression	Amygdala activity not modulated by task demands
Dalton et al. (2005)	Processing of facial expressions of emotions and face recognition	Positive correlation between level of amygdala activity and visual fixation on the eye region
Superior temporal sulcus		
Castelli et al. (2002)	Viewing animations of geometric shapes that elicit varying mental-state attributions	Reduced activity in the right superior temporal sulcus and reduced functional connectivity between the superior temporal sulcus and visual cortex
Boddaert et al. (2003)	Listening to human vocal sounds	Reversed hemispheric dominance and hypoactivation of left temporal regions for perception of speech
Gervais et al. (2004)	Listening to human vocal sounds	Reduced activity in the left and right superior temporal sulci and gyri
Pelphrey et al. (2005)	Analyzing intentions conveyed by eye-gaze shifts	Lack of contextual modulation in the right posterior superior temporal sulcus region for incongruent versus congruent gaze shifts
Fusiform gyrus		
Schultz et al. (2000)	Face versus object discrimination	Greater inferior temporal gyri and decreased right fusiform gyrus activation during face processing
Critchley et al. (2000)	Implicit and explicit processing of emotional facial expressions	Failed to activate amygdala in the implicit task and the fusiform gyrus in the explicit task
Pierce et al. (2001)	Viewing faces and objects	Reduced activity bilaterally in the fusiform gyrus, increased activity in idiosyncratic regions (e.g., frontal cortex, occipital cortex, anterior fusiform gyrus)
Hubl et al. (2003)	Viewing faces and complex patterns	Reduced activity in the fusiform gyrus during face processing and greater activity in the medial occipital gyrus
Hadjikhani et al. (2004)	Viewing faces and objects	Normal activity levels in the fusiform gyrus
Pierce et al. (2004)	Viewing familiar and unfamiliar faces	Normal activity levels in the fusiform gyrus
Dalton et al. (2005)	Processing of facial expressions of emotions and face recognition	Positive correlation between fusiform gyrus activity and visual fixation on the eye region

Note. Summary of key finding is made with reference to the primary reported difference between subjects with autism and those without autism.

however, this modulation did not occur for those with autism. Taken together, these studies suggest that the functioning of the amygdala is abnormal in people with autism during social perception, both in terms of levels of activation (most studies have found amygdala hypoactivation in autism) and with regard to modulation by the context established by varying task demands.

Neuropsychological marker tasks have been used to compare individuals with autism to those with amygdala lesions and have provided tantalizing, albeit indirect, evidence concerning the role of the amygdala in autism. Adolphs and colleagues (2001) compared high-functioning participants with autism to a woman with bilateral focal amygdala lesions (patient SM). The individuals with autism and patient SM were remarkably similar in exhibiting abnormal social judgments regarding the trustworthiness and approachability of others seen in photographs, overattributing these characteristics relative to judgments made by neurologically normal individuals. Also, judgments of facial expressions displaying negative affect were similarly poor, with particularly low performance on identification of fear and anger. The results of a later study by Adolphs and colleagues (2005) of patient SM's visual scanpaths, combined with data concerning abnormal scanpaths for faces in autism (Klin et al., 2002; Pelphrey et al., 2002), suggest a potential mechanism underlying these shared social perception abnormalities. The eye-tracking data demonstrated that patient SM failed to fixate on the eyes when viewing facial expressions of emotion (see their Figure 2). Similarly, Pelphrey and colleagues (2002) observed that individuals with autism did not make use of the eyes when judging facial expressions of emotion (see Plate 3.1). Notably, when Adolphs and colleagues instructed patient SM to look at the eyes, her deficit in recognizing fear temporarily disappeared, but it returned after the instruction was forgotten. It remains to be determined whether such an experimental manipulation would affect the emotion judgments of individuals with autism, but a study by Dalton and colleagues (2005) combined eye tracking and fMRI and found a strong positive correlation between the level of amygdala activity and gaze fixation upon the eye region in individuals with and without autism. Adolphs and colleagues interpreted their results as indicating that the amygdala is normally involved in directing the visual system to seek out and attend to the eyes as a socially important stimulus. Whether the amygdala fails to serve this purpose in autism remains to be tested.

SUPERIOR TEMPORAL SULCUS REGION

The role of the superior temporal sulcus region in social cognition and social perception has become the subject of intense investigation (see

Allison et al., 2000, for a review). As with the amygdala, work on this brain region has been conducted in both human and nonhuman primates. In monkeys, gaze direction can indicate dominance or submission and is integral to facial expressions (Emery, Lorincz, Perrett, Oram, & Baker, 1997). Campbell, Heywood, Cowey, Regard, and Landis (1990) found that monkeys were able to discriminate small shifts in gaze direction accurately, but monkeys with lesions of the superior temporal sulcus could not do so. Similarly, they found that human patients with prosopagnosia showed deficits on the task. Single neuron recordings performed by Perrett and colleagues have shown that portions of the superior temporal sulcus in the macaque respond to head and gaze direction (Perrett et al., 1985, 1989), hand movement (Perrett et al., 1989), head movement (Hasselmo, Rolls, Baylis, & Nalwa, 1989), and whole body motion (Oram & Perrett, 1996). This work also demonstrates that the superior temporal sulcus in monkeys is important for social attention because it processes where others' awareness is directed and the context within which their actions occur (Perrett, Hietanen, Oram, & Benson, 1992). Additional work in macaques has identified a region of the superior temporal sulcus—the superior temporal polysensory region—that integrates audio and visual components of complex social stimuli (Cusick, 1997).

In humans, the superior temporal sulcus region is a term used to describe the superior temporal sulcus proper, portions of the superior and middle temporal gyri, and areas of the angular gyrus near the ascending limb of the superior temporal sulcus (Allison et al., 2000). Functional neuroimaging studies in humans have implicated this area, particularly the posterior portion, in biological motion perception (for reviews see Allison et al., 2000; Decety & Grèzes, 1999). Below, we present work from our laboratory that has focused on identifying the role of the superior temporal sulcus region in the visual analysis of the actions and intentions of other humans as conveyed by different types of biological motion, including eye-gaze shifts (Pelphrey, Singerman, Allison, & McCarthy, 2003; Pelphrey, Viola, & McCarthy, 2004), walking (Pelphrey, Mitchell, et al., 2003), reaching (Pelphrey, Morris, & McCarthy, 2004), and audiovisual speech (Wright, Pelphrey, Allison, McKeown, & McCarthy, 2003).

In the first study of this series (Pelphrey, Mitchell, et al., 2003), we sought to determine whether the superior temporal sulcus region responded to biological motion more than to other types of complex coherent motion or random motion. As illustrated in the top panel of Plate 3.2, subjects viewed four types of animated stimuli: a walking human, a walking robot, a grandfather clock, and a disjointed mechanical figure. We established that the superior temporal sulcus region responded more strongly to biological motion (as conveyed by the walking robot or walking human) than to nonmeaningful but complex nonbiological motion (the disjointed mechanical figure) or complex and meaningful nonbiological motion (the movements of the grandfather clock). Importantly, not every brain region showed this pattern of effects. We observed a functional dissociation between the superior temporal sulcus region and an area corresponding to the functionally defined motion-sensitive visual area MT/V5 (McCarthy et al., 1995; Zeki et al., 1991). Whereas the superior temporal sulcus region preferred biological motion, MT/V5 responded equally to all four types of motion. This study allowed us to conclude that the superior temporal sulcus region is involved in social perception by representing perceived actions, but we could not yet determine whether this region was involved in deciphering the intentions, mental states, and goals conveyed by those actions. It remained possible that the posterior superior temporal sulcus region served as a simple biological motion detector and was not sensitive to the goals and intentions conveyed by the observed movements of actors.

Next, we conducted a study to determine whether the superior temporal sulcus region was sensitive to the intentionality or goal-directedness of observed gaze shifts (Pelphrey, Singerman, et al., 2003). During fMRI scanning, neurologically normal adults watched as a small checkerboard appeared and flickered in an animated character's visual field (see left panel of Plate 3.3). On congruent (goal-directed) trials, the character shifted her gaze toward the checkerboard, confirming the subject's expectations. On incongruent (non-goal-directed) trials, the character shifted her gaze toward empty space, violating the subject's expectations. We hypothesized that, if the superior temporal sulcus region is sensitive to the intentions conveyed by actions in this simple virtual social setting, then activity in the superior temporal sulcus region evoked by observation of gaze shifts would differentiate between congruent and incongruent trials. This differentiation, we reasoned, would reflect the ability of an adult to link the perception of the gaze shift with its mentalistic significance. We observed more activity in the posterior superior temporal sulcus region for incongruent than for congruent gaze, suggesting that additional processing was required of the superior temporal sulcus region when the character violated the subject's expectation. These initial findings have since been replicated in a sample of neurologically normal adults observing congruent and incongruent reaching-to-grasp movements (Pelphrey, Morris, & McCarthy, 2004) and using the same eye-gaze paradigm in 7- to 10-year-old typically developing children (Mosconi, Mack, McCarthy, & Pelphrey, 2005).

In a subsequent study, we examined whether the superior temporal sulcus region participated in the visual analysis of social information conveyed by gaze shifts in an overtly social and more complex virtual encounter: a stranger passing by the subject in a hallway (Pelphrey, Viola, &

McCarthy, 2004). Neurologically normal adults viewed an animated character who walked toward them and shifted his neutral gaze either toward (mutual gaze) or away (averted gaze) from them. We reasoned that, if gaze-related activity in the superior temporal sulcus region reflected the operation of a simple eye-movement detector (or more generally, a biological motion detector), the region should not respond differentially to mutual and averted gaze. The motion of the man walking toward the subject and the gaze shift evoked robust activity in the superior temporal sulcus and fusiform gyrus. Mutual gaze evoked greater activity in the superior temporal sulcus than did averted gaze (see bottom panel of Plate 3.2). In contrast, the fusiform gyrus responded equally to mutual and averted gaze, demonstrating a functional dissociation. This study extended our understanding of the role of the superior temporal sulcus region in social perception by demonstrating that it is highly sensitive to the social context in which a specific biological motion occurs, in this case, approach versus avoidance. Overall, the results of our studies of eye-gaze processing, together with the findings from the processing of intentions conveyed by reaching-to-grasp actions (Pelphrey, Morris, & McCarthy, 2004), strongly suggest that the posterior superior temporal sulcus region is involved in the visual analysis of the intentions underlying other people's actions.

Eye-gaze processing deficits, including failures to coordinate visual attention with others (i.e., initiating and responding to joint attention) and difficulties comprehending the mental states and social intentions of other people as conveyed by the eyes (Baron-Cohen, 1995; Dawson, Meltzoff, Osterling, Rinaldi, & Brown, 1998; Leekam, Hunnisett, & Moore, 1998; Leekam, Lopez, & Moore, 2000; Loveland & Landry, 1986; Mundy, Sigman, Ungerer, & Sherman, 1986), are key features of autism (Baron-Cohen, Wheelwright, Hill, Raste, & Plumb, 2001; Frith & Frith, 1999), and these impairments are identifiable early in the ontogeny of children with autism (Dawson et al., 1998; Mundy et al., 1986). Many affected children eventually learn to use joint attention in social interactions, but even higher-functioning adults exhibit impairments on tasks requiring subtle distinctions regarding intentions and mental states from viewing the eyes (Baron-Cohen et al., 2001). Eye-gaze processing deficits in autism are not the result of abnormal gaze discrimination but rather represent an inability to use gaze spontaneously to understand and predict other people's mental states and behaviors (Baron-Cohen, 1995; Baron-Cohen et al., 1999).

The nature of gaze processing deficits in autism combined with our prior neuroimaging findings led us to hypothesize that superior temporal sulcus dysfunction might be involved (Pelphrey, Morris, & McCarthy, 2005). To test this question, we employed our congruent-versus-incongruent eye-gaze paradigm (left panel of Plate 3.3). We predicted that, in autism, the superior temporal sulcus region would not be sensitive to intentions conveyed by the character's gaze shifts. As shown in the right panel of Plate 3.3, in neurologically normal control participants, "errors" (incongruent gaze shifts) again evoked more activity in the superior temporal sulcus and other regions involved in social perception, indicating a strong effect of intention (see Plate 3.3b). The same brain regions were activated during observation of gaze shifts in individuals with autism (see Plate 3.3c) but did not differentiate between congruent and incongruent trials (see Plate 3.3d), indicating that activity in these regions was not modulated by the context of the perceived gaze shift. This finding suggests that lack of modulation in activation of the superior temporal sulcus region is a potential mechanism underlying the eye-gaze processing deficits associated with autism. These findings are consistent with those of a prior positron emission tomography (PET) study conducted by Castelli, Frith, Happé, and Frith (2002) that found hypoactivation of the posterior superior temporal sulcus and reduced functional connectivity between the superior temporal sulcus and portions of the inferior occipital gyrus (visual area V3) in autism during tasks involving attribution of intentions to moving geometric figures.

Three other functional neuroimaging studies have explored the role of the superior temporal sulcus region in autism (see Table 3.1), focusing on the neural basis of speech perception deficits. A PET study reported abnormal laterality of responses and hypoactivation of the left superior temporal sulcus region (Boddaert et al., 2003) during speech perception. Similarly, an fMRI study reported abnormal responses to human voices in the superior temporal sulcus region (Gervais et al., 2004). A region of the superior temporal sulcus that had previously been shown to respond selectively to vocal sounds (Belin, Zatorre, Lafaille, Ahad, & Pike, 2000) failed to be activated by this stimulus category in individuals with autism (Gervais et al., 2004). These subjects showed normal auditory cortex activation to nonvocal sounds. Similarly, by comparing responses to various auditory and visual speech stimuli, we have explored the role of the superior temporal sulcus region in audiovisual speech perception in a small sample of individuals with autism and neurologically normal controls (Smith, Morris, & Pelphrey, 2005). The superior temporal sulcus region was activated bilaterally during audiovisual speech perception in both groups of subjects. For control subjects, responses from this region to matching audiovisual speech were greater than responses to the audio and visual components presented alone, and the mismatching audiovisual speech evoked a depressed response consistent with the inhibition that is generally observed in paradigms of this type (see Calvert, 2001, for a review). For the subjects with autism, there was overall hypoactivation in the superior temporal sulcus region, and this area responded equally to the matching and mismatching audiovisual stimuli, suggesting abnormal integration of the two sources of information.

FUSIFORM GYRUS

The fusiform gyrus is found in the ventral occipitotemporal cortex of humans (see Figure 3.2). When a neurologically normal individual is presented with faces versus non-face objects or scrambled images, face-evoked activity in the lateral portions of the fusiform gyrus is observed bilaterally, but typically more in the right than the left hemisphere (Kanwisher, McDermott, & Chun, 1997; McCarthy, Puce, Gore, & Allison, 1997; Puce, Allison, Asgari, Gore & McCarthy, 1996); thus, portions of this cortical region are specialized for processing faces (Kanwisher et al., 1997; McCarthy et al., 1997). Some of the clearest evidence for face specificity in the fusiform gyrus comes from studies during which electrodes inserted in the ventral occipitotemporal cortical surface during brain surgery displayed face-specific evoked activity within 200 ms of the presentation of a face stimulus (Allison, Puce, Spencer, & McCarthy, 1999; McCarthy, Puce, Belger, & Allison, 1999; Puce, Allison, & McCarthy, 1999), and electrical stimulation of this area led to transient prosopagnosia (Allison, McCarthy, Nobre, Puce, & Belger, 1994; see McCarthy, 1999, for a review). Models of the human face processing system emphasize the role of the fusiform gyrus in detecting faces and processing their static aspects, which are used for face identification (Haxby, Hoffman, & Gobbini, 2000; McCarthy, 1999).

In autism, behavioral studies have consistently demonstrated face processing deficits in affected individuals (e.g., Hobson, Ouston, & Lee, 1988; Loveland et al., 1997), although the specific mechanisms underlying these deficits remain elusive. Schultz and colleagues (2000) performed the first fMRI study of the fusiform gyrus response to faces and non-face objects in adolescents and adults with high-functioning autism and Asperger syndrome. They found that there was less face-evoked activation in this region and that areas typically recruited for non-face object perception were used for face perception in these individuals. Since this original study, three other fMRI studies have replicated the finding of fusiform gyrus hypoactivation in autism (Critchley et al., 2000; Hubl et al., 2003; Pierce, Mueller, Ambrose, Allen, & Courchesne, 2001). Schultz and colleagues (2000) and Dawson, Webb, and colleagues (2002; Dawson, Webb, & McPartland, 2005; see also Dawson & Bernier, Chapter 2, this volume) emphasize the importance of a developmental perspective and suggest a possible link between amygdala dysfunction and the lack of normal development of face-specific fusiform gyrus responsivity and, consequently, normal face perception (Schultz, 2005). In fleshing out the neurobiological basis for this developmental hypothesis, both Dawson, Webb, and colleagues (2002, 2005) and Schultz (2005) have argued that early amygdala disruption in autism leads to a lack of interest in faces. The corresponding lack of attention to faces throughout development leads to abnormalities in the functional pathways between the amygdala and the fusiform gyrus; these functional pathways are dependent upon ongoing input from the amygdala to develop fusiform gyrus face specificity. These hypotheses are supported by indirect evidence, such as the previously described findings by Adolphs and colleagues (2005) regarding the role of the amygdala in directing visual attention to the eyes (see Plate 3.1, bottom panel), but would be tested best in a longitudinal study of the development of face-specific responses in the fusiform gyrus and connectivity among the amygdala and other social brain structures.

It is important to note that the original findings by Schultz and colleagues (2000) have been contended. Some eye-tracking studies have found that individuals with autism do not look at faces in the same manner as do typically developing individuals, with this research reporting that affected individuals spend less time scanning the core features of the face (eyes, nose, and mouth—Dalton et al., 2005; Klin et al., 2002; Pelphrey et al., 2002; but see van der Geest, Kemner, Verbaten, & van Engeland, 2002, for contrasting results). These abnormal scanpaths could actually be the cause of the observed hypoactivation. For example, in a study by McCarthy and others (1999), the N200 response of the ERP waveform had the greatest amplitude for whole faces, followed by eyes, contours, lips, and noses, suggesting that attention to the eyes in face images could drive the fusiform gyrus response. To address the issue of visual attention to faces, Hadjikhani and colleagues (2004) added fixation points to the center of images of faces and objects and determined that people with autism exhibited enhanced fusiform gyrus activation under that condition. However, it is difficult to draw definitive conclusions from this study because the requirement to fixate on the crosshair would have altered scanpaths in both groups.

Dalton and colleagues (2005) directly explored the relationship between gaze fixation on the eyes and brain activation patterns in the fusiform gyrus and the amygdala in participants with and without autism. The participants with autism had significantly less gaze fixation on the eyes and showed greater activation than controls in the left amygdala and the left orbitofrontal gyrus when viewing emotional and neutral faces. In a second study, the participants viewed familiar and unfamiliar people. The neurologically normal group showed greater activation in the right occipital gyrus and fusiform gyrus for the familiar faces relative to the unfamiliar faces, and more activation for the familiar faces than did the group with autism. Again the participants with autism spent less time looking at the eyes and had less activation in the right and left fusiform gyri, but more activity in the right amygdala overall. Across both studies, the researchers found a strong positive correlation between the number and length of gaze fixations on the eyes of faces and the fusiform gyrus response in individuals with and without autism. Like Schultz and Dawson, they also implicated functional interactions between the amygdala and fusiform gyrus. However, unlike Schultz and Dawson, these authors interpreted this relationship from the perspective of social anxiety, suggesting that people with autism actively avoid eye gaze because of an autonomic hyperreactivity caused by dysregulation of affective processes in the amygdala in response to salient social stimuli. Notably, the amount of amygdala activation had a strong positive correlation with the amount of fixation on the eye region among the participants with autism.

An alternative explanation for the findings by Dalton and colleagues (2005) is that individuals with autism could be failing to marshal a social response to environmental cues even in the absence of anxiety. Rather than avoiding social situations in an active manner, as Schultz and Dawson argue, they instead might not appreciate the significance of the faces in their environments. In an effort to increase the probability that individuals with autism would find faces to be socially meaningful, Pierce, Haist, Sedaghat, and Courschesne (2004) showed participants with and without autism photographs of both very familiar people (friends and family members) and strangers. In the fusiform gyrus, both groups of subjects showed similar activation for the familiar faces. In response to the unfamiliar faces, the individuals with autism showed a significant, but much lower, level of activation. However, we note that this result and the findings from Dalton and colleagues regarding responses to familiar faces in subjects with and without autism are inconsistent. Further work is needed to explore potential reasons for these incompatible findings.

INTEGRATING THE SOCIAL BRAIN: FUTURE DIRECTIONS AND OUTSTANDING QUESTIONS

We have reviewed functional neuroimaging studies of individuals with and without autism that focused on identifying dysfunction in specific structures linked to particular aspects of social perception. We emphasized the unique contributions of three structures: the amygdala, the superior temporal sulcus region, and the fusiform gyrus. This analytic perspective was helpful in providing a framework for organizing our emerging understanding of social brain dysfunction in autism, but this approach does not fully reflect the complexity of interactions among these and other brain regions during social perception. These structures undoubtedly function in parallel and are better understood as components in a network of regions subserving social perception. For example, when encountering a socially ambiguous situation, such as when a person is approaching in a hallway, the amygdala will provide a rapid and automatic assessment of the potentially threatening aspects of the situation and, through its interconnections with the other structures, allocate processing resources accordingly. The fusiform gyrus will provide a perceptual representation of the face and will aid in identification of the person. The posterior superior temporal sulcus will conduct a visual analysis of the person's gait and other socially and communicatively important actions, including movements of facial features and shifts in eye gaze, while other sectors of this region incorporate auditory and visual components of speech. The rapid integration of the functions performed by each structure would guide social perception and the subsequent behavior of the observer. To date, disruption in each of the components of this system has been studied in autism, but their integration has generally been neglected, probably owing to the relative lack of techniques, until recently, for this type of analysis. A challenge for the future will be to offer a more precise account of the interplay between all of these different processes as a function of the detailed specification of the performance demands required by a given experimental task or by a given situation in real life.

A few studies have begun to examine functional interactions between brain regions and potential disruptions in functional connectivity in autism. For example, Just, Cherkassky, Keller, and Minshew (2004) reported lower levels of functional connectivity (defined as the correlation, over time, of activity in two brain regions) between Wernicke's and Broca's areas during sentence comprehension in individuals with autism relative to neurologically normal controls. In an earlier PET study, Castelli and colleagues (2002) reported reduced functional connectivity between the posterior superior temporal sulcus and the inferior occipital gyrus in individuals with autism during a task involving attribution of intentions to moving geometric figures. We conducted analyses of functional connectivity in our own research on the neural basis of eye-gaze processing deficits in autism (Pelphrey et al., 2005). Specifically, we reasoned that the lack of differential activity for incongruent versus congruent gaze in subjects with autism (see

Plate 3.3, right panel) could be caused by a functional disruption in the superior temporal sulcus region itself. On the other hand, the abnormal patterns of superior temporal sulcus activation could be the result of atypical connectivity between this and other brain regions involved in social perception. According to this hypothesis, the superior temporal sulcus could be activated during the initial perception of an action performed by another, creating a perceptual representation of the socially relevant information. These data are then sent to higher systems (possibly including prefrontal regions and/or the amygdala) for analysis of the intentions or goal orientations displayed, and these areas might maintain superior temporal sulcus activation in circumstances during which additional processing is required, such as violations of expectations. In autism, this connection could be faulty, leaving these higher areas incapable of sustaining activation in the superior temporal sulcus when needed. We explored this alternative by examining the temporal profile of the correlation between activity in the right posterior superior temporal sulcus and the right posterior middle temporal gyrus. In subjects without autism, there was a strong positive correlation between these regions, but this correlation was greatly reduced in the subjects with autism, suggesting abnormal functional connectivity during this social perception task.

Such analyses of fMRI data can provide indirect assessments of functional connectivity as revealed by correlations in temporal profiles of activity between two or more brain regions, but these correlation analyses do not provide direct information regarding connectivity in the living brain. The combined use of diffusion tensor imaging (DTI) and fMRI is promising for studying the role of abnormal connectivity in autism. DTI has emerged as a powerful method for the investigation of white matter architecture. By measuring the tensor associated with self-diffusion (Brownian motion) of endogenous water molecules in brain tissue—which diffuse less readily across, as compared to along, membranes—DTI permits investigators to measure aspects of connectivity and to trace the extent and direction of white matter tracts in the living brain. In future work, the use of DTI in autism to study connections between functional regions of interest will add to our understanding of dysfunction in the social brain in this disorder.

Another important future direction is the continued development of stimuli and tasks with more ecological validity. Progress has been limited by the lack of ecologically valid social situations that can be manipulated and presented with conditions adequately controlled within the constraints of an MRI scanner. Most functional imaging studies have used simple, static images; therefore, questions remain unanswered about the effects of context and motion on the social brain. After all, the perceived participation of the subject is an important element for successfully imaging social perception. Subtle but important social deficits are often most evident in high-functioning individuals with autism during unstructured social settings. As future studies begin to shift focus from single regions to networks involved in social perception, continued developments in imaging techniques will drive experimental innovation. We will see researchers more frequently combining data from complementary imaging techniques (i.e., multimodal imaging) to examine structure, function, and connectivity.

Autism is a neurodevelopmental disorder that has its onset in the earliest years of childhood, and its symptoms change over ontogeny. Although the core deficits persist throughout the lifespan, the specific manifestations shift across development. It will be very important to expand the body of research to include functional neuroimaging studies of young children with autism. Neuroimaging studies of autism that take into account psychological and behavioral continuities and discontinuities from childhood to adulthood would better inform us of the neurobiological mechanisms in autism than would studies that provide only a static picture in adults. We can thus incorporate a developmental perspective (i.e., a perspective involving early and longitudinal study of brain and behavioral development) into our analyses of the social brain.

A developmental perspective is important for understanding how higher-order deficits in aspects of social interactions might originate in primary impairments in joint attention, action understanding and imitation, and early language functioning. This stance could reveal that autism arises from subtle and more diffuse early neuropathology and ultimately affects multiple neural systems, directly and through compensatory experience-dependent reorganization, rather than being a disorder of a specific neuroanatomical structure. Neuroimaging studies focusing on changing brain–behavior relationships in the developing child may also provide clues to candidate genes in autism, as developmentally important genes begin to be linked to particular patterns of brain development, gene expression, and phenotypes.

Longitudinal studies of the social brain in neurologically normal children will be as important as developmental studies of children with autism. Currently, very little is known about the neural correlates of social perception in children or about the changes in brain function that underlie normative development in this domain. Fundamental scientific questions concerning the maturation of the brain and its relationship to changes in social perception in children without autism thus remain unanswered. This basic knowledge is essential to efforts aimed at understanding the neural basis of social perception deficits in autism.

UNDERSTANDING SOCIAL BRAIN DYSFUNCTION IN AUTISM: EDUCATION AND TREATMENT IMPLICATIONS

Techniques for earlier diagnosis of autism are still being improved. Unlike some other neurodevelopmental disorders (e.g., fragile X syndrome), we do not have a genetic test for autism, and the complexity of the interactive roles played by genes and environment makes it unlikely that such a test will be feasible. However, the analysis of functional brain correlates and networks could prove to be a useful tool in unambiguously identifying this disorder at an early age. Reliable and specific structural and/or functional differences in the brains of people with autism might serve as valuable neurobiological "markers" for the diagnosis of autism. In our own work, activity in the superior temporal sulcus offers a possible example of a neurobiological marker for the social perception deficits in autism. Currently, the Autism Diagnostic Observation Schedule—General (ADOS-G; Lord et al., 2000) and the Autism Diagnostic Interview—Revised (ADI-R; Lord, Rutter, & Le Couteur, 1994) are the most widely accepted tools for diagnosing autism. In a set of exploratory correlation analyses, we integrated information from the ADI-R with patterns of neural activity from the superior temporal sulcus region during an eye-gaze processing task (Pelphrey et al., 2005). As discussed previously, activity in the superior temporal sulcus region in the group of participants with autism did not differ significantly for incongruent and congruent gaze shifts, but individual differences in the patterns of activation were apparent. We wondered whether these individual differences might be related to the phenotypic variability in real-world social functioning seen in this disorder. To explore this question further, we correlated scores on several algorithmic domains of the ADI-R with the magnitude of differentiation in the right superior temporal sulcus region between stimulus conditions, predicting that the individuals with less severe behavioral deficits would show activity more similar to the participants without autism. We found a strong correlation between superior temporal sulcus activation patterns and the severity of impairments in the Reciprocal Social Interaction Domain, but correlations did not extend to the domains of Communication and Restricted–Repetitive–Stereotyped Behaviors. Notably, the patterns of brain activity obtained during the brief fMRI scan accounted for 61% of the variance in ADI-Reciprocal Social Interaction Domain scores. These findings suggest that the degree of neurofunctional impairment in the right superior temporal sulcus region is related to the severity of specific and relevant features of the autism phenotype. Future research using larger samples could elucidate the validity of this difference as a marker for autism severity.

It is generally accepted that earlier behavioral interventions are more effective for treating children with autism. Therefore, early diagnosis is pivotal to individual treatment outcomes for these children. A neurobiological marker, then, would be important not solely for improving early diagnosis but also for offering advantages in terms of earlier interventions. Moreover, based on research such as that described above, it could be that the marker would relate to the severity of specific deficits and might help us to understand better the heterogeneity in the core features of the autism phenotype. With this information, more targeted treatments could be developed on a child-by-child basis and implemented early in ontogeny, which might then guarantee the most effective course of intervention possible. In addition, the assessment of individual treatment needs could be far more efficient and standardized. Furthermore, functional neuroimaging techniques might actually provide a means to better, and more quantitatively, assess the effectiveness of treatment and reveal whether behavioral improvements correspond to compensatory changes in brain function or normalization of developmental pathways.

By defining functional brain phenotypes based on neurofunctional/behavioral developmental pathways and altered activation patterns, fMRI studies of children and adults with autism have the potential to dissect the heterogeneity present in autism as a behaviorally defined syndrome. Functional neuroimaging studies could reveal different brain phenotypes in the circuitry involved in social perception. This approach may allow us to partition this complex disorder, which is thought to be etiologically heterogeneous, into more homogenous subgroups. Thus a goal for future work is to identify developmental brain "endophenotypes" linking functioning in the social brain to clinically observed social perception and social cognition deficits. This link would be valuable because progress in understanding and treating autism has been hindered by its heterogeneity, which reduces the statistical power to (1) identify genes through linkage studies, (2) identify effective pharmacological treatments, and (3) describe the pathophysiology of autism. Early and longitudinal study will be critical in defining brain phenotypes in autism because the shape of developmental trajectories of brain functioning in specific circuits will provide more detail on the nature of the abnormalities in autism than will analysis of brain phenotypes in adults. These phenotypes might relate to behavioral outcomes and could suggest novel and more targeted intervention and treatment strategies. Knowledge of the development of the social brain could help geneticists search for abnormal genes or assist other researchers in the detection of possible environmental factors related to autism. A better understanding of abnormal and normal brain systems mapping onto behavioral strengths and weaknesses in the autism phenotype could help scientists and clinicians to develop strategies for assisting individuals with autism to utilize normally developing regions and circuits to compensate for abnormal function, and to create therapies targeted at training and reinforcing the abnormally functioning regions and circuits as early as possible in the ontogeny of affected individuals.

ACKNOWLEDGMENTS

Kevin A. Pelphrey is supported by a Career Development Award from the National Institutes of Health, National Institute of Mental Health Grant No. K01-MH071284. We gratefully acknowledge our collaborators Drs. Gregory McCarthy, James Morris, Truett Allison, Kevin LaBar, Joseph Piven, and Ralph Adolphs.

REFERENCES

Adolphs, R., Damasio, H., Tranel, D., Cooper, G., & Damasio, A. R. (2000). A role for somatosensory cortices in the visual recognition of emotion as revealed by three-dimensional lesion mapping. *Journal of Neuroscience, 20*(7), 2683–2690.

Adolphs, R., Gosselin, F., Buchanan, T. W., Tranel, D., Schyns, P., & Damasio, A. R. (2005). A mechanism for impaired fear recognition after amygdala damage. *Nature, 433*, 68–72.

Adolphs, R., Sears, L., & Piven, J. (2001). Abnormal processing of social information from faces in autism. *Journal of Cognitive Neuroscience, 13*(2), 232–240.

Adolphs, R., Tranel, D., & Damasio, A. R. (1998). The human amygdala in social judgment. *Nature, 393*, 470–474.

Adolphs, R., Tranel, D., Damasio, H., & Damasio, A. (1994). Impaired recognition of emotion in facial expressions following bilateral damage to the human amygdala. *Nature, 372*, 669–672.

Adolphs, R., Tranel, D., Hamann, S., Young, A. W., Calder, A. J., Phelps, E. A., et al. (1999). Recognition of facial emotion in nine individuals with bilateral amygdala damage. *Neuropsychologia, 37*(10), 1111–1117.

Allison, T., McCarthy, G., Nobre, A., Puce, A., & Belger, A. (1994). Human extrastriate visual cortex and the perception of faces, words, numbers, and colors. *Cerebral Cortex, 4*(5), 544–554.

Allison, T., Puce, A., & McCarthy, G. (2000). Social perception from visual cues: Role of the STS region. *Trends in Cognitive Science, 4*(7), 267–278.

Allison, T., Puce, A., Spencer, D. D., & McCarthy, G. (1999). Electrophysiological studies of human face perception I: Potentials generated in occipitotemporal cortex by face and non-face stimuli. *Cerebral Cortex, 9*(5), 415–430.

Amaral, D. G., & Insausti, R. (1992). Retrograde transport of d-[3h]-aspartate injected into the monkey amygdaloid complex. *Experimental Brain Research, 88*(2), 375–388.

Amaral, D. G., Veazey, R. B., & Cowan, W. M. (1982). Some observations on hypothalamo-amygdaloid connections in the monkey. *Brain Research, 252*(1), 13–27.

American Psychiatric Association. (1994). *Diagnostic and statistical manual of mental disorders* (4th ed., text rev.).Washington, DC: Author.

Anderson, A. K., & Phelps, E. A. (2000). Expression without recognition: Contributions of the human amygdala to emotional communication. *Psychological Science, 11*(2), 106–111.

Bachevalier, J. (1994). Medial temporal lobe structures and autism: A review of clinical and experimental findings. *Neuropsychologia, 32*(6), 627–648.

Bachevalier, J. (1996). Medial temporal lobe and autism: A putative animal model in primates. *Journal of Autism and Developmental Disorders, 26*(2), 217–220.

Bachevalier, J., & Mishkin, M. (1994). Effects of selective neonatal temporal lobe lesions on visual recognition memory in rhesus monkeys. *Journal of Neuroscience, 14*(4), 2128–2139.

Bailey, A., Le Couteur, A., Gottesman, I., Bolton, P., Simonoff, E., Yuzda, E., et al. (1995). Autism as a strongly genetic disorder: Evidence from a British twin study. *Psychological Medicine, 25*(1), 63–77.

Bailey, D. B., Jr., Hatton, D. D., Skinner, M., & Mesibov, G. (2001). Autistic behavior, fMR1 protein, and developmental trajectories in young males with fragile X syndrome. *Journal of Autism and Developmental Disorders, 31*(2), 165–174.

Baker, P., Piven, J., & Sato, Y. (1998). Autism and tuberous sclerosis complex: Prevalence and clinical features. *Journal of Autism and Developmental Disorders, 28*(4), 279–285.

Baron-Cohen, S. (1995). *Mindblindness: An essay on autism and theory of mind.* Cambridge, MA: MIT Press.

Baron-Cohen, S., Jolliffe, T., Mortimore, C., & Robertson, M. (1997). Another advanced test of theory of mind: Evidence from very high functioning adults with autism or Asperger syndrome. *Journal of Child Psychology and Psychiatry, 38*(7), 813–822.

Baron-Cohen, S., Ring, H. A., Wheelwright, S., Bullmore, E. T., Brammer, M. J., Simmons, A., et al. (1999). Social intelligence in the normal and autistic brain: An fMRI study. *European Journal of Neuroscience, 11*(6), 1891–1898.

Baron-Cohen, S., Wheelwright, S., Hill, J., Raste, Y., & Plumb, I. (2001). The "reading the mind in the eyes" test, revised version: A study with normal adults and adults with Asperger syndrome or high-functioning autism. *Journal of Child Psychology and Psychiatry, 42*(2), 241–251.

Belin, P., Zatorre, R. J., Lafaille, P., Ahad, P., & Pike, B. (2000). Voice-selective areas in human auditory cortex. *Nature, 403*, 309–312.

Blake, R., Turner, L. M., Smoski, M. J., Pozdol, S. L., & Stone, W. L. (2003). Visual recognition of biological motion is impaired in children with autism. *Psychological Science, 14*, 51–57.

Boddaert, N., Belin, P., Chabane, N., Poline, J. B., Barthélémy, C., Mouren-Simeoni, M. C., et al. (2003). Perception of complex sounds: Abnormal pattern of cortical activation in autism. *American Journal of Psychiatry, 160*(11), 2057–2060.

Breiter, H. C., Etcoff, N. L., Whalen, P. J., Kennedy, W. A., Rauch, S. L., Buckner, R. L., et al. (1996). Response and habituation of the human amygdala during visual processing of facial expression. *Neuron, 17*(5), 875–887.

Broks, P., Young, A. W., Maratos, E. J., Coffey, P. J., Calder, A. J., Isaac, C. L., et al. (1998). Face processing impairments after encephalitis: Amygdala damage and recognition of fear. *Neuropsychologia, 36*(1), 59–70.

Brothers, L. (1990). The social brain: A project for integrating primate behavior and neurophysiology in a new domain. *Concepts in Neuroscience, 1*, 27–51.

Brothers, L., Ring, B., & Kling, A. (1990). Response of neurons in the macaque amygdala to complex social stimuli. *Behavior and Brain Research, 41*, 199–213.

Brown, S., & Schafer, E. A. (1888). An investigation into the functions of the occipital and temporal lobes of the monkey's brain. *Philosophical Transactions of the Royal Society of London* (Series B: Biological Sciences), *179*, 303–327.

Calvert, G. A. (2001). Crossmodal processing in the human brain: Insights from functional neuroimaging studies. *Cerebral Cortex, 11*(12), 1110–1123.

Campbell, R., Heywood, C. A., Cowey, A., Regard, M., & Landis, T. (1990). Sensitivity to eye gaze in prosopagnosic patients and monkeys with superior temporal sulcus ablation. *Neuropsychologia, 28*(11), 1123–1142.

Castelli, F., Frith, C., Happé, F., & Frith, U. (2002). Autism, Asperger syndrome and brain mechanisms for the attribution of mental states to animated shapes. *Brain, 125*, 1839–1849.

Cook, E. H., Jr., Courchesne, R. Y., Cox, N. J., Lord, C., Gonen, D., Guter, S. J., et al. (1998). Linkage-disequilibrium mapping of autistic disorder, with 15q11–13 markers. *American Journal of Human Genetics, 62*(5), 1077–1083.

Critchley, H. D., Daly, E. M., Bullmore, E. T., Williams, S. C., Van Amelsvoort, T., Robertson, D. M., et al. (2000). The functional neuroanatomy of social behaviour: Changes in cerebral blood flow when people with autistic disorder process facial expressions. *Brain, 123*(11), 2203–2212.

Cross, H. A., & Harlow, H. F. (1965). Prolonged and progressive effects of partial isolation on the behavior of macaque monkeys. *Journal of Experimental Research in Personality, 1*, 39–49.

Cusick, C. G. (1997). The superior temporal polysensory region in monkeys. In K. S. Rockland, J. H. Kaas, & A. Peters (Eds.), *Cerebral cortex. Vol. 12: Extrastriate cortex in primates* (pp. 435–468). New York: Plenum Press.

Dalton, K. M., Nacewicz, B. M., Johnstone, T., Schaefer, H. S., Gernsbacher, M. A., Goldsmith, H. H., et al. (2005). Gaze fixation and the neural circuitry of face processing in autism. *Nature Neuroscience, 8*(4), 519–526.

Dawson, G., Meltzoff, A. N., Osterling, J., Rinaldi, J., & Brown, E. (1998). Children with autism fail to orient to naturally occurring social stimuli. *Journal of Autism and Developmental Disorders, 28*(6), 479–485.

Dawson, G., Munson, J., Estes, A., Osterling, J., McPartland, J., Toth, K., et al. (2002). Neurocognitive function and joint attention ability in young children with autism spectrum disorder versus developmental delay. *Child Development, 73*(2), 345–358.

Dawson, G., Webb, S. J., & McPartland, J. (2005). Understanding the nature of face processing impairment in autism: Insights from behavioral and electrophysiological studies. *Developmental Neuropsychology, 27*(3), 403–424.

Dawson, G., Webb, S., Schellenberg, G. D., Dager, S., Friedman, S., Aylward, E., et al. (2002). Defining the broader phenotype of autism: Genetic, brain, and behavioral perspectives. *Developmental Psychopathology, 14*(3), 581–611.

Decety, J., & Grezès, J. (1999). Neural mechanisms subserving the perception of human actions. *Trends in Cognitive Science, 3*(5), 172–178.

Dennett, D. C. (1987). *The intentional stance.* Cambridge, MA: MIT Press.

Emery, N. J., Capitanio, J. P., Mason, W. A., Machado, C. J., Mendoza, S. P., & Amaral, D. G. (2001). The effects of bilateral lesions of the amygdala on dyadic social interactions in rhesus monkeys (*macaca mulatta*). *Behavioral Neuroscience, 115*(3), 515–544.

Emery, N. J., Lorincz, E. N., Perrett, D. I., Oram, M. W., & Baker, C. I. (1997). Gaze following and joint attention in rhesus monkeys (*macaca mulatta*). *Journal of Computational Psychology, 111*(3), 286–293.

Fischer, K. W., & Bidell, T. R. (1998). Dynamic development of psychological structures in action and thought. In R. M. Lerner (Ed.), *Handbook of child psychology. Vol. 1: Theoretical models of human development* (5th ed., pp. 467–561). New York: Wiley.

Folstein, S. E., & Rosen-Sheidley, B. (2001). Genetics of autism: Complex aetiology for a heterogeneous disorder. *Nature Reviews Genetics, 2*(12), 943–955.

Folstein, S., & Rutter, M. (1977). Genetic influences and infantile autism. *Nature, 265*(5596), 726–728.

Fombonne, E. (1999). The epidemiology of autism: A review. *Psychological Medicine, 29*(4), 769–786.

Frith, C. D., & Frith, U. (1999) Interacting minds—biological basis. *Science, 286,* 1692–1695.

Gervais, H., Belin, P., Boddaert, N., Leboyer, M., Coez, A., Sfaello, I., et al. (2004). Abnormal cortical voice processing in autism. *Nature Neuroscience, 7*(8), 801–802.

Hadjikhani, N., Joseph, R. M., Snyder, J., Chabris, C. F., Clark, J., Steele, S., et al. (2004). Activation of the fusiform gyrus when individuals with autism spectrum disorder view faces. *NeuroImage, 22*(3), 1141–1150.

Hasselmo, M. E., Rolls, E. T., Baylis, G. C., & Nalwa, V. (1989). Object-centered encoding by face-selective neurons in the cortex in the superior temporal sulcus of the monkey. *Experimental Brain Research, 75*(2), 417–429.

Haxby, J. V., Hoffman, E. A., & Gobbini, M. I. (2000). The distributed neural system for face perception. *Trends in Cognitive Science, 4*(6),223–233.

Haxby, J. V., Horwitz, B., Ungerleider, L. G., Maisog, J. M., Pietrini, P., & Grady, C. L. (1994). The functional organization of human extrastriate cortex: A PET–RCBF study of selective attention to faces and locations. *Journal of Neuroscience, 14*(11), 6336–6353.

Hobson, R. P., Ouston, J., & Lee, A. (1988). What's in a face? The case of autism. *British Journal of Psychology, 79*(4), 441–453.

Hubl, D., Bèolte, S., Feineis-Matthews, S., Lanfermann, H., Federspiel, A., Strik, W., et al. (2003). Functional imbalance of visual pathways indicates alternative face processing strategies in autism. *Neurology, 61*(9), 1232–1237.

Hughes, C., Leboyer, M., & Bouvard, M. (1997). Executive function in parents of children with autism. *Psychological Medicine, 27*(1), 209–220.

Hughes, C., Plumet, M. H., & Leboyer, M. (1999). Towards a cognitive phenotype for autism: Increased prevalence of executive dysfunction and superior spatial span amongst siblings of children with autism. *Journal of Child Psychology and Psychiatry, 40*(5), 705–718.

Just, M. A., Cherkassky, V. L., Keller, T. A., & Minshew, N. J. (2004). Cortical activation and synchronization during sentence comprehension in high-functioning autism: Evidence of underconnectivity. *Brain, 127*(8), 1811–1821.

Kanner, L. (1943). Autistic disturbances of affective contact. *Nervous Child, 2*, 217–250.

Kanwisher, N., McDermott, J., & Chun, M. M. (1997). The fusiform face area: A module in human extrastriate cortex specialized for face perception. *Journal of Neuroscience, 17*(11), 4302–4311.

Klin, A., Jones, W., Schultz, R., & Volkmar, F. (2003). The enactive mind—from actions to cognition: Lessons from autism. *Philosophical Transactions of the Royal Society of London* (Series B: Biological Sciences), *358*, 345–360.

Klin, A., Jones, W., Schultz, R., Volkmar, F., & Cohen, D. (2002). Visual fixation patterns during viewing of naturalistic social situations as predictors of social competence in individuals with autism. *Archives of General Psychiatry, 59*(9), 809–816.

Kluver, H., & Bucy, P. (1938). An analysis of certain effects of bilateral temporal lobectomy in the rhesus monkey, with special reference to "psychic blindness." *Journal of Psychology, 5*, 33–54.

Kluver, H., & Bucy, P. (1939). Preliminary analyses of the functions of temporal lobes in monkeys. *Archives of Neurology and Psychiatry, 42*, 979–1000.

Landa, R., Piven, J., Wzorek, M. M., Gayle, J. O., Chase, G. A., & Folstein, S. E. (1992). Social language use in parents of autistic individuals. *Psychological Medicine, 22*(1), 245–254.

LeDoux, J. (1996). Emotional networks and motor control: A fearful view. *Progress in Brain Research, 107*, 437–446.

Leekam, S. R., Hunnisett, E., & Moore, C. (1998). Targets and cues: Gaze-following in children with autism. *Journal of Child Psychology and Psychiatry and Allied Disciplines, 39*(7), 951–962.

Leekam, S. R., Lopez, B., & Moore, C. (2000). Attention and joint attention in preschool children with autism. *Developmental Psychology, 36*, 261–273.

Lord, C., Pickles, A., McLennan, J., Rutter, M., Bregman, J., Folstein, S., et al. (1997). Diagnosing autism: Analyses of data from the Autism Diagnostic Interview. *Journal of Autism and Developmental Disorders, 27*(5), 501–517.

Lord, C., Risi, S., Lambrecht, L., Cook, E. H., Leventhal, B. L., DiLavore, P. C., et al. (2000). The Autism Diagnostic Observation Schedule—Generic: A standard measure of social and communication deficits associated with the spectrum of autism. *Journal of Autism and Developmental Disorders, 30*(3), 205–223.

Lord, C., Rutter, M., & Le Couteur, A. (1994). Autism Diagnostic Interview—Revised: A revised version of a diagnostic interview for caregivers of individuals with possible pervasive developmental disorders. *Journal of Autism and Developmental Disorders, 24,* 659–685.

Loveland, K. A., & Landry, S. H. (1986). Joint attention and language in autism and developmental language delay. *Journal of Autism and Developmental Disorders, 16*(3), 335–349.

Loveland, K. A., Tunali-Kotoski, B., Chen, Y. R., Ortegon, J., Pearson, D. A., Brelsford, K. A., et al. (1997). Emotion recognition in autism: Verbal and nonverbal information. *Developmental Psychopathology, 9*(3), 579–593.

Martin, A., Koenig, K., Scahill, L., Tierney, E., Porter, F. D., & Nwokoro, N. A. (2001). Smith–Lemli–Opitz syndrome. *Journal of the American Academy of Child and Adolescent Psychiatry, 40*(5), 506–507.

McCarthy, G. (1999). Physiological studies of face processing in humans. In M. S. Gazzaniga (Ed.), *The new cognitive neurosciences* (2nd ed., pp. 393–410). Cambridge, MA: MIT Press.

McCarthy, G., Puce, A., Belger, A., & Allison, T. (1999). Electrophysiological studies of human face perception II: Response properties of face-specific potentials generated in occipitotemporal cortex. *Cerebral Cortex, 9*(5), 431–444.

McCarthy, G., Puce, A., Gore, J. C., & Allison, T. (1997). Face-specific processing in the human fusiform gyrus. *Journal of Cognitive Neuroscience, 9*(5), 605–610.

McCarthy, G., Spicer, M., Adrignolo, A., Luby, M., Gore, J., & Allison, T. (1995). Brain activation associated with visual motion studied by functional magnetic resonance imaging in humans. *Human Brain Mapping, 2,* 234–243.

Morris, J. S., Frith, C. D., Perrett, D. I., Rowland, D., Young, A. W., Calder, A. J., et al. (1996). A differential neural response in the human amygdala to fearful and happy facial expressions. *Nature, 383,* 812–815.

Mosconi, M. W., Mack, P. B., McCarthy, G., & Pelphrey, K. A. (2005). Taking an "Intentional Stance" on eye-gaze shifts: A functional neuroimaging study of social perception in children. *NeuroImage, 27*(1), 247–252.

Mundy, P., Sigman, M., Ungerer, J., & Sherman, T. (1986). Defining the social deficits of autism: The contribution of non-verbal communication measures. *Journal of Child Psychology and Psychiatry, 27*(5), 657–669.

Murphy, M., Bolton, P. F., Pickles, A., Fombonne, E., Piven, J., & Rutter, M. (2000). Personality traits of the relatives of autistic probands. *Psychological Medicine, 30*(6), 1411–1424.

Oram, M. W., & Perrett, D. I. (1996). Integration of form and motion in the anterior superior temporal polysensory area (STPA) of the macaque monkey. *Journal of Neurophysiology, 76*(1), 109–129.

Pelphrey, K., Adolphs, R., & Morris, J. P. (2004). Neuroanatomical substrates of social cognition dysfunction in autism. *Mental Retardation and Developmental Disabilities Research Review, 10*(4), 259–271.

Pelphrey, K. A., Mitchell, T. V., McKeown, M. J., Goldstein, J., Allison, T., & McCarthy, G. (2003). Brain activity evoked by the perception of human walking: Controlling for meaningful coherent motion. *Journal of Neuroscience*, *23*(17), 6819–6825.

Pelphrey, K. A., Morris, J., & McCarthy, G. (2004). Grasping the intentions of others: The perceived intention of an action influences activity in the superior temporal sulcus during social perception. *Journal of Cognitive Neuroscience*, *16*, 1706–1716.

Pelphrey, K. A., Morris, J., & McCarthy, G. (2005). Neural basis of eye gaze processing deficits in autism. *Brain*, *128*(5), 1038–1048.

Pelphrey, K. A., Sasson, N. J., Reznick, J. S., Paul, G., Goldman, B. D., & Piven, J. (2002). Visual scanning of faces in autism. *Journal of Autism and Developmental Disorders*, *32*(4), 249–261.

Pelphrey, K. A., Singerman, J. D., Allison, T., & McCarthy, G. (2003). Brain activation evoked by perception of gaze shifts: The influence of context. *Neuropsychologia*, *41*(2), 156–170.

Pelphrey, K. A., Viola, R. J., & McCarthy, G. (2004). When strangers pass: Processing of mutual and averted social gaze in the superior temporal sulcus. *Psychological Science*, *15*(9), 598–603.

Perrett, D. I., Harries, M. H., Bevan, R., Thomas, S., Benson, P. J., Mistlin, A. J., et al. (1989). Frameworks of analysis for the neural representation of animate objects and actions. *Journal of Experimental Biology*, *146*, 87–113.

Perrett, D. I., Hietanen, J. K., Oram, M. W., & Benson, P. J. (1992). Organization and functions of cells responsive to faces in the temporal cortex. *Philosophical Transactions of the Royal Society of London* (Series B: Biological Sciences), *335*, 23–30.

Perrett, D. I., Smith, P. A., Potter, D. D., Mistlin, A. J., Head, A. S., Milner, A. D., et al. (1985). Visual cells in the temporal cortex sensitive to face view and gaze direction. *Proceedings of the Royal Society of London* (Series B: Biological Sciences), *223*, 293–317.

Pickles, A., Bolton, P., Macdonald, H., Bailey, A., Le Couteur, A., Sim, C. H., et al. (1995). Latent-class analysis of recurrence risks for complex phenotypes with selection and measurement error: A twin and family history study of autism. *American Journal of Human Genetics*, *57*, 717–726.

Pierce, K., Haist, F., Sedaghat, F., & Courchesne, E. (2004). The brain response to personally familiar faces in autism: Findings of fusiform activity and beyond. *Brain*, *127*(12), 2703–2716.

Pierce, K., Mueller, R. A., Ambrose, J., Allen, G., & Courchesne, E. (2001). Face processing occurs outside the fusiform "face area" in autism: Evidence from functional MRI. *Brain*, *124*, 2059–2073.

Piven, J. (2001). The broad autism phenotype: A complementary strategy for molecular genetic studies of autism. *American Journal of Medical Genetics*, *105*(1), 34–35.

Piven, J., & Palmer, P. (1997). Cognitive deficits in parents from multiple-incidence autism families. *Journal of Child Psychology and Psychiatry*, *38*(8), 1011–1021.

Piven, J., & Palmer, P. (1999). Psychiatric disorder and the broad autism pheno-type: Evidence from a family study of multiple-incidence autism families. *American Journal of Psychiatry, 156*(4), 557–563.

Piven, J., Palmer, P., Jacobi, D., Childress, D., & Arndt, S. (1997). Broader autism phenotype: Evidence from a family history study of multiple-incidence autism families. *American Journal of Psychiatry, 154*(2), 185–190.

Piven, J., Wzorek, M., Landa, R., Lainhart, J., Bolton, P., Chase, G. A., et al. (1994). Personality characteristics of the parents of autistic individuals. *Psychological Medicine, 24*(3), 783–795.

Prather, M. D., Lavenex, P., Mauldin-Jourdain, M. L., Mason, W. A., Capitanio, J. P., Mendoza, S. P., et al. (2001). Increased social fear and decreased fear of objects in monkeys with neonatal amygdala lesions. *Neuroscience, 106*(4), 653–658.

Puce, A., Allison, T., Asgari, M., Gore, J. C., & McCarthy, G. (1996). Differential sensitivity of human visual cortex to faces, letterstrings, and textures: A functional magnetic resonance imaging study. *Journal of Neuroscience, 16*(16), 5205–5215.

Puce, A., Allison, T., & McCarthy, G. (1999). Electrophysiological studies of human face perception III. Effects of top-down processing on face-specific potentials. *Cerebral Cortex, 9*, 445–448.

Risch, N., Spiker, D., Lotspeich, L., Nouri, N., Hinds, D., Hallmayer, J., et al. (1999). A genomic screen of autism: Evidence for a multilocus etiology. *American Journal of Human Genetics, 65*(2), 493–507.

Rogoff, B. (1990). *Apprenticeship in thinking: Cognitive development in social context*. New York: Oxford University Press.

Rolls, E. T. (1992). Neurophysiological mechanisms underlying face processing within and beyond the temporal cortical visual areas. *Philosophical Transactions of the Royal Society of London* (Series B: Biological Sciences), *335*, 11–20.

Schultz, R. T. (2005). Developmental deficits in social perception in autism: The role of the amygdala and fusiform face area. *International Journal of Developmental Neuroscience, 23*(2–3), 125–141.

Schultz, R. T., Gauthier, I., Klin, A., Fulbright, R. K., Anderson, A. W., Volkmar, F., et al. (2000). Abnormal ventral temporal cortical activity during face discrimination among individuals with autism and Asperger syndrome. *Archives of General Psychiatry, 57*(4), 331–340.

Sigman, M., Ruskin, E., Arbeile, S., Corona, R., Dissanayake, C., Espinosa, M., et al. (1999). Continuity and change in the social competence of children with autism, Down syndrome, and developmental delays. *Monographs of the Society for Research in Child Development, 64*(1), 1–114.

Smith, E. G., Morris, J. P., & Pelphrey, K. A. (2005, May). *Functional neuroimaging of audiovisual speech perception in autism*. Poster presented at the International Meeting for Autism Research, Atlanta, GA.

Sprengelmeyer, R., Young, A. W., Schroeder, U., Grossenbacher, P. G., Federlein, J., Buttner, T., et al. (1999). Knowing no fear. *Proceedings of the Royal Society of London* (Series B: Biological Sciences), *266*, 2451–2456.

Valsiner, J. (1987). *Culture and the development of children's action.* Chichester, UK: Wiley.

van der Geest, J. N., Kemner, C., Verbaten, M. N., & van Engeland, H. (2002). Gaze behavior of children with pervasive developmental disorder toward human faces: A fixation time study. *Journal of Child Psychology and Psychiatry, 43*(5), 669–678.

Veenstra-Vanderweele, J., Cook, E., Jr., & Lombroso, P. J. (2003). Genetics of childhood disorders: XLVI. Autism, Part 5: Genetics of autism. *Journal of the American Academy of Child and Adolescent Psychiatry, 42*(1), 116–118.

Vygotsky, L. S. (1978). *Mind and society: The development of higher mental processes.* Cambridge, MA: Harvard University Press.

Wang, A. T., Dapretto, M., Hariri, A. R., Sigman, M., & Bookheimer, S. Y. (2004). Neural correlates of facial affect processing in children and adolescents with autism spectrum disorder. *Journal of the American Academy of Child and Adolescent Psychiatry, 43*(4), 481–490.

Whalen, P. J., Kagan, J., Cook, R. G., Davis, F. C., Kim, H., Polis, S., et al. (2004). Human amygdala responsivity to masked fearful eye whites. *Science, 306,* 2061.

Whalen, P. J., Rauch, S. L., Etcoff, N. L., McInerney, S. C., Lee, M. B., & Jenike, M. A. (1998). Masked presentations of emotional facial expressions modulate amygdala activity without explicit knowledge. *Journal of Neuroscience, 18*(1), 411–418.

Wing, L. (1981). Sex ratios in early childhood autism and related conditions. *Psychiatry Research, 5,* 129–137.

Wing, L., & Gould, J. (1979). Severe impairments of social interaction and associated abnormalities in children: Epidemiology and classification. *Journal of Autism and Developmental Disorders, 9*(1), 11–29.

Winston, J. S., Strange, B. A., O'Doherty, J., & Dolan, R. J. (2002). Automatic and intentional brain responses during evaluation of trustworthiness of faces. *Nature Neuroscience, 5*(3), 277–283.

Wolff, S., Narayan, S., & Moyes, B. (1988). Personality characteristics of parents of autistic children: A controlled study. *Journal of Child Psychology and Psychiatry, 29*(2), 143–153.

Wright, T. M., Pelphrey, K. A., Allison, T., McKeown, M. J., & McCarthy, G. (2003). Polysensory interactions along lateral temporal regions evoked by audiovisual speech. *Cerebral Cortex, 13*(10), 1034–1043.

Yeargin-Allsopp, M., Rice, C., Karapurkar, T., Doernberg, N., Boyle, C., & Murphy, C. (2003). Prevalence of autism in a U.S. metropolitan area. *Journal of the American Medical Association, 289,* 49–55.

Zeki, S., Watson, J. D., Lueck, C. J., Friston, K. J., Kennard, C., & Frackowiak, R. S. (1991). A direct demonstration of functional specialization in human visual cortex. *Journal of Neuroscience, 11*(3), 641–649.

CHAPTER 4

Williams Syndrome

A MODEL DEVELOPMENTAL SYNDROME
FOR EXPLORING BRAIN–BEHAVIOR RELATIONSHIPS

Helen Tager-Flusberg
Daniela Plesa Skwerer

Williams syndrome (WS) is a relatively rare genetically based neuro-developmental disorder that was not described until the early 1960s (Williams, Barratt-Boyes, & Lowe, 1961; Beuren, 1972). Initial descriptions of WS focused on the medical and craniofacial characteristics. These clinically defining features include a specific heart defect (narrowing of the main aorta), gastrointestinal problems, hypercalcemia, hoarse voice, stellate iris, and "elfin" facies. Most people with WS have IQ scores in the mild to moderate range of mental retardation, or they have learning disabilities. We now know that WS is caused by a microdeletion of about 20 genes on one copy of the long arm of chromosome 7 (7q11.23), and current molecular genetic research is rapidly identifying the specific genes in this region (e.g., Korenberg et al., 2000; Stock et al., 2003; Tipney et al., 2004).

Ursula Bellugi was the first to introduce WS to the field of cognitive psychology (Bellugi, Sabo, & Vaid, 1988). Her early publications sparked great interest because children and adolescents with WS exhibited strikingly uneven performance across a range of cognitive and linguistic tests

ֱi, Marks, Bihrle, & Sabo, 1988; Bellugi, Sabo, & Vaid, 1988). These ֱl studies led to strong claims about the dissociation in WS between ֱct language and severely impaired cognition, and this profile was used ֱ garner support for the independence of a language module (e.g., Jackendoff, 1994; Pinker, 1994). As research progressed it became clear that, in fact, language was not intact in either children or adults with WS, but was generally commensurate with their lower mental age level (e.g., Volterra, Capirci, Pezzini, Sabbadini, & Vicari, 1996). Moreover, some studies demonstrated that children with WS who acquire languages that have complex morphology show specific problems in acquiring certain morphological features (e.g., Karmiloff-Smith et al., 1997), and young children with WS have semantic and pragmatic impairments as compared to typically developing children at the same level of grammatical development (Levy & Hermon, 2003). Based on these findings, global dissociations between "language" and "cognition" in WS have been replaced with increasingly focused sets of hypotheses that address more precisely defined deficits and strengths within these domains (for discussion, see Landau et al., 2006; Mervis, 2003). The prevalent new research approach, advanced by carefully designed and controlled experimental studies, is consistent with the view that even cognitive systems that appeared plausible candidates for specialization involve multiple mechanisms and develop in interaction with other systems, at multiple levels, and possibly with different rates of development (Thomas & Karmiloff-Smith, 2005).

In our view, WS is a model syndrome for exploring a fine-grained analysis of the development and organization of neurocognitive architecture and for mapping brain–gene relations. Unlike complex disorders such as autism or specific language impairment (see Dawson & Bernier, Chapter 2; Pelphrey & Carter, Chapter 3; Liegeois, Morgan, & Vargha-Khadem, Chapter 7, this volume), WS has a clearly defined genetic cause shared by almost all individuals who exhibit clinical features of the syndrome. This genetic consistency is reflected in specific cognitive and personality profiles that can be captured on standardized assessments (Klein-Tasman & Mervis, 2003; Mervis et al., 2000). Significant progress has been made over the past decade in mapping the functions of specific genes in the deleted region of WS in both human studies (e.g., Bellugi & St. George, 2000; Danoff, Taylor, Blackshaw, & Desiderio, 2004; Frangiskakis et al., 1996) and research using animal models (Meng et al., 2002; Zhao et al., 2005). In contrast to other genetic syndromes, such as Down syndrome or fragile X syndrome, many children and adults with WS have only mild mental retardation or learning deficits, which allow researchers to explore more directly the specific rather than global effects of genetic variation on brain and cognitive development. For these reasons, WS has fulfilled the expectations, initially promised by Bellugi (Bellugi & St. George, 2000; Bellugi, Wang, & Jernigan, 1994), that research on this unique syndrome would have a significant impact on the burgeoning field of developmental cognitive neuroscience (Mervis, 2003; Tager-Flusberg, 2004).

In this chapter, we focus on two domains that have been extensively investigated in WS: visual–spatial and social cognition. At first blush, it appears that visual–spatial cognition is extremely impaired on standardized testing in WS, whereas the socially engaging and superficially sophisticated social skills of children and adults with WS suggest spared social cognitive capacities. However, studies conducted over the past decade lead to a more complex and nuanced perspective on the relative strengths and limitations of visual–spatial and social information neural processing systems in WS. These studies of WS complement advances made in our understanding of the neurocognitive systems that underlie these domains, based on different populations and methodologies within cognitive neuroscience research, as we illustrate in our review of the literature on WS.

VISUAL–SPATIAL COGNITION IN WS

The most striking weakness in the cognitive profile of people with WS has been found consistently in the area of visual–spatial cognition (Bellugi et al., 1988; Bellugi, Bihrle, Neville, Jernigan, & Doherty, 1992; Farran & Jarrold, 2003; Morris & Mervis, 1999). Poor performance on psychometric measures such as the block design test (Wechsler, 1974) or the equivalent pattern construction test (Elliott, 1990) is considered a hallmark of the spatial deficit associated with WS. At the same time, many researchers have found that people with WS show relative strength in face recognition (Bellugi et al., 1988; Bellugi, Wang, & Jernigan, 1994; Tager-Flusberg, Plesa Skwerer, Faja, & Joseph, 2003; Wang, Doherty, Rourke, & Bellugi, 1995), obtaining scores within age norms or significantly higher than mental-age-matched controls on standardized measures such as the Benton Facial Recognition test (Benton, Hamsher, Varney, & Spreen, 1983). Proficiency in object recognition, assessed by the ability to name familiar objects displayed in noncanonical or unusual views, as well as sparing in other aspects of complex visual perception (e.g., biological motion) have also been reported in several studies (Hoffman & Landau, 2000; Jordan, Reiss, Hoffman, & Landau, 2002; Wang et al., 1995). Thus, performance on a variety of visual–spatial tasks is not uniformly impaired in WS but reflects the coexistence of strengths and extreme weaknesses within the visual perception domain, raising interesting questions about possibly genetically targeted specialization, selective preservation of cognitive structure, and the nature of the developmental processes involved in defining the profile of performances in this domain.

Clarifying the nature of the visual–spatial deficit in WS has proven to be a case in point for the need to understand the complex organization and the "normal" specialization of spatial cognitive systems, including the neural basis of visual–spatial processing and its potential relations to candidate genes. In our view, only the convergence of different methodologies, including the decomposition and analysis of behavioral performance, eye tracking, electrophysiological, and neuroimaging studies, can help reconcile and clarify apparently contradictory findings of extreme impairment in some tasks (e.g., pattern construction, copying, drawing) and relative proficiency in others (e.g., face and object recognition) found in people with WS.

Experimental Research

Cognitive research on the visual–spatial abilities of people with WS has revolved around three main hypotheses for explaining profiles of performance: (1) the local processing bias hypothesis (Bellugi et al., 1992, 1994), which suggests that the visual–spatial deficit stems from a deviant processing style characteristic of individuals with WS, specifically their focus on the parts of an image rather than its whole and their preferential processing of local features over global configurations; (2) the dorsal stream deficit hypothesis (Atkinson et al., 1997), which relates the visual–spatial deficit to a deficit in the parietal lobe, specifically to abnormalities in the functioning of the dorsal cortical stream of visual information, primarily involved in processing spatial relationships and the visual control of spatially directed actions; and (3) the hypothesis of visual short-term memory deficits (Landau et al., 2006), which suggests that impairments in visual short-term memory impact the acquisition and internal manipulation of spatial information, leading to selective deficits in the ability to use spatial representations appropriately in visual–spatial construction tasks.

Initial descriptions of the difficulties shown by people with WS on visual–spatial tasks emphasized the qualitative differences in the types of errors produced in block construction (Bellugi, Sabo, & Vaid, 1988) or copying tasks (Bellugi et al., 1994; Bihrle, Bellugi, Delis, & Marks, 1989) as compared to matched individuals with Down syndrome (DS): Children with WS tended to choose the correct parts on the block construction task but placed them incorrectly, producing broken configurations, whereas children with DS tended to capture the overall organization while making more errors in the internal details of their designs. Similarly, on other tests of spatial organization, such as the Developmental Test of Visuo–Motor Integration (Beery & Buktenica, 1967), which involves copying a series of figures of varying complexity, participants with WS often drew details of the figure quite accurately but failed to capture their global arrangement. These results have been interpreted by Bellugi and colleagues as reflecting a global representation deficit in which details appear preserved but the overall configuration is disrupted.

Several types of evidence argue against a pervasive local processing bias hypothesis in WS. First, people with WS show normal or near normal performance on some visual–spatial tasks that involve reliance on global or configural perceptual processes, such as face and object recognition (Atkinson et al., 1997; Hoffman & Landau, 2000; Mervis, Morris, Bertrand, & Robinson, 1999). Second, the use of configural processing by individuals with WS has been shown on tasks designed to tap perceptual grouping and on tests of visual closure (e.g., Mooney faces test, 1957), which require the ability to use fragmentary information to achieve a global percept. We also note that in typical development faster processing of information at the global compared to the local level becomes apparent only by late childhood (Farran, Jarrold, & Gatherole, 2003).

Using a visual search task that probed sensitivity to global configuration effects, Pani, Mervis, and Robinson (1999) found that visual grouping mechanisms facilitated search in adults with WS in the same way as in the typical control group. Both groups were influenced strongly by gestalt grouping more than by display size. Recently, Deruelle, Rondan, Mancini, and Livet (2006) tested children and adolescents with WS on a battery of four tasks tapping configural abilities and found that individuals with WS performed as well as mental-age-matched typical controls on all tasks and at the same level and in the same manner as age-matched typical controls on three of the tasks.

Close inspection of performance on tasks that probe sensitivity to both global and local organization of stimuli indicates that people with WS can process visual information at both global and local levels when primed to do so, and that processing biases are dependent on the type of task administered (Farran et al., 2003). This lack of evidence for either a local or a global processing preference suggests that the local processing bias hypothesis likely cannot explain the profound deficits on complex visual construction tasks, such as block design, which require the processing and storing of spatial representations, and the ability to use spatial information to guide motor actions. Indeed, as Farran and Jarrold (2003) point out, a local processing bias would enhance the ability to analyze the component parts of the block design stimulus and lead to improved, rather than impaired, performance.

Given that visual construction tasks involve spatial working memory, attentional, planning, and executive functions, it becomes clear that only a detailed componential analysis of performance can help disentangle the possible sources of difficulty shown by people with WS. Such an analysis was carried out by Hoffman, Landau, and Pagani (2003), who examined eye fixation and error patterns in solving simple and complex visual–spatial tasks using a computerized block construction task. On simple puzzles, in which block designs contained a single color, children with WS and mental-age-matched controls were comparable in performance and showed similar eye-fixation patterns, indicating that basic executive processes and some aspects of perceptual organization were intact in WS. However, on more complex block designs, the performance of the WS children dropped abruptly because they fixated models and checked partial solutions less often than the controls and attempted fewer repairs when detecting errors. The authors concluded that in WS a persistent deficit in representing spatial relationships influences how intact executive processes are deployed, producing increasingly impoverished performance as the complexity of a task increases. This explanation is an example of "cascading" processes (e.g., Thelen & Smith, 1994), in which one aspect of a breakdown can lead to changes in other processes within a task as well as over the course of development (Hoffman et al., 2003). The implication is that only understanding the exact points of breakdown can clarify the nature of the visual–spatial deficit in WS and possibly advance our understanding of the organization of spatial cognitive systems in typical development.

Atkinson and her colleagues have related performance profiles on visual–spatial tasks in WS to a possible deficit of the cortical dorsal stream function, which encodes information about spatial relations and the visual control of action (Atkinson et al., 1997). In this view, the dissociations in relatively spared performance on tasks of object and face recognition, in contrast to impairments on tasks of visual construction, map onto the functional distinction between a preserved ventral stream (occipitotemporal lobes), principally involved in processing object properties, and an impaired dorsal stream (occipitoparietal lobes) involved in spatial processes such as object localization and movement detection (Ungerleider & Mishkin, 1982). Anatomical findings reported by Galaburda and Bellugi (2000), based on autopsied brains from four children and adults with WS, appear to be consistent with this hypothesis: Across all brains they found a curtailment in the posterior parietal and occipital regions, and a short central sulcus, bringing attention to a possible developmental anomaly affecting the dorsal part of the hemispheres.

Targeting the dissociation between dorsal and ventral cortical stream function, Atkinson and colleagues (1997, 2003) tested children with WS on global motion coherence thresholds, compared to an analogous form-coherence test, and on a visual manual task of posting a card through a slot, compared with a task of perceptually matching the slot orientation. In addition, a set of inhibition tasks tapping frontal lobe functions was administered to the children. Patterns of performance differed among the children with WS, with a small group showing essentially normal performance on most tasks, and other subgroups showing a range of difficulties, especially with tasks involving frontoparietal circuits (e.g., frontal control processes associated with spatially directed responses). These findings were interpreted as consistent with "a persisting immaturity of global visual processing, which shows a similar balance of dorsal and ventral function to that seen in other impaired or immature systems" (Atkinson et al., 2003, p. 166). It appears from the lack of consistency in the results on these tasks that generalized dorsal-stream impairment cannot account for the extreme weakness in visual–spatial constructive cognition in WS, and that further specification of the neural basis of this deficit is needed. Moreover, Reiss, Hoffman, and Landau (2003) showed that individuals with WS performed at normal levels on both biological and motion coherence tasks—two tasks mediated by a key dorsal area (V5)—suggesting that any dorsal-stream damage must be selective.

Given the evidence of impoverished spatial representations as one potential source of difficulty with block construction tasks (Hoffman et al., 2003), several authors have suggested that deficits in visual–spatial memory are involved in selective deficits in the ability to acquire, maintain, and manipulate spatial information in WS (Jarrold, Baddeley, & Hewes, 1999; Vicari, Bellucci, & Carlesimo, 2003). Dilks, Landau, Hoffman, and Oberg (2003) administered a similar set of "posting" (action/dorsal stream) versus "matching slot orientation" (perception/ventral stream) tasks as those used by Atkinson and her colleagues, with and without a delay between viewing the slot and providing a response. Participants with WS performed the same as controls in the matching condition when there was no delay but significantly worse than controls in both conditions when there was a delay, providing support for the view that visual short-term memory plays a significant role in the visual–spatial deficits in WS.

In summary, findings from research on the visual–spatial skills of individuals with WS provide a complex picture of variability in performance as a function of specific task demands (e.g., perceptual or constructional) and suggest several different interpretations for the source and nature of the severe difficulties shown by people with WS in selective aspects of visual–spatial cognition. Further investigations of the developmental path of visual–spatial skills and of the neural mechanisms involved in spatial cognition are needed to better understand the unusual pattern of sparing and impairment within the visual–spatial domain in WS.

Developmental Research

Fewer studies have explored developmental aspects of visual–spatial cognition in WS, and conflicting claims of atypical developmental trajectories versus typical but delayed or arrested developments in this domain remain largely unresolved. Early studies contrasting performance by children with WS and children with DS were taken as evidence for deviant rather than delayed development (Bellugi, Sabo, & Vaid, 1988; Bellugi et al., 1994). However, subsequent research using different contrast groups and including analyses of performance profiles in typically developing children has demonstrated that developmental models are more appropriate for characterizing the deficits evidenced by children with WS on a range of visual construction tasks. For example, on pattern construction tasks, young, typically developing children tend to produce solutions where the configurations are broken, as seen in people with WS (Akshoomof & Stiles, 1996), and children with WS show significant improvements in performance as they get older, with the majority of adults producing no broken configurations (Mervis et al., 1999). Similar clear improvements with age were found in longitudinal analyses of drawing abilities in people with WS (Bertrand & Mervis, 1996).

A recent investigation of copying abilities (Georgeopoulos, Georgeopoulos, Kurz, & Landau, 2004) compared children with WS to mental-age-matched, typically developing children. Similar to reports of the development of drawing ability in WS (Bertrand, Mervis, & Eisenberg, 1997), the figure copies of the children with WS resembled those of typically developing children at a much earlier developmental point, suggesting that the deficit in WS reflected arrested development rather than a deviant copying style.

Nevertheless, claims of aberrant or atypical development of abilities in WS persist in the literature, despite a paucity of longitudinal studies or studies involving infants and very young children with WS. One study involving toddlers with WS (23–37 months) examined saccade planning based on a "double-step saccade paradigm" used to probe the spatial representations underlying simple visually guided actions (Brown et al., 2003). The control groups of mental-age-matched toddlers with DS and typically developing children executed saccades within body-centered spatial coordinates. The toddlers with WS were not able to combine extraretinal information with retinal information to the same extent as the other groups in orienting to a target, and displayed deficits in saccade planning indicative of greater reliance on subcortical processing mechanisms than controls. Although these differences in the spatial representations underlying visually guided actions early in life may have the potential to impact the developmental trajectories of visual–spatial abilities, more research, especially using longitudinal designs, is needed to demonstrate whether such abilities develop in aberrant or normative ways in WS.

So far, the majority of experimental evidence suggests that, in WS, spatial abilities develop normally but at a slower rate than verbal abilities (Atkinson et al., 2001; Jarrold, Baddeley, & Hewes, 1998), and in some areas, they do not develop beyond the level achieved by a typical 6-year-old. Thus, it may be the case that WS leads to selective sparing and breakdown of spatial systems along the lines of normal cognitive architecture (Landau et al., 2006), suggesting that neurocognitive development of visual–spatial cognition is a highly constrained process.

Brain Imaging Research

As revealed in our review of behavioral research, the nature of the visual–spatial deficit associated with WS remains elusive in light of persisting contradictory findings or interpretations of experimental results. Recently, a group of researchers (Meyer-Lindenberg et al., 2004) investigated the neural concomitants and underpinnings of the visual–spatial construction deficit in WS, using multiple converging methods: (1) multimodal neuroimaging to identify functional activation patterns, (2) regional volumetric measures to identify underlying morphological abnormalities, as well as (3) an analysis of the pathways connecting the hierarchical levels in the dorsal stream of the visual system. Simple but elegantly designed functional magnetic resonance imaging (fMRI) tasks were used to delineate the ventral and dorsal visual streams. One task required comparison (match condition) or assembly into a square (construction condition) of pairs of shapes with a boundary of elementary line segments (see Plate 4.1A and 4.1C), whereas another task involved directed attention to either the location (i.e., whether the pictures on the left and right were at the same vertical position relative to a fixation cross) or the content (i.e., house, face) of pairs of images shown sequentially (see Plate 4.1E). A group of adults with WS but within normal-range intelligence scores was matched with typical controls on age, sex, handedness, and IQ, thus assuring that any group differences found would be directly attributable to WS and not to general cognitive functioning.

On the first fMRI task, in the construction minus match comparison, participants with WS showed significant hypoactivation in dorsal stream areas, whereas normal controls activated the dorsal stream bilaterally (Plate 4.1D); however, both groups activated the ventral stream equally well. On the second fMRI task, there were no group differences for either faces or houses in the content (ventral) condition; however, in the location condition, the WS group showed significant hypoactivation in the parietal portion of the dorsal stream (Plate 4.1F). Voxel-based morphometric analyses revealed reduced gray matter volume in the immediately adjacent parietal–occipital–intraparietal sulcus in WS, and path analysis showed that the functional abnormalities in the dorsal stream could be attributed to impaired input from this structurally altered region. This study demonstrates effects of a highly localized abnormality on visual information processing in the dorsal visual stream and provides a systems-level phenotype for potentially mapping the genetic determinants of visual–spatial construction.

The same research team recently used multimodal neuroimaging to characterize hippocampal structure, function, and metabolic integrity in the same WS adults and controls (Meyer-Lindenberg, Mervis, et al., 2005). The hippocampal formation (HF) is of great interest because of its role in both declarative memory and processing of spatial navigational information. Recent studies of murine models, in which key genes in the WS region linked to the visual–spatial deficits in WS were eliminated (LIMK1 and CYLN2), showed significant functional and metabolic abnormalities but grossly normal structure in the HF of the knockout mice. Consistent with the findings from the murine models in the above-referenced study, Meyer-Lindenberg, Mervis, and colleagues (2005) found that positron emission tomography (PET) and fMRI studies on adults with WS revealed significant metabolic and functional abnormalities of the anterior portion of the HF (profound reduction in resting blood flow and absent differential response to visual stimuli in the anterior HF) compared to controls. The converging evidence from this study for depressed hippocampal energy metabolism and synaptic activity in WS provides a neurobiological correlate for the difficulties in long-term memory and spatial navigation prominent in WS and points to the involvement of specific genes deleted in WS that are important in human hippocampal function.

Summary of Research on Visual–Spatial Cognition in WS

This review of research that has been conducted on visual–spatial cognition in WS reveals that visual–spatial abilities in WS are not impaired across the board, as once thought. Moreover, the more fine-grained within-domain deficits that have been found are associated with specialized structures that are potentially identifiable at the neural systems level. Studies currently underway, involving individuals with atypical genetic deletions or duplications, as well as murine models, target the potential genetic determination of the abnormalities found in the neural basis of certain behavioral pheno-types, including the visual–spatial construction deficit in WS.

SOCIAL COGNITION IN WS

One of the most striking and endearing aspects of children and adults with WS is their social profile. Children with WS have a strong interest in other people, including strangers. They show empathic concern and are highly sociable, as documented in parental anecdotes, clinical reports, and system-atic investigations (Jones et al., 2000; Mervis & Klein-Tasman, 2000). Indeed, these characteristics in conjunction with relatively spared language abilities, highly expressive verbal communication (Reilly, Klima, & Bellugi, 1990), and an outgoing, affectionate personality (Gosch & Pankau, 1994), led some to propose that, in contrast to autism, WS represented a syndrome in which social-cognitive capacities were intact (Karmiloff-Smith, Klima, Bellugi, Grant, & Baron-Cohen, 1995; Tager-Flusberg, Boshart, & Baron-Cohen, 1998). However, despite their sociable disposition, children with WS have problems making friends and the majority of adults with WS experience difficulties in social interactions, with many developing high lev-els of anxiety and social isolation (Davies, Udwin, & Howlin, 1998; Dykens & Rosner, 1999; Udwin & Yule, 1991). Thus, as we saw in the visual–spatial domain, the social profile of WS presents a more complex picture of positive and negative features. Research on social cognition in WS has focused on delineating the unusual social phenotype to determine the neurocognitive mechanisms that underlie the social strengths and impairments that characterize this population.

Experimental Research

Initial studies on social-cognitive abilities in WS focused on theory-of-mind skills: the ability to predict and explain other people's actions based on inferences about their mental states, such as intentions, knowledge, or beliefs. One early study by Karmiloff-Smith and her colleagues (Karmiloff-Smith et al., 1995) reported that the majority of the participants with WS in their study passed standard first-order and higher-order belief tasks, leading them to conclude that theory of mind may be an "islet of preserved ability" in WS (Karmiloff-Smith et al., 1995, p. 202). Later studies, how-ever, demonstrated that theory-of-mind skills are not spared in WS. Tager-Flusberg and Sullivan (2000) investigated performance on false belief and other theory-of-mind tasks in younger children with WS who were matched on age, IQ, and standardized language measures to two comparison groups, children with Prader–Willi syndrome, and children with nonspecific mental retardation. Prader–Willi syndrome is a rare genetic disorder caused by the hemizygous loss of paternally donated genes in the q11–13 region of chromosome 15. The IQ distribution among individuals with Prader–Willi syndrome is very similar to that found in WS, but the typical cognitive profile of people with Prader–Willi syndrome does not include the unusual "peaks and valleys" in verbal and nonverbal abilities characteristic of people with WS. Thus, individuals with Prader–Willi syndrome provide a good match for the participants with WS on general cognitive measures but, at the same time, allow researchers to capture the distinctive social phenotype of people with WS.

On three different first-order theory-of-mind tasks the children with WS performed no better than the matched comparison groups (Plesa Skwerer & Tager-Flusberg, 2006; Tager-Flusberg & Sullivan, 2000). In another series of studies, higher-order theory-of-mind tasks were administered to adolescents with WS and matched groups of adolescents with Prader–Willi syndrome and mental retardation. Again, no differences were found among these groups in second-order belief reasoning (Sullivan & Tager-Flusberg, 1999), distinguishing between lies and jokes (Sullivan, Winner, & Tager-Flusberg, 2003), or in using trait information to attribute intentionality (Plesa Skwerer & Tager-Flusberg, 2006). Across these higher-order tasks, most of the participants with WS, as well as those in the comparison groups, had difficulty passing test questions, especially in justifying their answers by correctly referring to mental states. Thus, studies on theory of mind in WS provide no evidence of relative sparing in this domain for either children or adolescents with WS. On the contrary, children and adolescents with WS exhibit problems in social-cognitive abilities that involve making inferences from narratives to interpret mental state information.

More direct information about other people may be inferred from perceiving cues in social stimuli, including faces, voices, and body movements. Research on these social-perceptual skills in WS has produced a mixed picture of preserved and impaired abilities. As noted earlier, children and adults with WS generally perform within the normal range and better than mental-age-matched controls on standardized tests of face recognition (Bellugi, Marks, et al., 1988; Bellugi et al., 1994; Karmiloff-Smith, 1997; Tager-Flusberg et al., 2003; Udwin & Yule, 1991). Some researchers have argued that despite their good performance on standardized measures, people with WS recognize faces using atypical piecemeal strategies, instead of processing faces holistically (Deruelle, Mancini, Livet, Cassé-Perrot, & de Schonen, 1999; Elgar & Campbell, 2001; Gagliardi et al., 2003; Karmiloff-

Smith, 1997; Karmiloff-Smith, Scerif, & Thomas, 2002). Tager-Flusberg and her colleagues (Tager-Flusberg et al., 2003) tested this hypothesis using the whole–part method introduced by Tanaka and Farah (1993), which compares recognition of face features presented in the context of whole faces or in isolation for both upright and inverted faces. Adolescents and adults with WS showed the same patterns of performance across the different conditions, performing significantly better in the whole-face condition for upright faces, but not for inverted faces, as did age-matched controls, although their overall performance was lower. The whole-face advantage only in the upright condition provides strong evidence that people with WS encode and recognize faces holistically, in the same way as unimpaired controls, and confirms the relative preservation of face-processing skills in this population. Similar findings have been obtained in other experiments using different paradigms to test holistic face processing in WS (Schofield, Verbalis, Plesa Skwerer, Faja, & Tager-Flusberg, 2004).

Several experimental studies have examined emotion recognition in people with WS. Tager-Flusberg and colleagues (1998) reported that adults with WS were significantly better than a matched group of adults with Prader–Willi syndrome on Baron-Cohen's eyes task (Baron-Cohen, Jolliffe, Mortimore, & Robertson, 1997), which tests the ability to recognize subtle and fairly complex mental states from photographs taken only of the eye region of faces. However, using a more rigorous, revised version of the task (Baron-Cohen, Wheelwright, Hill, Raste, & Plumb, 2001), performance by a different, substantially larger group of adults with WS was significantly worse than that of the age-matched typical controls and no different from the age- and IQ-matched participants with mental retardation or learning disabilities (Plesa Skwerer, Verbalis, Schofield, Faja, & Tager-Flusberg, 2006).

Other studies have also found that children and adults with WS are no better than well-matched controls at discriminating, matching, or labeling facial expressions of basic emotions. Tager-Flusberg and Sullivan (2000) administered an emotion-matching task, developed by Hobson, Ouston, and Lee (1988), to children with WS, children with Prader–Willi syndrome, and children with nonspecific mental retardation, matched on age, IQ, and language. The children with WS were as proficient, but no better than, the control groups in discriminating and matching facial expressions of emotion. Similar results were reported by Gagliardi and colleagues (2003), who used an animated facial expression comprehension test.

Plesa Skwerer, Faja, Schofield, Verbalis, and Tager-Flusberg (2006) compared adolescents and adults with WS to matched groups of individuals with typical development and individuals with mental retardation/learning disabilities (LD) on a standardized measure of emotion recognition: the

Diagnostic Analysis of Nonverbal Accuracy test (Nowicki & Duke, 1994). This computerized task requires the participant to select the appropriate emotion label (*happy, sad, angry, fearful*) for each face or voice presented. The participants with WS were less accurate than age-matched normal control participants, but were similar to the age- and IQ-matched LD comparison group on both the faces and voices subtests. All three groups showed the same pattern of performance, across both modalities and all emotions, suggesting that the same mechanisms underlie the ability to perceive emotions across populations. At the same time, the WS group in this study showed spared face recognition skills but impaired facial expression recognition skills, supporting other research in the cognitive neuroscience literature on the separable mechanisms that subserve the identification of faces and emotions (e.g., Haxby, Hoffman, & Gobbini, 2002). According to the model developed by Haxby and his colleagues, face perception is mediated by a distributed neural system that involves a distinction between the representation of invariant aspects of faces, which is crucial for face identification, and the representation of changeable aspects, such as facial expression, which underlies the perception of information that facilitates social communication.

A different social-perceptual task that has been used with adults with WS taps the ability to judge the approachability and trustworthiness of strangers from facial cues. Bellugi, Adolphs, Cassady, and Chiles (1999) administered such a task, developed by Adolphs (Adolphs, Tranel, & Damasio, 1998), to adults with WS, who were compared to and age- and gender-matched normal controls. The adults with WS gave abnormally positive ratings overall, judging the stimulus people as more approachable and more trustworthy than did matched controls. These findings have been interpreted as evidence for specific deficits in WS in processing the social and psychological significance of facial displays of social cues; these deficits have been attributed to amygdala dysfunction (Adolphs, Sears, & Piven, 2001). More recently, Frigerio and colleagues (2006) administered a similar task, using a series of faces taken from the Ekman and Friesen (1976) set, including faces with positive and negative emotional expressions. On this task, the group with WS only rated the *happy* faces as more approachable than the matched controls. Faces expressing negative emotions (*anger, disgust, fear, sadness*) were rated as less approachable by the WS group compared to the controls. Frigerio and colleagues argue that people with WS can discriminate people's faces on the basis of approachability, but they cannot inhibit their compulsion to interact with strangers, whether or not they appear approachable. One problem with this study, however, is that the WS ratings may have been based on different facial cues than the ratings obtained by Adolphs and colleagues (1998). Specifically, the WS participants may simply have rated their reactions to the emotional expressions rather than making more complex social judgments of approachability and trustworthiness, which depend on subtle cues that are independent of emotional expression.

Taken together, the studies reviewed here suggest that people with WS are better than IQ-matched controls (i.e., other individuals with mental retardation) at recognizing faces, are equally impaired in their ability to recognize emotional expressions or understand and interpret other mental states, but may show atypical social judgments that relate to their unique interest in, and attention to, people. These experimental studies complement findings from studies that have used parent-report measures, which document the focused attention of children with WS toward people, their intense social engagement and empathy coupled with difficulties with friendship and inappropriate behavior, and their indiscriminate friendliness to strangers (e.g., Davies et al., 1998; Dykens & Rosner, 1999; Klein-Tasman & Mervis, 2003).

Developmental Research

Studies of infants and young children with WS have explored the origins of the unusual attention to people, sociability, and empathic responsiveness that define the personality profile of WS (Klein-Tasman & Mervis, 2003; Tager-Flusberg & Plesa Skwerer, in press). Mervis and colleagues (2003) reported on two observational studies examining the attention behavior of infants and toddlers with WS. The first study compared the looking behavior of one toddler with WS to typically developing infants in free-play interaction with the mother and with unfamiliar partners. The toddler with WS differed from the controls in the greater amount of time spent looking at the play partner's face and in the unusual intensity of her gaze toward faces. The second study compared a group of infants and toddlers with WS observed during a medical evaluation to a large sample of age-matched children assessed in a similar setting. The children with WS in all age groups looked primarily at the physician throughout the session, and the majority of them, especially those younger than 30 months, evidenced *intense* looking behavior, whereas none of the control participants ever looked intensely at the physician. Mervis and colleagues explain these findings in terms of highly increased arousal during social interaction in the infants and toddlers with WS.

Experimental studies have also found atypical patterns of social attention in toddlers with WS. Laing and her colleagues (Laing et al., 2002) administered the Early Social Communication Scales (ESCS; Mundy & Hogan, 1996) to a group of toddlers with WS and to a group of normal toddlers matched on developmental age. The toddlers with WS showed fewer object-related behaviors (pointing, reaching, requesting toys) and more social-interactive behaviors (requests for tickling, turn-taking behaviors, eye contact not related to objects) than the control group. Overall, the WS group scored higher on dyadic social-interactive behaviors, whereas the control group scored higher on all joint-attention-related behaviors, especially initiating requesting and producing more triadic eye contact. The findings from this study confirmed earlier research by Mervis and Bertrand (1997) showing that, in contrast to normally developing children, in children with WS there is no predictive relationship between social–communication behaviors such as joint attention and measures of language acquisition.

Studies of temperament in toddlers and young children with WS using parent-report measures found that many fall into the category of "difficult" children, although unlike other difficult children, they show more approach, rather than withdrawal, behavior (e.g., Tomc, Williamson, & Pauli, 1990). Jones, Anderson, Reilly, and Bellugi (1998) conducted an experimental study of temperament in children with WS and comparison groups of typically developing controls using a subset of the Laboratory Temperament Assessment Battery to code emotional responses during a parental separation task. The children with WS showed less negative facial and vocal affect than controls and a lower intensity of distress, whereas children in control groups showed clear signs of frustration or distress in the parent's absence. The children with WS also recovered more quickly and needed less consoling than the controls. It is difficult to conclude from this study whether young children with WS experience negative emotions during parental separation but manage to regulate their expression in anticipation of resuming social interaction upon the parent's return, or whether they show an abnormal pattern of attachment, possibly related to their indiscriminate approach behavior toward strangers.

The capacity of children with WS to empathize with a person in distress has been tested experimentally in two investigations using a simulated distress paradigm. Tager-Flusberg and Sullivan (1999) coded the responses of children with WS and a matched comparison group of children with Prader–Willi syndrome as they observed an experimenter feigning distress after banging her knee. Although both groups spent most of the time during the distress scene looking at the experimenter, the children with WS showed significantly greater empathy, as evidenced by their comforting behavior, expressions of sympathy, and overall concern. Similar findings were reported by Rowe, Beccera, and Mervis (2002), who used the same procedure with preschoolers with WS in comparison to matched groups of normal children and children with developmental delays. The young children with WS showed higher levels of empathic behavior relative to both comparison groups, suggesting that this distinctive personality characteristic is evident by age 4 and is manifest to a greater degree than in typically developing children of similar age. Taken together, these studies of infants and toddlers with WS demonstrate that their unusual attention and responsiveness toward other people is evident from the earliest stages of development.

Brain Imaging Research

The neural bases for both the intact and atypical components of the social phenotype of WS have been studied using several different methodologies. As noted earlier, in the behavioral literature there is controversy over whether preserved face recognition skills are related to normal or aberrant cognitive mechanisms. Mills and colleagues (2000) used electrophysiological recordings of event-related potentials (ERPs) to investigate the timing of the neural response to face identity in adults with WS and age-matched controls. Participants judged whether two faces, presented in either upright or inverted orientations, were the same or different. The adults with WS showed an unusually small N100 component but large N200 peaks to all the face stimuli. Mills and her colleagues suggested that the larger N200 peak reflected the increased attention that people with WS pay to faces. On the later N320 component, which is linked to face recognition processes, the ERP patterns found among the adults with WS were similar to those found among younger typically developing adolescents, but were somewhat larger and delayed relative to the age-matched adults. The authors concluded that "in WS, the brain systems that mediate face recognition might be normally organized but developmentally delayed" (Mills et al., 2000, p. 59).

Research using fMRI has demonstrated that there are specialized brain mechanisms that support face processing, primarily the so-called fusiform face area (FFA) located on the underside of the temporal lobes along the fusiform gyrus (Damasio, Tranel, & Damasio, 1990; Haxby et al., 1994; Kanwisher, Tong, & Nakayama, 1998). In a preliminary study, Schultz and his colleagues (Schultz, Grelotti, & Pober, 2001) investigated FFA activation to faces in adults with WS. They found that these adults had normal activation patterns in both location and intensity of activation in the right and left hemisphere FFA, and that activity in the FFA was selective to faces in adults with WS.

A more recent study by Mobbs and colleagues (2004) compared adults with WS to age- and gender-matched controls in a paradigm that required participants to monitor eye-gaze direction in faces presented at different orientations. Mobbs and colleagues reported numerous significant differences in brain activation patterns between the WS and control groups; however, these differences are not easy to interpret, given the complex nature of the task and stimuli used in their study. Nevertheless, the study highlighted three main regions of interest selected on the basis of their known connection to face and gaze processing: fusiform gyrus, superior temporal sulcus, and the amygdala. There were no significant differences between the groups in activation patterns in any of these regions. Thus, these findings replicate those reported by Schultz and colleagues (2001) and confirm that in WS, the same areas of the brain are used to process faces as in controls. These functional imaging studies support the conclusions drawn earlier from the cognitive studies: In WS, the same cognitive and neurobiological mechanisms are involved in processing and recognizing faces as in normally developing individuals.

Studies using high-resolution structural magnetic resonance imaging (MRI) have focused on the size of specific neural areas, relative to overall brain size, in adults and children with WS as compared to controls. Two regions that have been studied in relation to the unusual social phenotype of WS are the cerebellar vermis and the superior temporal gyrus (STG). Following up on earlier small-scale reports in the literature (Jernigan & Bellugi, 1990, 1994), Schmitt, Eliez, Warsofksy, Bellugi, and Reiss (2001) compared the neuroanatomical structure of the cerebellar vermis and related neocerebellar structures in adults with WS and age- and gender-matched controls. They found that the neocerebellum in the WS group was relatively enlarged. They speculated that the neocerebellum sparing may relate to the relative sparing of language (cf. Schmahmann, 1991) and especially social–emotional behavior in WS, because in autism, a neuro-developmental disorder characterized by significant impairments in social–emotional behavior, the neocerebellum is reduced in size. Jones and colleagues (2002) found similar evidence of an enlarged cerebellum in MRI scans from infants and toddlers with WS. These findings suggest that the atypical cerebellar enlargement is present from a very early age; however, there is no clear evidence for a relationship between cerebellar size and social functioning.

Another area that has been identified as relatively preserved in size in WS is the STG, which has been associated with perception of biological motion and with auditory, language, and music processing (Reiss et al., 2000). Reiss and his colleagues compared adults with WS to age- and gender-matched controls. They found that when they controlled for overall cerebral gray matter, the volumes for STG were proportionally larger in the group with WS (see also Hickok et al., 1995). Reiss and his colleagues suggest that the preservation of STG may relate to the strong language abilities and emotional responsiveness to music that characterize people with WS, and are closely linked to the social–affective responsiveness toward other people that defines the social phenotype of WS.

Current interest in the neurobiological substrate for the atypical social responsiveness of people with WS is focused on the role of the amygdala. Bellugi and her colleagues (Bellugi et al., 1999) highlight the similarity of the atypical performance of the adults with WS on the approachability/ trustworthiness task to patients with bilateral amygdala damage (Adolphs et al., 1998, 2001). These individuals share the same behavior patterns as people with WS—approaching strangers and acting in an overly friendly manner—and they also have intact face recognition skills but impaired recognition of negative facial emotional expressions. However, structural MRI studies have yielded inconsistent findings on the relative size of the amygdala in WS. Earlier studies, which compared WS to DS, found that the size of the amygdala was preserved, relative to total brain size (e.g., Jernigan & Bellugi, 1994). This finding was replicated in a recent study conducted in Australia (Martens, Wilson, & Reuters, n.d.), which found no differences between children and adults with WS and matched controls in the absolute volumes of either the left or right amygdala. Furthermore, this unpublished study reported a significant correlation between the volume of the right amygdala and the participants' approachability ratings on a modified version of the Adolph's task.

In contrast to these structural MRI studies, Galaburda and Bellugi (2000) investigated amygdala size in a WS autopsy specimen and found that the overall volume of the amygdala was significantly smaller compared to matched controls. The dorsal portion of the lateral nucleus was especially small and abnormal in shape compared to the control amygdalae. Galaburda and Bellugi speculate that since this nucleus of the amygdala receives connections from the visual cortex, perhaps in WS a reduction in connectivity between these brain regions means that sensory experiences fail to acquire the appropriate emotional valence, including the danger associated with unfamiliar people. This neuroanatomical difference could account for the unusual approach and overfriendliness toward strangers demonstrated by people with WS. It is not clear how to interpret the contradictory findings on amygdala volumes in WS; however, comprehensive MRI studies of typically developing children have highlighted significant sex differences and age-related changes in amygdala size, which need to be taken into consideration in designing future MRI studies of WS (Giedd, 2004; Schumann et al., 2004).

More direct evidence for the role of the amygdala in the atypical social responsiveness of people with WS comes from a recent functional imaging study. Meyer-Lindenberg, Hariri, and colleagues (2005) used fMRI to investigate amygdala function in response to threatening social and nonsocial stimuli. They compared activation patterns in nonretarded adults with WS to controls who were asked to match photographs of angry and fearful faces or threatening scenes. The adults with WS showed significantly lower amygdala activation to the faces but significantly higher amygdala activation to the scenes. The authors also found differences in activation between the groups in the prefrontal regions, which are densely connected to the amygdala. In contrast to the controls, the WS group did not show activation of the orbitofrontal cortex to the face stimuli; instead, these participants showed equivalent activation to the social and nonsocial stimuli in both medial and dorsolateral prefrontal regions, suggesting that the neurobiological substrate for the atypical social phenotype in WS may lie in the abnormal regulation or modulation of amygdala function from the orbitofrontal cortex (Meyer-Lindenberg, Hariri, et al., 2005).

Summary of Research on Social Cognition in WS

Beginning in infancy, individuals with WS are unusually interested in other people, attending and responding to people in an exuberant and indiscriminate way. Children and adults with WS appear very sociable and engaging and although they are good at recognizing people, they are not spared in their ability to read social–affective cues or in theory-of-mind skills. Studies using neuroimaging methods, especially the exciting findings reported by Meyer-Lindenberg, Hariri, and colleagues (2005), highlight a possible neural basis for the social-cognitive phenotype of WS that eventually will lead to the discovery of specific genes associated with this component of human cognition.

CLINICAL AND EDUCATIONAL IMPLICATIONS

Children and adults with WS are not like other people with mental retardation. In everyday interactions, they seem quite able, linguistically fluent, and socially engaging. This appearance masks both general intellectual disability as well as more significant deficits in many areas of cognition. In this chapter, we have focused on visual–spatial and social cognition, identifying the neurocognitive abnormalities that underlie the deficits that require behavioral interventions beginning early in childhood, when these deficits are already apparent. The possibility of developing efficient intervention and educational strategies to improve certain skills in people with WS depends on the quality of the research that aims to explain the nature of the deficits and sparing in specific cognitive domains in WS. Thus, distinguishing the different aspects of visual–spatial cognition that are severely impaired from those that are relatively spared could lead to finding strategies for helping people with WS compensate for their impairments by building on their relatively spared abilities. In the domain of social cognition, the strong interest in other people exhibited in people with WS at all ages could be used to motivate remediation of their limitations in social perception and social cognition.

Weaknesses in visual–spatial abilities in WS are related to daily difficulties that may be manifested at the level of large-scale motor movements, such as walking on uneven surfaces or down stairs; in terms of spatial navigation; and in terms of fine-motor skills, such as learning handwriting, holding and using a pencil, or tying shoelaces. Semel and Rosner (2003) describe several forms of intervention that may be suited for improving perceptual and motor skills in children with WS. The same principles can also be used in the design of interventions for the social deficits in WS.

One approach is to design task-specific interventions that involve targeted training and guided learning experiences in a particular area of weakness. This type of intervention might build on the plasticity of brain connections, potentially leading to a gradual improvement in those brain circuits deficient in WS (cf. Meyer-Lindenberg et al., 2004; Meyer-Lindenberg, Hariri, et al., 2005). Another approach involves the guided use of compensatory strategies, especially verbal mediation, thus building on the relative strength in verbal abilities and the spontaneous tendency of children with WS to "talk themselves through activities" (Mervis et al., 1999). Teaching individuals with WS to use verbal self-direction and words to remember places or the succession of steps in completing activities that involve spatial and temporal aspects can help them find alternative ways to overcome difficulties in areas of weakness, such as motor tasks and spatial memory. Similarly, verbal labels for emotional expressions or other types of subtle social cues could be taught and then used to compensate for the deficits in social cognition in children and adults with WS, an approach that is often taken in the treatment of children with autism spectrum disorders. Future research should systematically investigate and compare the efficacy of these and other types of interventions in the treatment of visual–spatial and social-cognitive impairments in WS, using both behavioral and neuroimaging outcome measures. Moreover, the development of novel interventions that could be implemented during infancy for these domains of impairment could be especially important, given what is known about the greater efficacy of very early intensive intervention and the opportunities for identification of WS at birth using genetic testing.

CONCLUSIONS

Although the study of people with WS may not ultimately resolve contro-versial theoretical debates about the architecture of the mind, it will con-tinue to focus interest on the kind of complex questions, amenable to empirical research, that can provide insights into the organization of the mind and brain in connection to our genetic endowment: Do impairments in a cognitive domain reflect genetically targeted specialization, and if so, at what level of organization are these effects found? The specific questions to be asked then become whether the genetic deletion impacts the cortex dif-fusely or focally (Reiss et al., 2004) and whether performance reflects qual-itatively different architecture that has evolved from an altered genetic potential (Karmiloff-Smith, 1998) or reflects normal cognitive structure "which evolves from an architecture that is so highly constrained that it survives despite altered genetic potential" (Landau et al., 2006, p. 3). How can we determine the links between behavior, neural processes, and, ulti-mately, specific genes when genetic-to-behavior causation is extremely complex and indirect (Karmiloff-Smith et al., 2006)? These are just a few of the fascinating questions that may find at least partial answers from contin-uing to explore what such "experiments of nature" as WS have to offer.

ACKNOWLEDGMENTS

Preparation of this chapter was supported by Grant No. R01 HD 33470 from the National Institute of Child Health and Human Development.

REFERENCES

Adolphs, R., Sears, L., & Piven, J. (2001). Abnormal processing of social informa-tion from faces in autism. *Journal of Cognitive Neuroscience, 13,* 232–240.

Adolphs, R., Tranel, D., & Damasio, A. R. (1998). The human amygdala in social judgment. *Nature, 393,* 470–475.

Akshoomoff, N., & Stiles, J. (1996). The influence of pattern type on children's block design performance. *Journal of the International Neuropsychological Society, 2,* 392–402.

Atkinson, J., Anker S., Braddick, O., Nokes, L., Mason, A., & Braddick, F. (2001). Visual and visuospatial development in young children with Williams syn-drome. *Developmental Medicine and Child Neurology, 43*(5), 330–337.

Atkinson, J., Braddick, O., Anker, S., Curran, W., Andrew, R., Wattam-Bell, J., et al. (2003). Neurobiological models of visuospatial cognition in children with Williams syndrome: Measures of dorsal stream and frontal function. *Develop-mental Neuropsychology, 23,* 139–172.

Atkinson, J., King, J., Braddick, O., Nokes, L., Anker, S., & Braddick, F. (1997). A specific deficit of dorsal stream function in Williams syndrome. *NeuroReport, 8*, 1919–1922.

Baron-Cohen, S., Jolliffe, T., Mortimore, C., & Robertson, M. (1997). Another advanced test of theory of mind: Evidence from very high-functioning adults with autism or Asperger syndrome. *Journal of Child Psychology and Psychiatry, 38*, 813–822.

Baron-Cohen, S., Wheelwright, S., Hill, J., Raste, Y., & Plumb, I. (2001). The "Reading the Mind in the Eyes" Test revised version: A study with normal adults, and adults with Asperger syndrome or high-functioning autism. *Journal of Child Psychology and Psychiatry, 42*, 241–251.

Beery, K. E., & Buktenica, N. A. (1967). *Developmental test of visual–motor integration.* Cleveland, OH: Modern Curriculum Press.

Bellugi, U., Adolphs, R., Cassady, C., & Chiles M. (1999). Towards the neural basis for hypersociability in a genetic syndrome. *NeuroReport, 10*(8), 1653–1657.

Bellugi, U., Bihrle, A., Neville, H., Jernigan, T., & Doherty, S. (1992). Language, cognition, and brain organization in a neurodevelopmental disorder. In M. Gunnar & C. Nelson (Eds.), *Developmental behavioral neuroscience: The Minnesota symposium* (pp. 201–232). Hillsdale, NJ: Erlbaum.

Bellugi, U., Marks, S., Bihrle, A., & Sabo, H. (1988). Dissociation between language and cognitive functions in Williams syndrome. In D. Bishop & K. Mogford (Eds.), *Language development in exceptional circumstances* (pp. 177–189). London: Churchill Livingstone.

Bellugi, U., Sabo, H., & Vaid, J. (1988). Spatial deficits in children with Williams syndrome. In J. Stiles-Davis, M. Kritchevsky, & U. Bellugi (Eds.), *Spatial cognition: Brain bases and development* (pp. 273–298). Hillsdale, NJ: Erlbaum.

Bellugi, U., & St. George, M. (Eds.). (2000). Linking cognitive neuroscience and molecular genetics: New perspectives from Williams syndrome. *Journal of Cognitive Neuroscience, 12*(1), 1–107.

Bellugi, U., Wang, P., & Jernigan, T. L. (1994). Williams syndrome: An unusual neuropsychological profile. In S. Broman & J. Grafman (Eds.), *Atypical cognitive deficits in developmental disorders: Implications for brain function* (pp. 23–56). Hillsdale, NJ: Erlbaum.

Benton, A. L., Hamsher, K. de S., Varney, N. R., & Spreen, O. (1983). *Contributions to neuropsychological assessment.* New York: Oxford University Press.

Bertrand, J., & Mervis, C. B. (1996). Longitudinal analysis of drawings by children with Williams syndrome: Preliminary results. *Visual Arts Research, 22*, 19–34.

Bertrand, J., Mervis, C. B., & Eisenberg, J. D. (1997). Drawing by children with Williams syndrome: A developmental perspective. *Developmental Neuropsychology, 13*, 41–67.

Beuren, A. J. (1972). Supravalvular aortic stenosis: A complex syndrome with and without mental retardation. *Birth Defects, 8*, 45–46.

Bihrle, A. M., Bellugi, U., Delis, D., & Marks, S. (1989). Seeing either the forest or the trees: Dissociation in visuospatial processing. *Brain and Cognition, 11*, 37–49.

Brown, J., Johnson, M. H., Paterson, S., Gilmore, R. O., Gsödl, M., Longhi, E., et al. (2003). Spatial representation and attention in toddlers with Williams syndrome and Down syndrome. *Neuropsychologia, 41*(8), 1037–1046.

Damasio, A. R., Tranel, D., & Damasio, H. (1990). Face agnosia and the neural substrates of memory. *Annual Review of Neuroscience, 13*, 89–109.

Danoff, S. K., Taylor, H. E., Blackshaw, S., & Desiderio, S. (2004). TFII-I, a candidate gene for Williams syndrome cognitive profile: Parallels between regional expression in mouse brain and human phenotype. *Neuroscience, 123*, 931–938.

Davies, M., Udwin, O., & Howlin, P. (1998). Adults with Williams syndrome. *British Journal of Psychiatry, 172*, 273–274.

Deruelle, C., Mancini, J., Livet, M., Cassé-Perrot, C., & de Schonen, S. (1999). Configural and local processing of faces in children with Williams syndrome. *Brain and Cognition, 41*, 276–298.

Deruelle, C., Rondan, C., Mancini, J., & Livet, M. O. (2006). Do children with Williams syndrome fail to process visual configural information? *Research in Developmental Disabilities, 27*, 243–253.

Dilks, D., Landau, B., Hoffman, J., & Oberg, P. (2003, March). *Vision for action vs. perception in Williams syndrome: Evidence for developmental delay in the dorsal stream.* Poster presented at the annual meeting of the Cognitive Neuroscience Society, New York.

Dykens, E. M., & Rosner, B. (1999). Refining behavioral phenotypes: Personality–motivation in Williams and Prader–Willi syndromes. *American Journal on Mental Retardation, 104*(2), 158–169.

Ekman, P., & Friesen, W. V. (1976). *Pictures of facial affect.* Palo Alto, CA: Consulting Psychological Press.

Elgar, K., & Campbell, R. (2001). Annotation: The cognitive neuroscience of face recognition: Implications for developmental disorders. *Journal of Child Psychology and Psychiatry 42*(6), 705–717.

Elliott, C. D. (1990). *Differential ability scales: Introductory and technical handbook.* New York: Psychological Corporation.

Farran, E. K., & Jarrold, C. (2003). Visuospatial cognition in Williams syndrome: Reviewing and accounting for the strengths and weaknesses in performance. *Developmental Neuropsychology, 23*(1–2), 173–200.

Farran, E. K., Jarrold, C., & Gatherole, S. (2003). Divided attention, selective attention and drawing: Processing preferences in Williams syndrome are dependent on the task administered. *Neuropsychologia, 41*(6), 676–687.

Frangiskakis, J. M., Ewart, A., Morris, C. A., Mervis, C. B., Bertrand, J., Robinson, B. F., et al. (1996). LIM-kinase 1 hemizygosity implicated in impaired visuospatial constructive cognition. *Cell, 86*, 59–69.

Frigerio, E., Gagliardi, C., Burt, D. M., Cazzaniga, I., Perrett, D., & Borgatti, R. (in press). Is everybody always my friend? Perception of approachability in Williams syndrome. *Neuropsychologia, 44*, 254–259.

Gagliardi, C., Frigerio, E., Burt, D. M., Cazzaniga, I., Perrett, D., & Borgatti, R. (2003). Facial expression recognition in Williams syndrome. *Neuropsychologia, 41*, 733–738.

Galaburda, A. M., & Bellugi, U. (2000). Multi-level analysis of cortical neuroanatomy in Williams syndrome. *Journal of Cognitive Neuroscience, 12*(Suppl.), 74–88.

Galaburda, A. M., Schmitt, E., Atlas, S. W., Eliez, S., Bellugi, U., & Reiss, A. L. (2001). Dorsal forebrain anomaly in Williams syndrome. *Archives of Neurology, 58,* 1865–1869.

Georgeopoulos, M. A., Georgeopoulos, A. P., Kurz, N., & Landau, B. (2004). Figure copying in Williams syndrome and normal subjects. *Experimental Brain Research, 157*(2), 137–146.

Giedd, J. N. (2004). Structural magnetic resonance imaging of the adolescent brain. *Annals of the New York Academy of Sciences, 1021,* 77–85.

Gosch A., & Pankau, R. (1994). Social–emotional and behavioral adjustment in children with Williams–Beuren syndrome. *American Journal of Medical Genetics, 52,* 291–296.

Haxby, J. V., Hoffman, E. A., & Gobbini, M. I. (2002). Human neural systems for face recognition and social communication. *Biological Psychiatry, 51*(1), 59–67.

Haxby, J. V., Horwitz, B., Ungerleider, L. G., Maisog, J. M., Pietrini, P., & Grady, C. L. (1994). The functional organization of human extrastriate cortex: A PET–rCBF study of selective attention to faces and locations. *Journal of Neuroscience, 14,* 6336–6353.

Hickok, G., Neville, H., Mills, D., Jones, W., Rossen, M., & Bellugi, U. (1995). Electrophysiological and quantitative MR analysis of the cortical auditory system in Williams syndrome. *Cognitive Neuroscience Society Abstracts, 2,* 66.

Hobson, R. P., Ouston, J., & Lee, A. (1988). What's in a face?: The case of autism. *British Journal of Psychiatry, 79,* 441–453.

Hoffman, J. E., & Landau, B. (2000). *Spared object recognition with profound spatial deficits: Evidence from children with Williams Syndrome.* Poster presented at the annual meeting of the Cognitive Neuroscience Society, San Francisco.

Hoffman, J. E., Landau, B., & Pagani, B. (2003). Spatial breakdown in spatial construction: Evidence from eye fixations in children with Williams syndrome. *Cognitive Psychology, 46*(3), 260–301.

Jarrold, C., Baddeley, A., & Hewes, A. K. (1998). Verbal and nonverbal abilities in the Williams syndrome phenotype: Evidence for diverging developmental trajectories. *Journal of Child Psychology and Psychiatry, 39,* 511–523.

Jarrold, C., Baddeley, A. D., & Hewes, A. K. (1999). Genetically dissociated components of working memory: Evidence from Down's and Williams syndrome. *Neuropsychologia, 37,* 637–651.

Jackendoff, R. (1994). *Patterns in the mind: Language and human nature.* New York: Basic Books.

Jernigan, T. L., & Bellugi, U. (1990). Anomalous brain morphology on magnetic resonance images in Williams syndrome and Down syndrome. *Archives of Neurology, 47,* 529–533.

Jernigan, T. L., & Bellugi, U. (1994). Neuroanatomical distinctions between Williams and Down syndromes. In S. Broman & J. Grafman (Eds.), *Atypical cog-

nitive deficits in developmental disorders: Implications for brain function (pp. 57–66). Hillsdale, NJ: Erlbaum.

Jones, W., Anderson, D., Reilly, J., & Bellugi, U. (1998). Emotional expression in infants and children with Williams syndrome: A relationship between temperament and genetics? *Journal of the International Neuropsychological Society, 4*, 56.

Jones, W., Bellugi, U., Lai, Z., Chiles, M., Reilly, J., Lincoln, A., et al. (2000). Hypersociability in Williams syndrome. *Journal of Cognitive Neuroscience, 12*(Suppl.), 30–46.

Jones, W., Hesselink, J., Courchesne, E., Duncan, T., Matsuda, K., & Bellugi, U. (2002). Cerebellar abnormalities in infants and toddlers with Williams syndrome. *Developmental Medicine and Child Neurology, 44*, 688–694.

Jordan, H., Reiss, J. E., Hoffman, J. E., & Landau, B. (2002). Intact perception of biological motion in the face of profound spatial deficits: Williams syndrome. *Psychological Science, 13*, 162–167.

Kanwisher, N., Tong, F., & Nakayama, K. (1998). The effect of face inversion on the human fusiform face area. *Cognition, 68*, B1–B11.

Karmiloff-Smith, A. (1997). Crucial differences between developmental cognitive neuroscience and adult neuropsychology. *Developmental Neuropsychology, 13*, 513–524.

Karmiloff-Smith, A. (1998). Development itself is the key to understanding developmental disorders. *Trends in Cognitive Sciences, 2*, 389–398.

Karmiloff-Smith, A., Ansari, D., Campbell, L., Scerif, G., & Thomas. M. (2006). Theoretical implications of studying cognitive development in genetic disorders: The case of Williams–Beuren syndrome. In C. Morris, H. Lenhoff, & P. Wang (Eds.), *Williams–Beuren syndrome: Research and clinical perspectives* (pp. 254–273). Baltimore: Johns Hopkins University Press.

Karmiloff-Smith, A., Grant, J., Berthoud, I., Davies, M., Howlin, P., & Udwin, O. (1997). Language and Williams syndrome: How intact is "intact"? *Child Development, 68*, 246–262.

Karmiloff-Smith, A., Klima, E., Bellugi, U., Grant, J., & Baron-Cohen, S. (1995). Is there a social module? Language, face processing and theory of mind in individuals with Williams syndrome. *Journal of Cognitive Neuroscience, 7*, 196–208.

Karmiloff-Smith, A., Scerif, G., & Thomas, M. S. C. (2002). Different approaches to relating genotype to phenotype in developmental disorders. *Developmental Psychobiology, 40*, 311–322.

Klein-Tasman, B. P., & Mervis, C. B. (2003). Distinctive personality characteristics of 8-, 9-, and 10-year-olds with Williams syndrome. *Developmental Neuropsychology, 23*(1–2), 269–290.

Korenberg, J. R., Chen, X.-N., Hirota, H., Lai, Z., Bellugi, U., Burian, D., et al. (2000). Genome structure and cognitive map of Williams syndrome. *Journal of Cognitive Neuroscience, 12*(Suppl.), 89–107.

Laing, E., Butterworth, G., Ansari, D., Gsodl, M., Longhi, E., Panagiotaki, G., et al. (2002). Atypical development of language and social communication in toddlers with Williams syndrome. *Developmental Science, 5*(2), 233–246.

Landau, B., Hoffman, J. E., Reiss, J. E., Dilks, D., Lakusta, L., & Chunyo, G. (2006). Specialization, breakdown, and sparing in spatial cognition: Lessons from Williams syndrome. In C. Morris, H. Lenhoff, & P. Wang (Eds.), *Williams–Beuren syndrome: Research and clinical perspectives* (pp. 207–236). Baltimore: Johns Hopkins University Press.

Levy, Y., & Hermon, S. (2003). Morphological abilities of Hebrew-speaking adolescents with Williams syndrome. *Developmental Neuropsychology, 23*(1–2), 59–83.

Martens, M., Wilson, S., & Reutens, D. (n.d.). *The amygdala and the development of sociability: Insights from Williams syndrome.* Unpublished manuscript, Monash University, Victoria, Australia.

Meng, Y., Zhang, Y., Tregoubov, V., Janus, C., Cruz, L., Jackson, M., et al. (2002). Abnormal spine morphology and enhanced LTP in LIMK-1 knockout mice. *Neuron, 35*(1), 121–133.

Mervis, C. B. (2003). Williams syndrome: 15 years of psychological research. *Developmental Neuropsychology, 23*(1–2), 1–12.

Mervis, C. B., & Bertrand, J. (1997) Developmental relations between cognition and language: Evidence from Williams syndrome. In L. B. Adamson & M. A. Romski (Eds.), *Research on communication and language disorders: Contributions to theories of language development* (pp. 75–106). New York: Brookes.

Mervis, C. B., & Klein-Tasman, B. P. (2000). Williams syndrome: Cognition, personality, and adaptive behavior. *Mental Retardation and Developmental Disabilities Research Reviews, 6*(2), 148–158.

Mervis, C. B., Morris, C. A., Bertrand, J., & Robinson, B. F. (1999). Williams syndrome: findings from an integrated program of research. In H. Tager-Flusberg (Ed.), *Neurodevelopmental disorders* (pp. 65–110). Cambridge, MA: MIT Press.

Mervis, C., Morris, C. A., Klein-Tasman, B. P., Bertrand, J., Kwitny, S., Appelbaum, L. G., et al. (2003). Attentional characteristics of infants and toddlers with Williams syndrome during triadic interactions. *Developmental Neuropsychology, 23*(1–2), 243–268.

Mervis, C. B., Robinson, B. F., Bertrand, J., Morris C. A., Klein-Tasman, B. P., & Armstrong, S. C. (2000). The Williams syndrome cognitive profile. *Brain and Cognition, 44*, 604–628.

Meyer-Lindenberg, A., Hariri, A. R., Munoz, K. E., Mervis, C. B., Mattay, V. S., Morris, C. A., et al. (2005). Neural correlates of genetically abnormal social cognition in Williams syndrome. *Nature Neuroscience, 8*(8), 991–993.

Meyer-Lindenberg, A., Kohn, P., Mervis, C. B., Kippenhan, J. S., Olsen, R. K., Morris, C. A., et al. (2004). Neural basis of genetically determined visuospatial construction deficit in Williams syndrome. *Neuron, 43*, 623–631.

Meyer-Lindenberg, A., Mervis, C. B., Sarpal, D., Koch, P., Steele, S., Kohn, P., et al. (2005). Functional, structural, and metabolic abnormalities of the hippocampal formation in Williams syndrome. *Journal of Clinical Investigation, 115*(7), 1888–1895.

Mills, D. L., Alvarez, T. D., St. George, M., Appelbaum, L. G., Bellugi, U., &

Neville, H. (2000). Electrophysiological studies of face processing in Williams syndrome. *Journal of Cognitive Neuroscience, 12*(Suppl.), 47–64.

Mobbs, D., Garrett, A. S., Menon, V., Rose, F. E., Bellugi, U., & Reiss, A. L. (2004). Anomalous brain activation during face and gaze processing in Williams syndrome. *Neurology, 62*, 2070–2076.

Mooney, C. M. (1957). Age in the development of closure ability in children. *Canadian Journal of Psychology, 11*, 219–310.

Morris, C. A., & Mervis, C. B. (1999). Williams syndrome. In S. Goldstein & C. R. Reynolds (Eds), *Handbook of neurodevelopmental and genetic disorders in children* (pp. 555–590). New York: Guilford Press.

Mundy, P., & Hogan, A. (1996). *A preliminary manual for the abridged Early Social Communication Scales (ESCS).* Coral Gables, FL: University of Miami.

Nowicki, S., Jr., & Duke, M. P. (1994). Individual differences in the nonverbal communication of affect: The Diagnostic Analysis of Nonverbal Accuracy Scale. *Journal of Nonverbal Behavior, 18*(1), 9–35.

Pani, J., Mervis, C. B., & Robinson, B. F. (1999). Global spatial organization by individuals with Williams syndrome. *Psychological Science, 10*, 453–458.

Pinker, S. (1994). *The language instinct.* London: Penguin.

Plesa Skwerer, D., Faja, S., Schofield, C., Verbalis, A., & Tager-Flusberg, H. (2006). Perceiving facial and vocal expression of emotion in Williams syndrome. *American Journal on Mental Retardation, 111*(1), 15–26.

Plesa Skwerer, D., & Tager-Flusberg, H. (2006). Social cognition in Williams–Beuren syndrome. In C. A. Morris, H. M. Lenhoff, & P. Wang (Eds.), *Williams–Beuren syndrome: Research and clinical perspectives* (pp. 237–253). Baltimore: Johns Hopkins University Press.

Plesa Skwerer, D., Verbalis, A., Schofield, C., Faja, S., & Tager-Flusberg, H. (2006). Social-perceptual abilities in adolescents and adults with Williams syndrome. *Cognitive Neuropsychology, 23*, 338–348.

Reilly, J., Klima, E., & Bellugi, U. (1990). Once more with feeling: Affect and language in atypical populations. *Development and Psychopathology, 2*, 367–391.

Reiss, A. L., Eckert, M. A., Rose, F. E., Karchemisky, A., Kesler, S., Chang, M., et al. (2004). An experiment of nature: Brain anatomy parallels cognition and behavior in Williams syndrome. *Journal of Neuroscience, 24*, 5009–5015.

Reiss, A., Eliez, S., Schmitt, J. E., Strous, E., Lai, Z., Jones, W., et al. (2000). Neuroanatomy of Williams syndrome: A high-resolution MRI study. *Journal of Cognitive Neuroscience, 12*(Suppl.), 67–73.

Reiss, J. E., Hoffman, J. E., & Landau, B. (2003). Motion processing in Williams syndrome: Evidence against a general dorsal stream deficit [Abstract]. *Journal of Vision, 3*(9), 288a. Retrieved from *http://journalofvision.org/3/9/288.*

Rowe, M., Beccera, A., & Mervis, C. B. (2002, July). *The development of empathy in 4-year-old children with Williams syndrome.* Paper presented at the 9th International Professional Conference on Williams Syndrome, Long Beach, CA.

Schmahmann, J. D. (1991). An emerging concept: The cerebellar contribution of higher function. *Archives of Neurology, 48*, 1178–1187.

Schmitt, J. E., Eliez, S., Warsofksy, I., Bellugi, U., & Reiss, A. L. (2001). Enlarged cerebellar vermis in Williams syndrome. *Journal of Psychiatric Research, 35,* 225–229.

Schofield, C., Verbalis, A., Plesa Skwerer, D., Faja, S., & Tager-Flusberg, H. (2004, July). *Perceptual processes in face and object recognition in Williams syndrome.* The 10th International Professional Conference on Williams Syndrome, Grand Rapids, MI.

Schultz, R. T., Grelotti, D. J., & Pober, B. A. (2001). Genetics of childhood disorders: XXVI. Williams syndrome and brain–behavior relationships. *Journal of the American Academy of Child and Adolescent Psychiatry, 40*(5), 606–609.

Schumann, C. M., Harustra, J., Goodlin-Jones, B. L., Lotspeich, L. J., Kwon, H., Buonocore, M. H., et al. (2004). The amygdala is enlarged in children but not adolescents with autism; the hippocampus is enlarged at all ages. *Journal of Neuroscience, 24,* 6392–6401.

Semel, E., & Rosner, S. (2003). *Understanding Williams syndrome.* Hillsdale, NJ: Erlbaum.

Stock, D. A., Spallone, P. A., Dennis, T. R., Netski, D., Morris, C. A., Mervis, C. B., et al. (2003). Heat shock protein 27 gene: Chromosomal and molecular location and relationship to Williams syndrome. *American Journal of Medical Genetics, 120A,* 320–325.

Sullivan, K., & Tager-Flusberg, H. (1999). Second-order belief attribution in Williams syndrome: Intact or impaired? *American Journal on Mental Retardation, 104,* 523–532.

Sullivan, K., Winner, E., & Tager-Flusberg, H. (2003). Can adolescents with Williams syndrome tell the difference between lies and jokes? *Developmental Neuropsychology, 23,* 87–105.

Tager-Flusberg, H. (2004). Fulfilling the promise of the cognitive neurosciences. *Neuron, 43,* 595–596.

Tager-Flusberg, H., Boshart, J., & Baron-Cohen, S. (1998). Reading the windows to the soul: Evidence of domain-specific sparing in Williams syndrome. *Journal of Cognitive Neuroscience, 10*(5), 631–639.

Tager-Flusberg, H., & Plesa Skwerer, D. (in press). Social engagement in Williams syndrome. In P. J. Marshall & N. A. Fox (Eds.), *The development of social engagement: Neurobiological perspectives.* New York: Oxford University Press.

Tager-Flusberg, H., Plesa Skwerer, D., Faja, S., & Joseph, R. M. (2003). People with Williams syndrome process faces holistically. *Cognition, 89,* 11–24.

Tager-Flusberg, H., & Sullivan, K. (1999, April). *Are children with Williams syndrome spared in theory of mind?* Paper presented at the biennial meeting of the Society for Research in Child Development, Albuquerque, NM.

Tager-Flusberg, H., & Sullivan, K. (2000). A componential view of theory of mind: Evidence from Williams syndrome. *Cognition, 76,* 59–89.

Tanaka, J. W., & Farah, M. J. (1993). Parts and wholes in face recognition. *Quarterly Journal of Experimental Psychology, 46A,* 225–245.

Thelen, E., & Smith, L. B. (1994). *A dynamic systems approach to the development of cognition and action.* Cambridge, MA: MIT Press.

Thomas, M. S. C., & Karmiloff-Smith, A. (2005). Can developmental disorders reveal the component parts of the human language faculty? *Language Learning and Development, 1*(1), 65–92.

Tipney, H. J., Hinsley, T. A., Brass, A., Metcalfe, K., Donnai, D., & Tassabenji, M. (2004). Isolation and characterisation of GTF2IRD2, a novel fusion gene and member of the TFII-I family of transcription factors, deleted in Williams–Beuren syndrome. *European Journal of Human Genetics, 12*(7), 551–560.

Tomc, S. A., Williamson, N. K., & Pauli, R. M. (1990). Temperament in Williams syndrome. *American Journal of Medical Genetics, 36*, 345–352.

Udwin, O., & Yule, W. (1991). A cognitive and behavioural phenotype in Williams syndrome. *Journal of Clinical and Experimental Neuropsychology, 13*, 232–244.

Ungerleider, L. D., & Mishkin, M. (1982). Two cortical visual systems. In D. Ingle, M. Goodale, & R. Mansfield (Eds.), *Analysis of visual behavior* (pp. 549–586). Cambridge, MA: MIT Press.

Vicari, S., Bellucci, S., & Carlesimo, G. A. (2003). Visual and spatial working memory dissociation: Evidence from Williams syndrome. *Developmental Medicine and Child Neurology, 45*(4), 269–273.

Volterra, V., Capirci, O., Pezzini, G., Sabbadini, L., & Vicari, S. (1996). Linguistic abilities in Italian children with Williams syndrome. *Cortex, 32*, 663–677.

Wang, P. P., Doherty, S., Rourke, S. B., & Bellugi, U. (1995). Unique profile of visuo-perceptual skills in a genetic syndrome. *Brain and Cognition, 29*, 54–65.

Wechsler, D. (1974). *Wechsler Intelligence Scale for Children—Revised*. New York: Psychological Corporation.

Williams, J. C., Barratt-Boyes, B. G., & Lowe, J. B. (1961). Supravalvular aortic stenosis. *Circulation, 23*, 1311–1318.

Zhao, C., Aviles, C., Abel, R. A., Almli, C. R., McQuillen, P., & Pleasure, S. J. (2005). Hippocampal and visuospatial learning defects in mice with a deletion of frizzled 9, a gene in the Williams syndrome deletion interval. *Development, 132*(12), 2917–2927.

CHAPTER 5

Triangulating Developmental Dyslexia

BEHAVIOR, BRAIN, AND GENES

Elena L. Grigorenko

Many volumes of work have been published on the topic of developmental dyslexia, and the scope of the field is truly breathtaking. A simple search for the keyword *dyslexia*—limited only to the last decade—returns 1,702 titles in PsycLIT and 1,663 titles in Medline. The complexity of the field is underscored by its varied names: *dyslexia, developmental dyslexia* (347 records in PsycLIT and 217 records in Medline), and *reading disability* (413 records in PsycLIT and 199 records in Medline). Some authors use all three concepts interchangeably; others preserve the specificity of each term. But whichever term is used, even a simple list of these publications exceeds the page limit for this chapter! Correspondingly, this review is inevitably selective. I structure the chapter around the following discussion topics: (1) the converging definition of developmental dyslexia; (2) definition-based hypotheses of the etiological bases of developmental dyslexia and, in more detail, evidence supporting the hypotheses of its genetic bases; (3) various theoretical models that have attempted to account for the observed pattern of genetic influences; and (4) our current understanding of the impact of the main effects and interactions of etiological forces contributing to the manifestation of developmental dyslexia.

TERMINOLOGY AND DEFINITION:
WHAT *IS* DEVELOPMENTAL DYSLEXIA?

It is important to note that in this chapter the terms *dyslexia, developmental dyslexia* (DD), *reading disability/difficulty* (RD), and *specific reading disability/difficulty* (SRD) are used interchangeably. The only distinction among the types of dyslexia important in the context of this chapter is between the terms above and the term *acquired dyslexia* (or *acquired reading disability/difficulty*, a type of dyslexia caused by extensive left-hemispheric brain damage resulting from brain trauma, stroke, or some other traumatic event); acquired dyslexia will not be discussed here, although research on that topic has made fundamental theoretical and empirical contributions to the field of DD.

With that said, what is meant by DD, RD, or SRD (hereafter, DD)? Nowadays, the definition of the phenomenon underlying these concepts is typically six-faceted.

1. The *first* facet assumes the experience of *unexpected* difficulty in mastering reading (e.g., Shaywitz & Shaywitz, 2005). This facet of the definition embodies a number of assumptions. Specifically, it is assumed that (1) development in other domains of cognitive functioning progresses normally within *expected* developmental norms (i.e., a horizontal developmental comparison with other skills is made), and (2) this difficulty becomes noticeable when the child begins to learn how to read at an appropriate developmental stage (i.e., a vertical comparison with the rate of acquisition of other skills is made). In short, DD can be established only as specific to reading, that is, with all other skills preserved, and only when a child starts mastering reading, not earlier in development.

2. The *second* facet of the definition points to the basis of DD that is assumed to be *linguistic (phonological)* in origin (e.g., Lyon, Shaywitz, & Shaywitz, 2003; see also Goswami, Chapter 6, this volume). Although there are other theories of DD that collectively view the disorder as a general sensorimotor syndrome (for a review, see Ramus, 2003), the phonological theory of DD has predominated for the last 25 years or so, and there is no evidence of a decline in its power, credibility, or popularity. Yet there is a substantial body of literature suggesting the importance of other points of view on DD; other researchers have defined the disorder through lenses of specific deficiencies in auditory processing (e.g., Tallal, 1980; Tallal, Miller, & Fitch, 1993), visual processing (e.g., Livingstone, Rosen, Drislane, & Galaburda, 1991; Lovegrove, Bowling, Badcock, & Blackwood, 1980), cerebellar function (e.g., Nicolson & Fawcett, 1990;

Nicolson, Fawcett, & Dean, 2001), and common dysfunction of magno-cells in sensory pathways (Stein, 2001).

3. The *third* facet of the definition assumes that DD is a *lifetime* condition (Felton, Naylor, & Wood, 1990; Gottesman, Bennett, Nathan, & Kelly, 1996) diagnosable only when the individual is confronted with printed letters (as per the first facet of the definition). However, both prospective (e.g., Gallagher, Frith, & Snowling, 2000; van Alphen et al., 2004) and retrospective (e.g., Catts, Fey, & Proctor-Williams, 2000; Feldman et al., 1993; Snowling, Bishop, & Stothard, 2000) longitudinal studies point to pre-reading-age precursors of DD (e.g., Lyytinen, Poikkeus, Laakso, Eklund, & Lyytinen, 2001; Scarborough, 1991; see also Molfese, Molfese, & Molfese, Chapter 8, this volume).

4. The *fourth* facet defines DD as a *complex common* condition, with an estimated prevalence of 12–17% (http://www.interdys.org, Fact Sheet #62-05/00). This commonly observed disorder appears to be best explained by a componential model of complex traits, similar to those successfully employed with a number of medical conditions (e.g., cardiovascular conditions and diabetes). There are two relevant assumptions for this facet: (1) DD is multidimensional, that is, it arises from a combination of traits (see also facet 2 of the definition); and (2) DD appears to be continuously distributed in the population, so that deficiencies in multiple related processes can give rise to a holistic manifestation of DD, and complex combinations of these deficiencies might be related to the severity or degree of affectedness by the disorder.

5. The *fifth* facet of the definition is most critical to this chapter; this facet attests to the etiology of DD. It is commonly recognized that DD is a disorder that has *biological* bases (e.g., Definition of Dyslexia adopted by the Board of Directors, November 12, 2002, http://www.interdys.org; Lyon et al., 2003). An explicit discussion of this facet can be found later in this chapter.

6. Finally, the *sixth* facet of the definition is exclusionary rather than inclusive. Specifically, as stated in "facts on dyslexia" presented by the International Dyslexia Association, "15–20% of the population has a reading disability.[1] Of those, 85% has [*sic*] dyslexia" (www.interdys.org, Fact Sheet #62-05/00). In other words, about 15% of reading problems[2] can be attributed to other causes, such as a developmental disability in which reading problems are either part of the diagnosis (e.g., mental retardation) or can be attributed to poor schooling (e.g., impoverished schooling in economically disadvantaged developing countries or poor teaching in developed countries) or the unavailability of schooling (e.g., as for Sudanese children in Darfur, a region fraught with current ethnic and political con-

flict). Thus, not everyone who has reading difficulties has DD: Phenotypically similar reading-related processes and attributes can originate for different etiological reasons.

It is important to note the division of opinions about every single facet of the hexagonal definition of DD discussed above. Yet consensus is a powerful force in science and, driven by an agreement among the majority, the definition of DD used in this chapter has emerged as follows: *Dyslexia refers to a complex, componential, common, biologically grounded, lifetime condition that is marked by early signs of atypicality in linguistic development, is fully manifested in serious unexpected difficulty in mastery and automatization of the skill of reading, is present in the absence of other developmental disorders and in spite of adequate instruction, and is often characterized by comorbid developmental conditions and negative developmental outcomes.*[3] With this definition in place, I now proceed to the discussion of definition-based hypotheses regarding the etiological bases of DD and the research-based evidence supporting these hypotheses.

ETIOLOGICAL BASES OF DD:
A CAPSULE REVIEW OF MAIN EFFECTS

The reason for providing a definition of DD was to preface the discussion of its etiological factors. Specifically, the discussion in this section is based on facets 2, 4, 5, and 6 of the hexagonal definition of DD. To reiterate, "true" DD is viewed as a multivariate phenomenon (facets 2 and 4 of the definition) with an unknown biological basis that is detectable through the deficient functioning of brain networks (facets 5 and 6). In an attempt to understand the texture of the biological bases of DD, many researchers in the field study genes. It is no leap of the imagination to assume that genes involved with brain development and maturation, especially in those neural areas that appear to be related to reading, form the biological bases for DD. Yet, currently, no single theory accounts for the full construction of DD. These days, there is significant appreciation of the complexity of the links between the genome, the brain, behavior, and the crucial role of the environment that contextualize the development of a single cell into a human being. To steer this discussion toward the presentation of some models that might underlie these links in dyslexia, I briefly review main points of the literature on brain, genetic, and environmental findings with regard to DD.

Reading-Related Processes

So far, there have been only generic references to the disruption of both the acquisition and mastery of reading skills that constitute the texture of DD. When this generic reference is closely considered, another massive body of literature materializes: (1) cognitive psychology literature on the types of representation of information involved in reading (i.e., reading involves the translation of meaningful symbolic visual codes [orthographical representation] into pronounceable and distinguishable sounds of language [phonological representation] so that a meaning [semantic representation] arises; e.g., Harm & Seidenberg, 2004); (2) developmental psychology literature on when these representations develop and what might cause the development of a dysfunctional representational system (e.g., Karmiloff-Smith, 1998); and (3) educational psychology literature on how the formation of functional representations can be aided or corrected when at risk for malfunction (e.g., Blachman et al., 2004).

Because of space limitations I comment here only on four points in this literature that are relevant to the discussion of the etiological factors of DD. Today, given the predominance of the phonology-based connectionist account of DD, the phenotype (i.e., behavioral manifestation) of DD is captured through a collection of highly correlated traits. Although different researchers use different terms for specific traits, these traits can be loosely structured into groups aimed at capturing different types of information representation, for example: (1) performance on orthographic choice or homonym choice judgment tasks for quantifying parameters of orthographical representation; (2) phonemic awareness, phonological decoding, and phonological memory for quantifying phonological representation; and (3) vocabulary and indices of comprehension at different levels of linguistic processing for quantifying semantic representation. Correspondingly, in studies of the etiology, development, and educational malleability of DD, the quantification of the disorder is carried out through these various phenotypes (often referred to as componential phenotypes or endophenotypes of DD). Thus, many studies attempt to subdivide DD into its components and explore their etiological bases, developmental trajectories, and susceptibility to pedagogical interventions separately as well as jointly.

DD Is Biologically Grounded

The definition of DD, as stated earlier, acknowledges the biological foundations of the disorder. More specifically, it states that the very presence of this foundation defines DD—if there is no detectable biological foundation, there is no disorder (facet 6 of the definition). Thus, not all reading difficulties can be called DD, only those that have a biological foundation. So, what is meant when it is said that DD is biologically grounded? Two lines of evidence for the biological foundation of DD are typically cited.

The first line goes back to early skull and brain damage and trepanation surgeries carried out in ancient Greece (as evidenced in the writings of Hippocrates, c. 460–355 B.C.). Even those first documented observations implied the link between damage to the brain and loss of function of reading, and subsequent centuries of clinical cases and psychological experiments established the unequivocal brain–reading skill link (Simos, Billingsley-Marshall, Sarkari, & Papanicolaou, in press).

Multiple methodological techniques (e.g., EEG, ERP, fMRI, MEG, PET, and TMS,[4] to name a few) have been used to investigate brain–reading relationships. When data from multiple sources are combined, it appears that a developed, automatized skill of reading engages a widespread, bilateral (but predominantly left-hemispheric) network of brain areas, passing activation from the occipitotemporal regions through temporal (posterior) areas and toward the frontal (precentral and inferior frontal gyri) lobes (e.g., Fiez & Petersen, 1998; Mechelli, Gorno-Tempini, & Price, 2003; Petersen, Fox, Posner, Mintun, & Raichle, 1988; Price & Mechelli, 2005; Price, Wise, & Frackowiak, 1996; Pugh et al., 2001; Snyder, Abdullaev, Posner, & Raichle, 1995; Turkeltaub, Gareau, Flowers, Zeffiro, & Eden, 2003). Clearly, the process of reading is multifaceted and involves evocation of orthographic, phonological, and semantic (Fiez, 1997; Poldrack et al., 1999; Pugh et al., 1996; Tagamets, Novick, Chalmers, & Friedman, 2000) representations that, in turn, call for the activation of brain networks participating in visual, auditory, and conceptual processing (for a review, see Turkeltaub, Eden, Jones, & Zeffiro, 2002). Correspondingly, it is expected that the areas of activation observed in reading studies serve as anatomic substrates supporting all these types of representations and processing.[5]

However, possibly somewhat surprisingly, per recent reviews (e.g., Price & Mechelli, 2005; Shaywitz & Shaywitz, 2005; Simos et al., in press), there appear to be only four areas of the brain of particular, specific interest with regard to reading. These areas are the fusiform gyrus (i.e., the occipitotemporal cortex in the ventral portion of Brodmann's area [BA] 37), the posterior portion of the middle temporal gyrus (roughly BA 21, but possibly more specifically, the ventral border with BA 37 and the dorsal border of the superior temporal sulcus), the angular gyrus (BA 39), and the posterior portion of the superior temporal gyrus (BA 22). It is also important to note that developmental changes in patterns of brain functioning occur with increased mastery of reading skill: progressive, behaviorally modulated development and increased engagement of left-hemispheric "versions" of these areas and progressive disengagement of homologous right-hemispheric areas (Eden et al., 2004; Gaillard, Balsamo, Ibrahim, Sachs, & Xu, 2003; Pugh et al., 2001; Turkeltaub et al., 2003).

The second line of evidence pertains to a now well-established fact: DD is a heritable condition. This statement originates from years of research into the familiality of DD (i.e., similarity on the skill of reading among relatives of different degree), characterized by studies that have engaged multiple genetic methodologies, specifically, twin (e.g., Byrne et al., 2005; Cardon et al., 1994, 1995), family (e.g., Cope et al., 2005; Grigorenko, Wood, Meyer, & Pauls, 2000; Wolff & Melngailis, 1994), and sib-pair (e.g., Francks et al., 2004; Ziegler et al., 2005) designs. Although each of these methodologies has its own resolution power with regard to explaining similarities among relatives by means of referring to genes and environments as sources of these similarities and obtaining corresponding estimates of relative contributions of genes and environments, *all* methodologies have produced data that unanimously point to genetic similarities as the main source of the familiality of DD.

There are multiple comprehensive reviews of the literature on the genetic bases of DD (e.g., Barr & Couto, in press; Fisher & DeFries, 2002; Grigorenko, 2005). Though delivered in different words, voices, and often under different assumptions, three main conclusions can be deduced from this literature.

The *first* is that, even though the genetic basis of DD is extremely important, *genes, at best, explain only a portion, although substantial, of the relevant variance* (e.g., Grigorenko, 2004). Merely to provide an illustration, let me cite a few specific figures here. For example, the heritability estimates for word reading range from .19 (Stevenson, Graham, Fredman, & McLoughlin, 1987) to .55–.59 (Harlaar, Spinath, Dale, & Plomin, 2005). The estimates for phonemic awareness also leave a lot of room for environmental influences: .52 (Hohnen & Stevenson, 1999) and .83 (Gayan & Olson, 2003).

In other words, even if we fully understand the genetic machinery behind DD, we will be only halfway there. We will still need to identify which factors account for the rest of the variance. Needless to say, researchers in the field have a great many guesses as to what these factors might be. Years of research into individual differences in reading skill point to the importance of three environmental (outside-the-child) factors: a child's (1) socioeconomic strata at large (e.g., a child's country, community, and school, and his or her economic well-being); (2) teachers (e.g., global pedagogical approach of teachers and teacher-specific pedagogical techniques); and (3) home environment (e.g., availability of relevant materials to practice the skill and motivate its further development).

The *second* conclusion refers to the realization that *multiple genes appear to form the genetic bases for DD*. Three lines of research are relevant here:

a. The first line originates from quantitative genetics (Falconer & Mackay, 1996) and suggests that, to reach the appearance of uninterrupted, continuous distributions of a behavioral trait, many genes, each of which is responsible for a definable, discrete contribution, should form the genetic basis of this trait. This tradition has been very successful in contributing to the understanding of complex continuous phenotypes such as cholesterol concentration (Reed, Nanthakumar, North, Bell, & Price, 2001) and bone density (Karasik et al., 2002), and appears to be highly relevant to the literature on DD.

The field has certainly enjoyed the quantitative nature of all reading-related traits, at least at some developmental periods (i.e., many phonemic awareness tasks trigger significant individual variability among preschoolers and show a ceiling effect after primary school), and no researcher will argue that reading-related traits are continuously distributed in the general population, although not everyone will agree on the nature of these distributions with regard to the number of modes and other characteristics of distributional moments. Thus, looking at which behavioral traits the field of DD works with, it is only natural to assume that many genes are involved in forming these traits.

b. The second line of research is found in the literature that attempts to fit different genetic models to behavioral data in an effort to estimate the number of genes contributing to the manifestation of different reading-related skills (e.g., Marlow et al., 2003; Wijsman et al., 2000). The point of interest here is to model the observed familiality of reading-related componential processes by assuming various models of inheritance (e.g., dominant, recessive, additive), the number of genes involved, and the constellations of genes with regard to common and specific genes contributing to specific reading-related traits. Although there are disagreements about whether the genes contribute to *all versus some* reading-related processes, there is consensus that there are many genes, and likely genes of fairly small effects, contributing to DD-related processes.

c. Finally, the third line of research is traceable to the 1983 paper by Smith and colleagues that triggered the development of the molecular–genetic field of DD (Smith, Kimberling, Pennington, & Lubs, 1983). In that paper, the field got its first candidate region for DD, a region somewhere around the centromere on chromosome 15. The precision of genetic mapping was so low at that time that the boundaries of the region were huge, by genetic standards, and subsequent attempts to work with chromosome 15 resulted in both replications and nonreplications simply because researchers looked at various subregions of this initially flagged piece of the chromosome. Little did we know that it was only the beginning! The current state of affairs is quite remarkable: The field has nine candidate regions to entertain (Grigorenko, 2005)! These regions are recognized as DD candidate regions; they are abbreviated as *DYX1-9* and refer to the regions on chromosomes 15q, 6p, 2p, 6q, 3cen, 18p, 11p, 1p, and Xq, respectively. Each of these regions harbors dozens of genes, so, clearly, the field offers empirical validation that multiple genes contribute to the manifestation of DD.

The *third* conclusion refers to the *putative function* of the contributing genes. A number of different research groups work on these loci in an attempt to identify plausible candidate genes. Four successful attempts have been announced in the literature: one for the 15q region—the candidate gene known as *DYX1C1* (Taipale et al., 2003); two for the 6p region—the candidate gene known as *KIAA0319* (Cope et al., 2005) and the candidate gene *DCDC2* (Meng et al., 2005); and one for the 3cen region, *ROBO1* (Hannula-Jouppi et al., 2005). Yet after the first presentation of the *DYX1C1* gene, somewhat controversial evidence followed that challenged the association between *DYX1C1* and dyslexia (Cope et al., 2004; Scerri et al., 2004). The association between *KIAA0319* also awaits further confirmation, because there is at least one nonreplication (Barr, 2005), but there is some promising supporting evidence for *DCDC2* (Schumacher et al., 2006). To my knowledge, no replications of *ROBO1* have yet been attempted. Although the field has not yet converged on "firm" candidates, it is remarkable and of great scientific interest that all three current candidate genes for DD are involved with biological functions of neuronal migration and axonal development. It is possible that these genes are related to the establishment and dynamic development of the connectivity networks forming the brain bases for typical and atypical reading.

It is also important to note in the context of this discussion that there is a growing body of literature specifically attesting to the universality versus specificity of biological mechanisms underlying reading failure in different populations and across different languages (e.g., Grigorenko, Ngorosho, Jukes, & Bundy, 2006; Paulesu et al., 2001; see also Goswami, Chapter 6, this volume). Although relatively few in number, these studies suggest that (a) the current dominant cognitive model of different, differentially damaged types of representations involved in reading (especially with regard to phonological representation) appears to hold across languages with very different characteristics (e.g., Goulandris, 2003); and (b) these representations appear to have universal bases in both the brain (e.g., Paulesu et al., 2001) and the genome (e.g., Grigorenko et al., 1997; Marino et al., 2004; Morris et al., 2000; Schulte-Körne et al., 1998). In summary, the biological risks predisposing a child to the manifestation of DD appear to be influential and powerful regardless of the child's natal linguistic system. Depending on the stress (degree of challenge) imposed by a particular linguistic system on the maturing brain, these risk factors might result in different manifestations of DD.[6]

DD Is Environmentally Sensitive

Throughout the chapter, there have been references to reading difficulties outside the scope of DD (i.e., reading difficulties that appear to manifest *without* biological bases). In the still very prevalent, but far from valid, tradition of separating biological and environmental bases of human traits, I briefly reference another substantial body of literature that must be acknowledged here. This literature covers research on environmental risk and protective factors relevant to academic learning, in general, and mastery of reading, in particular. Multiple comprehensive reviews cover the latest frontiers of this research (e.g., Vellutino, Fletcher, Snowling, & Scanlon, 2004). In general, this research finds that the odds of preventing and remediating the manifestation of DD are higher for (1) children from families of higher levels of socioeconomic status (SES; e.g., Nicholson, 1997); (2) individuals who have had more schooling (e.g., D'Angiulli, Siegel, & Hertzman, 2004); (3) children who are taught to read by directed methods of teaching reading and who are trained in meta-linguistic skills, especially phonemic awareness (e.g., Snowling, 1996); (4) children whose early home environments are enriched by literacy-relevant materials (e.g., Kamhi & Laing, 2001); and (5) children with diets that are adequately nutritious rather than nutrient and microelement impoverished (e.g., Ames, 2004). This is by no means a complete list of environmental factors that may prevent or remediate the manifestation of the biological risk factors for DD. The point I would like to make here is that *none* of these factors is *deterministic*. Even when all of these risk factors are present, the manifestation of reading difficulties is still linked only to odds, not outcomes. And *none* of these factors, when viewed in isolation (as if there were such a thing!) from biological factors, can explain DD. Again, in the context of the definition of DD used here (facets 5 and 6), these environmental factors can only moderate, mediate, or have some other type of *interactive* influence on the impact of the biological bases (hereafter, genes) of DD.

THEORETICAL MODELS OF GENETIC INFLUENCES

Having defined the phenomenon and briefly discussed the special characteristics of etiological studies of DD, I now turn to the third section of the chapter, which offers a speculative discussion of possible underlying mechanisms of DD. In this section, the biological bases of DD are equated with genetic bases of DD. This is not to say that I do not allow for the identification of other, nongenetic, biological factors influencing the manifestation of DD. I make the distinction simply to limit the scope of the discussion in this chapter.

A number of thinkers have highlighted characteristic signatures of the influences imposed by genetic factors in attempts to develop models of etiological mechanisms of common complex disorders (e.g., Merikangas & Risch, 2003; Sing & Reilly, 1993; Thompson, 1994). Collectively, these models incorporate the following considerations: (1) the continuous and quantitative nature of a liability distribution for a given disorder, with a disorder status categorization based on a somewhat arbitrary threshold; (2) difficulty in identifying, measuring, and characterizing holistic phenotypes for disorders and therefore the need to rely on endophenotypes (Gottesman & Gould, 2003)—phenotypic traits that may capture intermediate states between the pattern of expression of underlying genes and the disorder; (3) an abundance of evidence concerning the importance of environmental contributions to complex genetically based diseases, resulting in a hypothesis that environmental exposure is often a *prerequisite* to a disorder (Merikangas & Risch, 2003); (4) the determination of a particular manifestation and severity of a disorder by a complex interaction of genetic and environmental risk and protective factors; (5) the pleiotropic foundation of genetic and environmental risk factors prohibiting exclusive gene–disorder connections and establishing "many genes–many disorders" connections that, in turn, form the bases of comorbidity among multiple disorders; and (6) the knowledge that risk factors are typically shared among a number of disorders and, therefore, comorbidity of common disorders is the rule rather than exception.

Following other researchers (Morton & Frith, 1995; Pennington, 2002), in presenting the models below, I distinguish between (1) observed behavioral phenotypes (i.e., a constellation of symptoms specifying a disorder), (2) cognitive or other processes underlying these phenotypes (i.e., endophenotypes), (3) neurological processes associated with both cognitive processes and behavioral phenotypes, and (4) etiological mechanisms of these neurological processes. Similar and relevant ideas have been discussed in a variety of writings on complex phenotypes related to developmental disorders (Pennington, 2002; Pennington & Lefly, 2001; Snowling, Gallagher, & Frith, 2003).

At the level of integration, the considerations described above permit the general formulation of a set of theoretical causal models that need to be tested empirically. These models can be summarized in four broadly conceptualized diagrams (Figure 5.1A–5.1D), which, by necessity, omit details, given that more information needs to be collected to further exemplify the models. The models are based on the assumption (as per facet 4 of our definition) that DD is a holistic state of functioning that can be further dissected into deficient cognitive processes. Thus, it is assumed here that DD is a multivariate phenomenon, emerging from co-function (or, rather, co-dysfunction) of multiple underlying processes engaged in phonological, orthographic, and semantic representation. Here are brief descriptions of these four models connecting genes, brains, and behaviors.

Model 1 (in Figure 5.1A) is based on the following assumptions. There is an underlying "generalized" genetic deficiency (G) that results in a deviation from a typical pattern of brain development. This deficiency manifests itself early and results in challenging first-order brain-based information-

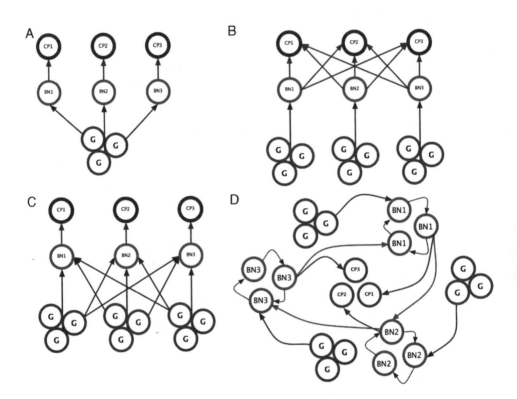

FIGURE 5.1. Models of multilevel influences for biological bases of DD.

processing neuronal network deficiencies (BN for brain networks, BN1–BN3) underlying the neurological and cognitive foundation for atypical development of cognitive processes (CP for cognitive processes, CP1–CP3). Note that it is assumed here that the genetic bases are common for all disrupted neuronal networks, but each network provides an independent cause for a disordered cognitive process. For example, a disrupted neuronal migration (which can be caused by genetic malfunction) might result in brain miswiring, which, in turn, might lead (as a secondary cause) to the formation of disordered (dysfunctional) cognitive functions, reflective of dysfunctional neuronal networks. The impact of this genetic deficiency factor undermines the whole domain of functioning of the developing individual. A proximal analogy here is Spearman's g-factor model of cognitive functioning (Spearman, 1927). A distal analogy of this impact is the crack in the foundation of a building, where the structural damage in the foundation results in problems in the whole building, but the specific nature of these problems is not predictable and is characterized by the presence of random factors, for example, environmental influences. Within this model, the observed correlations of deficient cognitive processes characteristic of DD (i.e., the processes descriptive of phonological, orthographic, and semantic representations) are secondary and reflect the causal links between the brain networks and deficient information processing at the phenotypic, not genotypic, levels. This model assumes a search for a common g-factor governed by the generalist gene(s) (Plomin & Kovas, 2005).

The following models (2 and 3, in Figures 5.1B and 5.1C, respectively) are quite similar and assume the presence of a set of genes influencing specific brain networks, which in turn contribute to the manifestation of the challenged cognitive phenotypes in unique or overlapping fashion. To illustrate these models, we can think of a "latent variable" model, often used in the DD literature (Wagner, Torgesen, & Rashotte, 1994). A proximal analogy of models 2 and 3 is the Thurstone model of cognitive functioning[7] (Thurstone, 1938). A distal analogy is multiple operations malfunctioning in our hypothetical building (electricity, heating, and water systems), each for specific overlapping or unique reasons. The difference between models 2 and 3 occurs at the level of genetic etiology and brain bases of cognitive processing: Model 2 specifies unique sets of genes influencing specific brain networks, but overlapping brain networks contributing to different cognitive phenotypes, whereas model 3 specifies both network-specific and network-shared genes influencing more than one process, but each cognitive process is governed by a specific network only.

Specifically, in model 2 (in Figure 5.1B) it is assumed that a set of distinct genes affects the development or functioning of a particular neuronal network that, in turn, forms the foundation for a cognitive process. Thus, the formation and functioning of a particular brain network is governed by a set of specific genes (G), and each network (BN1–BN3) contributes to the manifestation of multiple dysfunctional cognitive processes (CP1–CP3). The observed phenotypic correlation between cognitive processes CP1–CP3 is not due to shared genetic etiology, but rather, because of overlapping contributions of the brain's neuronal networks, reflects the engagement of overlapping networks with more than one cognitive process (e.g., different types of attention; Fan & Posner, 2004), or arises as a property of a complex system in which many independent elements are involved in a common function.

Model 3 (Figure 5.1C) is a modification of model 2 in that it assumes that (1) the development and functioning of particular brain networks are influenced by sets of partially overlapping genes—that is, there are general and specific genes (G) for each brain network (BN); and (2) each network contributes uniquely to a particular dysfunctional cognitive process (CP). In this model, the phenotypic correlation between cognitive processes is due to shared genetic factors mediated by a particular neuronal network.

Finally, model 4 (in Figure 5.1D) assumes that multiple unrelated genetic factors influence the many neuronal networks recruited into the systems of complex architecture that form the foundation for cognitive functioning. In this model, no shared or general factors are assumed, and the appearance of commonalities is attributed to epiphenomenological manifestations. A proximal analogy of this model is Thompson's model of cognitive functioning[8] (Thompson, 1939). A distal analogy is the behavior of a complex system constructed of independent "particles" (as in Crichton's *Prey* [2002]), where the common factor is the characteristic of the system, not of its separate elements, which can arise only when a critical mass of elements is present. At the phenotypic level, model 4 calls for the use of multivariate models, and at the genetic level, calls not only for the analysis of the mutations in single genes (i.e., linkage and association analyses), but also for the analysis of the context (the genome as a whole) in which these genes are expressed.

Clearly, these four models are only a sample of possible models. They are intended to capture the importance of considering multiple levels of causal influences and the lack of one-to-one and the abundance of one-to-many, many-to-one, and many-to-many correspondences. Thus, by varying the number of genes influencing the emerging neuronal networks, the number of neuronal networks influencing cognitive processes, and the number of shared and unique connections between these levels, a fairly large number of models can be created. To appreciate the number, just reflect for a moment on the thought that, of the ~30,000 genes in the human genome, ~5,000 are supposedly expressed in the brain. If we follow the estimates obtained in segregation analyses of DD and related traits (e.g., Wijsman et al., 2000) and assume that, on average, 4 genes contribute to a reading-related trait, we face $26,010,428,123,750^9$ possible unique combinations. Thus, to understate the case, there are many possibilities, and we are talking about the lowest level of hierarchy considered in these causal models.

It must be noted, of course, that I did not include the impact of environmental factors in the models discussed above. That is because these factors do not operate within the models and do not form a separate layer of influences; they act across all four levels of the models considered above. To illustrate, consider the impact of SES. SES has been shown to influence dietary choices (Monteiro, Moura, Conde, & Popkin, 2004), which, in turn, have been shown to result in altered gene expression (Li et al., 2005). Different levels of SES are also associated with differences in brain networking and functioning (Noble, McCandliss, & Farah, in press). There are robust correlations linking SES and variability in cognitive functioning (Bornstein & Bradley, 2003). Finally, the manifestation and remediation of DD itself is likely to be linked to SES: the higher the level of SES, in general, the more remediation and support services the family can afford, and the better the outcome (Kelman & Lester, 1998). In fact, in considering these relationships, it becomes clear that environment is inseparable from "biological" influences. Environmental influences have an impact on what is considered biological at the next level of hierarchy in the model (e.g., proteins formed under the influence of different diets [i.e., *environmentally modified proteins*] are still viewed as *biological* factors in processes utilizing these proteins [e.g., neuronal signal transduction]). With this remark, I move to the last section of the chapter, a discussion that attempts to summarize the current state of the field with regard to our understanding of the impact of main effects and interactions of etiological forces contributing to the manifestation of DD.

The Etiology of Developmental Dyslexia: Main Effects and Interactions

I opened the chapter with a discussion of the hexagonal definition of DD, progressed through brief descriptions of bodies of literature associated with different facets of this definition, and focused specifically on the brief characterization of biological bases of DD. A summary of various points that have been covered so far is presented in Figure 5.2, illustrating the known genetic and environmental risk factors for DD.

In essence, Figure 5.2 represents a two-by-two table, with one dimension of the table separating etiological influences into genetic and environmental factors, and another dimension subdividing risk and protective fac-

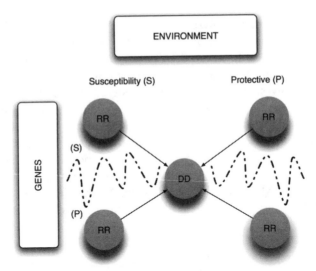

FIGURE 5.2. A diagram of influences of genetic and environmental factors in DD.

tors. The cells then capture risk ratios (RR) for the manifestation of DD. Clearly, the highest risk ratios are expected for the cell at the cross-section of genetic and environmental susceptibility factors. The presence of two sources of risk typically works multiplicatively, not additively. The presence of protective factors, either genetic or environmental, is expected to diminish the risk. The last cell indicates the absence of risk factors, either genetic or environmental, as main effects. The risk ratio associated with this cell is expected to be the lowest. Several additional aspects of this figure warrant discussion.

First, it is important to note that, at this time, there are no known deterministic factors for DD, either for genetic or environmental effects. With regard to genetic factors, it is possible that these factors have not been discovered yet. Based on the field's experience with complex human traits, it is possible that as-yet-undiscovered genetic factors cause DD deterministically. However, if that is the case, it will most likely be of great importance for only a relatively small number of families. In other words, there might be deterministic genes for DD that will account for an uncommon subset of DD. An illustrative example comes from the literature on genetic bases of Alzheimer's disease. There are known deterministic genes for the manifestation of this disease (ß-amyloid precursor protein and presenilin-1 and -2); however, although the risk for an individual with these mutations is high (inheriting mutated copies of these genes is associated with a near-

100% likelihood of developing the disease), these mutations are very rare and thus the population risk is low. There is also a known genetic susceptibility factor, the ε4 allele of the *APOE* gene; it appears that the risk of developing Alzheimer's varies with the number of copies of the ε4 allele. Specifically, it has been reported that one copy of the ε4 allele is associated with 2.5–3.2 odds (i.e., the proportion of having the disease versus not having the disease) and two copies of the ε4 allele are associated with 14.9 odds of the manifestation of the disease (Farrer et al., 1997). The frequency of this allele is relatively high in the general population (although it varies substantially for different ethnic groups), and, although the associated individual risks are probabilistic rather than deterministic, the ε4 allele has a very high population attributable risk. For DD, there are currently no known deterministic genes, but a number of genes are currently being evaluated as susceptibility genes (as noted, *DCDC2, DYX1C1, KIAA0319, ROBO1*).

Listing the currently investigated candidate genes for DD is relevant to the *second* point of this discussion. Although the genes listed above are considered to be susceptibility factors for DD, it is possible that some alleles of these genes can act as risk factors and others as protective factors. To illustrate, let us consider the *APOE* gene again. As discussed earlier, the ε4 allele of this gene has a high population attributable risk. However, two other alleles of this gene, ε2 and ε3, when forming the ε2/ε3 genotype, appear to act as a protective factor (Farrer et al., 1997). Although the candidate genes for DD have not yet been confirmed as susceptibility factors, there is an interesting inconsistency in the literature with regard to the alleles of the *DYX1C1* gene. The first presentation of this gene as a susceptibility gene named the A allele of the 3G-to-A change in the promoter region of the *DYX1C1* gene as a risk factor (Taipale et al., 2003). The first attempt to replicate this finding suggested that an alternative allele (G) was associated with DD (Wigg et al., 2004); thus, it is possible that the G allele is a protective factor. These intriguing results are yet to be sorted out in large, phenotypically well-characterized, preferably population-based samples. To my knowledge, there are currently no such samples available. Thus, one of the field's many tasks on the road to understanding genetic population risks for DD will be to build such samples.

The *third* important point is that, from what we know from the developmental literature at large, there are virtually no factors among environmental influences that are typically considered by developmentalists as truly deterministic. However, there are countless environmental factors that can be named as susceptibility (e.g., poverty, printed-material-impoverished home environment, low level of parental education) and protective (e.g., amount of schooling, high-quality teaching, presence of mentors and role models, positive peer networking) factors for the manifestation of DD. The impact of all these environmental factors is probabilistic by nature. Yet, as is true for development in general and maladaptive behavior in particular (e.g., Sameroff & Mackenzie, 2003), an accumulation of risk factors changes the odds of the manifestation of DD, most likely in a bidirectional and nonlinear manner.

The *fourth* point brings us back to the definition of DD (facet 6). How, in this diagram, is the risk ratio conceived when genetic protective factors and environmental susceptibility factors are considered? Facet 6 of the hexagonal definition of DD assumes that *only* the presence of biological bases qualifies reading difficulties to be referred to as DD. Does the presence of protective alleles in a gene whose alleles are also risk alleles etiologically connect DD and high reading performance? The answer is yes—there is a significant possibility of allele heterogeneity with regard to DD, and understanding this heterogeneity will be a major task of molecular–genetic research on DD even after candidate genes for DD are identified and confirmed. The protective gene/environmental susceptibility cell in Figure 5.2 calls for a discussion of an interesting paradox: If the same gene, through its differential alleles, forms differential genetic backgrounds (disadvantageous and advantageous) for DD, how might this consideration influence the field's sampling strategies? Does this consideration, among others, suggest the necessity of recruiting individuals with high and very high performance on reading and reading-related tasks? Although the detailed consideration of the issue of sampling in genetic studies of DD is a very interesting topic in its own right (e.g., Grigorenko et al., 2006; Ziegler et al., 2005), here I simply want to stress the importance of considering all kinds of samples (e.g., large rare families with high incidence of DD, small nuclear families with a DD proband, sib-pairs ascertained through a single proband with a reading deficit, as well as through sib-pairs [i.e., double proband selection] concordant for deficit or high performance and highly discordant), because each of these sampling strategies will contribute to our understanding of the intricacies of gene–environment co-action in DD.

The *fifth* point of discussion involves an exploration of risk and protective genetic and environmental factors. As noted earlier, the current state of affairs suggests a multilevel causality model of *biological* (i.e., gene–brain-based) *predisposition* for DD that is alterable by environmental factors at all levels. There are no convergent data just yet that are powerful enough to establish a preference for one of the models suggested above, connecting genes and the brain in the etiological pathway so as to result in the manifestation of DD. Yet the emerging evidence suggests that, most likely, the model will engage multiple genes that will contribute probabilistically in unique and shared fashions to the formation of neuronal networks, which, in turn, will probabilistically contribute to the establishment of cognitive processes involved in forming different types of information representation. It appears that the manifestation of DD, mostly likely, is a product of complex probabilistic machinery that has no single deterministic factor, but rather many factors involved in many possible interactive ways.

Now, to conclude, where does this discussion leave us with regard to public health policies and considerations?

The link between biomedical research and public health is in forming policies that ultimately result in the reduction of morbidity and mortality through prevention and treatment. The link between biomedical research and education is in providing informed summaries to educational authorities, whose outreach to children is unprecedented in terms of its potential effectiveness. What other civic institution but school has the power to establish policies that reach every boy and girl between the ages of 5 and 17? There is none. So, what might this summary be? It appears that it might be inclusive of the following components.

First, at this point, the genomic priorities for DD are related to *finding* the genes and genetic pathways underlying the biological bases of DD. As compared with research in other developmental disorders, it is quite possible that researchers will discover both rare variants with high level of penetrance (i.e., a high, possibly deterministic, correlation between genetic predisposition and the disorder) and probabilistic genetic risk factors, each of which, in isolation, will be associated with lower individual risk but might be associated with high population risk. Identification of both rare (high individual risk/lower population risk) and common (low individual risk/high population risk) genetic risk factors is very important for two reasons. With regard to rare families in which DD accumulates at high rates and is transmitted from generation to generation, the identification of causal genetic factors segregating in these families will result in the option of informed genetic counseling; the development of drug therapies; and the development of specialized, intensive remediation programs for children who carry these rare genetic variants and for whom this intense education will be delivered, under federal laws and regulation, upon proper diagnoses or screening. With regard to the identification of common genetic risk factors, it is important to understand the extent of their "riskiness" and to determine the environmental forces that are able to diminish the risk. For example, it has been established that for carriers of the ε4 allele, one of the major protective factors against developing Alzheimer's disease is level of education: The more schooling individuals at genetic risk had, the lower their odds ratios were in developing the disease, as compared with risk allele carriers with lower levels of education (Farrer et al., 1997). However, the identification of education as a protective factor became possible only when the risk allele was identified and its impact studied by methods of genetic epidemiology in large, unselected samples of both affected and unaffected individuals. Thus, understanding the genetic machinery underlying biological bases of DD is a *critical*, not optional, step in finding ways to accommodate children in need of services under the Individuals with Disabilities Education Act (IDEA).

Second, this summary should include a comprehensive account of ongoing integration of advances in neuroscience and genetics. Specifically, the majority of neuroscience literature on DD today is focused on discovering and discussing correlates rather than presenting causal pathways (e.g., Price & Mechelli, 2005). Because the brain is an organ whose development and maturation is, at least initially, preprogrammed in genes, understanding the links between brain neuronal pathways, their patterns of activation, and their malleability is as important, if not more important, than understanding the connection between the brain and behavior. As of today, in the field of DD, the ratio of research articles describing studies addressing the gene–brain link and those addressing the brain–behavior link is 0 to many. Clearly, the next step forward should be not in changing "many" to innumerable, but in changing "0" to a positive number.

Finally, and most importantly, it is crucial for educators to understand that our attempt to decode biological bases of DD is aimed at strengthening everyday educational practices. As I hope to have shown throughout this chapter, even under the most liberal estimate, the genetic contribution accounts only for a portion (most likely, the smallest portion) of individual differences in reading. I have also tried to make it clear that environment (described as temperature that changes as part of human emotion, diet that is a part of cultural belonging, oxygen concentration that is an outcome of exercise schedule, and so forth) is a part of any biological function, no matter how conservatively preprogrammed that function is. Despite the amazing advances in human genome research that have unfolded within the last few years, it is unlikely that any radical transformation of medical practices (Varmus, 2002) for either adults and children, or the upbringing and education of children, will take place any time soon, if at all. Thus, the lethal weapon against DD is still the protective environmental factor of good teaching. It is, without a doubt, our most effective public health policy.

ACKNOWLEDGMENTS

Preparation of this chapter was supported by Grant Nos. REC-9979843 from the National Science Foundation; R206R00001 from the Javits Act Program administered by the Institute for Educational Sciences, U.S. Department of Education; and

TW006764 from the National Institutes of Health. Grantees undertaking such projects are encouraged to express freely their professional judgment. This chapter, therefore, does not necessarily represent the position or policies of the National Science Foundation, the Institute for Educational Sciences, or the National Institutes of Health, and no official endorsement should be inferred. I express sincere gratitude to Ms. Robyn Rissman for her editorial assistance and to Mr. Adam Naples for preparing the figures.

NOTES

1. *Difficulty* would be a preferred word here.
2. These estimates are imprecise and are used by the IDA generally. The reference to 15% here is an average of the 12–17% prevalence rate cited above.
3. This definition assumes the primacy of DD as an initial diagnosis. This means that manifested reading difficulties cannot be attributed to other developmental disorders (e.g., autism), but there could be secondary comorbid manifestations of other developmental conditions (e.g., DD is often comanifested with ADHD, dyscalculia, and conduct disorder).
4. EEG: electroencephalogram; ERP: event-related potential; fMRI: functional magnetic resonance imaging; MEG: magnetoencephalography; PET: positron emission tomography; TMS: transcranial magnetic stimulation.
5. Though accurate in terms of broad generalization, this statement should be interpreted differentially with regard to what Price and Mechelli called "the conspicuous absence of brain areas that are dedicated to orthography" (2005, p. 236).
6. To illustrate, spelling and automatization problems are more indicative of DD in German than in English; phonemic awareness deficits are more indicative of DD in English than in German. German and English vary on a number of parameters capturing linguistic diversity, two of which are phonological transparency (i.e., English is more phonologically complex) and morphological richness (i.e., German is more complex morphologically) of language.
7. In opposition to Spearman, Thurstone formulated a model of intelligence centered around "Primary Mental Abilities," which were independent group factors of intelligence that different individuals possessed in varying degrees. Thurstone distinguished seven primary mental abilities: verbal comprehension, verbal fluency, inductive reasoning, spatial visualization, number computation, memory, and perceptual speed.
8. Thompson stated that general intelligence could be thought of as including a large number of independent structural "bonds" (e.g., reflexes, habits, learned associations). Correspondingly, a large number of bonds are activated while a task is performed. When overlapping tasks are performed (e.g., those on an intelligence test), many sets of bonds activated for a given task will overlap as well. This overlap will result in manifested "closeness" captured by a factor analysis. Thus, although a factor analysis might form an impression of a single factor, Thompson argues that the communality among tests cannot be

attributed to a unitary source (e.g., mental energy), but should be attributable to a multiplicity of sources where each source is of relatively small magnitude, but many of the same sources contribute to different tasks in an overlapping manner.

9. http://mathforum.org/dr.math/faq/faq.comb.perm.html.

REFERENCES

Ames, B. N. (2004). A role for supplements in optimizing health: the metabolic tune-up. *Archives of Biochemistry and Biophysics, 423*, 227–234.

Barr, C. L. (2005, June). *Linkage studies of reading disabilities and ADHD in the chromosome 6p and 15q regions*. Paper presented at the annual meeting of the Society for Scientific Studies of Reading, Toronto.

Barr, C. L., & Couto, J. M. (in press). Molecular genetics of reading. In E. L. Grigorenko & A. Naples (Eds.), *Single-word reading: Cognitive, behavioral and biological perspectives*. Mahwah, NJ: Erlbaum.

Blachman, B. A., Schatschneider, C., Fletcher, J. M., Francis, D., Clonan, S. M., Shaywitz, B. A., et al. (2004). Effects of intensive reading remediation for second and third graders and a 1–year follow-up. *Journal of Educational Psychology, 96*, 444–461.

Bornstein, M. H., & Bradley, R. H. (2003). *Socioeconomic status, parenting, and child development*. Mahwah, NJ: Erlbaum.

Byrne, B., Wadsworth, S., Corley, R., Samuelsson, S., Quain, P., DeFries, J. C., et al. (2005). Longitudinal twin study of early literacy development: Preschool and kindergarten phases. *Scientific Studies of Reading, 9*, 219–235.

Cardon, L. R., Smith, S. D., Fulker, D. W., Kimberling, W. J., Pennington, B. F., & DeFries, J. C. (1994). Quantitative trait locus for reading disability on chromosome 6. *Science, 226*, 276–279.

Cardon, L. R., Smith, S. D., Fulker, D. W., Kimberling, W. J., Pennington, B. F., & DeFries, J. C. (1995). Quantitative trait locus for reading disability: Correction. *Science, 268*, 1553.

Catts, H. W., Fey, M. E., & Proctor-Williams, K. (2000). The relationship between language and reading. Preliminary results from a longitudinal investigation. *Logopedics, Phoniatrics, Vocology, 25*, 3–11.

Cope, N., Harold, D., Hill, G., Moskvina, V., Holmans, P., Owen, M. J., et al. (2005). Strong evidence that KIAA0319 on chromosome 6p is a susceptibility gene for developmental dyslexia. *American Journal of Human Genetics, 76*, 581–591.

Cope, N., Hill, G., van den Bree, M., Harold, D., Moskvina, V., Green, E. K., et al. (2004). No support for association between Dyslexia Susceptibility 1 Candidate 1 and developmental dyslexia. *Molecular Psychiatry, 10*, 237–238.

Crichton, M. (2002). *Prey*. New York: HarperCollins.

D'Angiulli, A., Siegel, L. S., & Hertzman, C. (2004). Schooling, socioeconomic context and literacy development. *Educational Psychology, 24*, 867–883.

Eden, G. F., Jones, K. M., Cappell, K., Gareau, L., Wood, F. B., Zeffiro, T. A., et al.

(2004). Neural changes following remediation in adult developmental dyslexia. *Neuron, 44*, 411–422.

Falconer, D. S., & Mackay, T. F. C. (1996). *Introduction to quantitative genetics* (4th ed.). New York: Longman.

Fan, J., & Posner, M. (2004). Human attentional networks. *Psychiatrische Praxis, 31*(Suppl. 2), S210–S214.

Farrer, L. A., Cupples, L. A., Haines, J. L., Hyman, B., Kukull, W. A., Mayeux, R., et al. (1997). Effects of age, sex, and ethnicity on the association between apolipoprotein E genotype and Alzheimer disease: A meta-analysis. APOE and Alzheimer Disease Meta Analysis Consortium. *Journal of the American Medical Association, 278*, 1349–1356.

Feldman, E., Levin, B. E., Lubs, H., Rabin, M., Lubs, M. L., Jallad, B., et al. (1993). Adult familial dyslexia: A retrospective developmental and psychosocial profile. *Journal of Neuropsychiatry and Clinical Neurosciences, 5*, 195–199.

Felton, R. H., Naylor, C. E., & Wood, F. B. (1990). Neuropsychological profile of adult dyslexics. *Brain and Language, 39*, 485–497.

Fiez, J. A. (1997). Phonology, semantics, and the role of the left inferior prefrontal cortex. *Human Brain Mapping, 5*, 79–83.

Fiez, J. A., & Petersen, S. E. (1998). Neuroimaging studies of word reading. *Proceedings of the National Academy of Sciences USA, 95*, 914–921.

Fisher, S. E., & DeFries, J. C. (2002). Developmental dyslexia: Genetic dissection of a complex cognitive trait. *Nature Reviews: Neuroscience, 3*, 767–780.

Francks, C., Paracchini, S., Smith, S. D., Richardson, A. J., Scerri, T. S., Cardon, L. R., et al. (2004). A 77–kilobase region on chromosome 6p22.2 is associated with dyslexia in families from the United Kingdom and from the United States. *American Journal of Human Genetics, 75*, 1046–1058.

Gaillard, W. D., Balsamo, L. M., Ibrahim, Z., Sachs, B. C., & Xu, B. (2003). fMRI identifies regional specialization of neural networks for reading in young children. *Neurology, 60*, 94–100.

Gallagher, A., Frith, U., & Snowling, M. J. (2000). Precursors of literacy delay among children at genetic risk of dyslexia. *Journal of Child Psychology and Psychiatry and Allied Disciplines, 41*, 203–213.

Gayan, J., & Olson, R. K. (2003). Genetic and environmental influences on individual differences in printed word recognition. *Journal of Experimental Child Psychology, 84*, 97–123.

Gottesman, I. I., & Gould, T. D. (2003). The endophenotype concept in psychiatry: Etymology and strategic intentions. *American Journal of Psychiatry, 160*, 636–645.

Gottesman, R. L., Bennett, R. E., Nathan, R. G., & Kelly, M. S. (1996). Inner-city adults with severe reading difficulties: A closer look. *Journal of Learning Disabilities, 29*, 589–597.

Goulandris, N. (Ed.). (2003). *Dyslexia in different languages: Cross-linguistic comparisons*. London: Whurr.

Grigorenko, E. L. (2004). Genetic bases of developmental dyslexia: A capsule review of heritability estimates. *Enfance, 3*, 273–287.

Grigorenko, E. L. (2005). A conservative meta-analysis of linkage and linkage-association studies of developmental dyslexia. *Scientific Studies of Reading, 9,* 285–316.

Grigorenko, E. L., Ngorosho, D., Jukes, M., & Bundy, D. (2006). Reading in able and disabled readers from around the world: Same or different? An illustration from a study of reading-related processes in a Swahili sample of siblings. *Journal of Research in Reading, 29,* 104–123.

Grigorenko, E. L., Wood, F. B., Meyer, M. S., Hart, L. A., Speed, W. C., Shuster, A., et al. (1997). Susceptibility loci for distinct components of developmental dyslexia on chromosomes 6 and 15. *American Journal of Human Genetics, 60,* 27–39.

Grigorenko, E. L., Wood, F. B., Meyer, M. S., & Pauls, D. L. (2000). Chromosome 6p influences on different dyslexia-related cognitive processes: Further confirmation. *American Journal of Human Genetics, 66,* 715–723.

Hannula-Jouppi, K., Kaminen-Ahola, N., Taipale, M., Eklund, R., Nopola-Hemmi, J., Käänäinen, H., et al. (2005). The axon guidance receptor gene *ROEO1* is a candidate gene for developmental dyslexia. *PLoS Genetics, 1*(4), e50.

Harlaar, N., Spinath, F. M., Dale, P. S., & Plomin, R. (2005). Genetic influences on early word recognition abilities and disabilities: A study of 7–year-old twins. *Journal of Child Psychology and Psychiatry, 46,* 373–384.

Harm, M. W., & Seidenberg, M. S. (2004). Computing the meanings of words in reading: Cooperative division of labor between visual and phonological processes. *Psychological Review, 111,* 662–720.

Hohnen, B., & Stevenson, J. (1999). The structure of genetic influences on general cognitive, language, phonological, and reading abilities. *Developmental Psychology, 35,* 590–603.

Kamhi, A. G., & Laing, S. P. (2001). The path to reading success or failure: A choice for the new millennium. In J. L. Harris, A. G. Kamhi, & K. E. Pollock (Eds.), *Literacy in African American communities* (pp. 127–145). Mahwah, NJ: Erlbaum.

Karasik, D., Myers, R. H., Cupples, L. A., Hannan, M. T., Gagnon, D. R., Herbert, A., et al. (2002). Genome screen for quantitative trait loci contributing to normal variation in bone mineral density: The Framingham Study. *Journal of Bone and Mineral Research, 17,* 1718–1727.

Karmiloff-Smith, A. (1998). Development itself is the key to understanding developmental disorders. *Trends in Cognitive Sciences, 2,* 389–398.

Kelman, M., & Lester, G. (1998). *Jumping the queue: An inquiry into the legal treatment of students with learning disabilities.* Cambridge, MA: Harvard University Press.

Li, Y., Hou, M. J., Ma, J., Tang, Z. H., Zhu, H. L., & Ling, W. H. (2005). Dietary fatty acids regulate cholesterol induction of liver CYP7alpha1 expression and bile acid production. *Lipids, 40,* 455–462.

Livingstone, M. S., Rosen, G. D., Drislane, F. W., & Galaburda, A. M. (1991). Physiological and anatomical evidence for a magnocellular defect in developmental dyslexia. *Proceedings of the National Academy of Sciences USA, 88,* 7943–7947.

Lovegrove, W. J., Bowling, A., Badcock, D., & Blackwood, M. (1980). Specific reading disability: Differences in contrast sensitivity as a function of spatial frequency. *Science, 210,* 439–440.

Lyon, G. R., Shaywitz, S. E., & Shaywitz, B. A. (2003). A definition of dyslexia. *Annals of Dyslexia, 53,* 1–14.

Lyytinen, P., Poikkeus, A. M., Laakso, M. L., Eklund, K., & Lyytinen, H. (2001). Language development and symbolic play in children with and without familial risk for dyslexia. *Journal of Speech Language and Hearing Research, 44,* 873–885.

Marino, C., Giorda, R., Vanzin, L., Nobile, M., Lorusso, M. L., Baschirotto, C., et al. (2004). A locus on 15q15–15qter influences dyslexia: Further support from a transmission/disequilibrium study in an Italian speaking population. *Journal of Medical Genetics, 41,* 42–48.

Marlow, A. J., Fisher, S. E., Francks, C., MacPhie, I. L., Cherny, S. S., Richardson, A. J., et al. (2003). Use of multivariate linkage analysis for dissection of a complex cognitive trait. *American Journal of Human Genetics, 72,* 561–570.

Mechelli, A., Gorno-Tempini, M. L., & Price, C. J. (2003). Neuroimaging studies of word and pseudoword reading: Consistencies, inconsistencies, and limitations. *Journal of Cognitive Neuroscience, 15,* 260–271.

Meng, H., Smith, S. D., Hager, K., Held, M., Liu, J., Olson, R. K., et al. (2005). DCDC2 is associated with reading disability and modulates neuronal development in the brain. *Proceedings of the National Academy of Sciences USA, 102,* 17053–17058.

Merikangas, K. R., & Risch, N. (2003). Genomic priorities and public health. *Science, 302,* 599–601.

Monteiro, C. A., Moura, E. C., Conde, W. L., & Popkin, B. M. (2004). Socioeconomic status and obesity in adult populations of developing countries: A review. *Bulletin of the World Health Organization, 82,* 940–946.

Morris, D. W., Robinson, L., Turic, D., Duke, M., Webb, V., Milham, C., et al. (2000). Family-based association mapping provides evidence for a gene for reading disability on chromosome 15q. *Human Molecular Genetics, 9,* 843–848.

Morton, J., & Frith, U. (1995). Causal modeling: A structural approach to developmental psychopathology. In D. Cicchetti & D. J. Cohen (Eds.), *Developmental psychopathology* (Vol. 2, pp. 357–390). New York: Wiley.

Nicholson, T. (1997). Social class and reading achievement: Sociology meets psychology. *New Zealand Journal of Educational Studies, 32,* 105–108.

Nicolson, R. I., & Fawcett, A. J. (1990). Automaticity: A new framework for dyslexia research? *Cognition, 35,* 159–182.

Nicolson, R. I., Fawcett, A. J., & Dean, P. (2001). Developmental dyslexia: The cerebellar deficit hypothesis. *Trends in Neurosciences, 24,* 508–511.

Noble, K. G., McCandliss, B. D., & Farah, M. (in press). Socioeconomic gradients predict individual differences in neurocognitive abilities. *Developmental Science.*

Paulesu, E., Demonet, J. F., Fazio, F., McCrory, E., Chanoine, V., Brunswick, N., et al. (2001). Dyslexia: Cultural diversity and biological unity. *Science, 291,* 2165–2167.

Pennington, B. F. (2002). *The development of psychopathology: Nature and nurture.* New York: Guildford Press.

Pennington, B. F., & Lefly, D. L. (2001). Early reading development in children at family risk for dyslexia. *Child Development, 72,* 816–833.

Petersen, S. E., Fox, P. T., Posner, M. I., Mintun, M., & Raichle, M. E. (1988). Positron emission tomographic studies of the cortical anatomy of single-word processing. *Nature, 331,* 585–589.

Plomin, R., & Kovas, Y. (2005). Generalist genes and learning disabilities. *Psychological Bulletin, 131,* 592–617.

Poldrack, R. A., Wagner, A. D., Prull, M. W., Desmond, J. E., Glover, G. H., & Gabrieli, J. D. (1999). Functional specialization for semantic and phonological processing in the left inferior prefrontal cortex. *NeuroImage, 10,* 15–35.

Price, C. J., & Mechelli, A. (2005). Reading and reading disturbance. *Current Opinion in Neurobiology, 15,* 231–238.

Price, C. J., Wise, R. J., & Frackowiak, R. S. (1996). Demonstrating the implicit processing of visually presented words and pseudowords. *Cerebral Cortex, 6,* 62–70.

Pugh, K. R., Mencl, W. E., Jenner, A. R., Katz, L., Frost, S. J., Lee, J. R., et al. (2001). Neurobiological studies of reading and reading disability. *Journal of Communication Disorders, 34,* 479–492.

Pugh, K. R., Shaywitz, B. A., Shaywitz, S. E., Constable, R. T., Skudlarski, P., Fulbright, R. K., et al. (1996). Cerebral organization of component processes in reading. *Brain, 119,* 1221–1238.

Ramus, F. (2003). Developmental dyslexia: Specific phonological deficits or general sensorimotor dysfunction? *Current Opinion in Neurology, 13,* 212–218.

Reed, D. R., Nanthakumar, E., North, M., Bell, C., & Price, R. A. (2001). A genome-wide scan suggests a locus on chromosome 1q21–q23 contributes to normal variation in plasma cholesterol concentration. *Journal of Molecular Medicine, 79,* 262–269.

Sameroff, A. J., & Mackenzie, M. J. (2003). Research strategies for capturing transactional models of development: The limits of the possible. *Development and Psychopathology, 15,* 613–640.

Scarborough, H. S. (1991). Antecedents to reading disability: Preschool language development and literacy experiences of children from dyslexic families. *Reading and Writing: An Interdisciplinary Journal, 3,* 219–233.

Scerri, T. S., Fisher, S. E., Francks, C., MacPhie, I. L., Paracchini, S., Richardson, A. J., et al. (2004). Putative functional alleles of DYX1C1 are not associated with dyslexia susceptibility in a large sample of sibling pairs from the UK. *Journal of Medical Genetics, 41,* 853–857.

Schulte-Körne, G., Grimm, T., Nöthen, M. M., Müller-Myhsok, B., Cichon, S., Vogt, I. R., et al. (1998). Evidence for linkage of spelling disability to chromosome 15. *American Journal of Human Genetics, 63,* 279–282.

Schumacher, J., Anthioni, H., Dahdouh, F., Konig, I. R., Hillmer, H. M., Kluck, N., et al. . (2006). Strong evidence of DCDC2 as a susceptibility gene for dyslexia. *American Journal of Human Genetics, 78,* 52–62.

Shaywitz, S. E., & Shaywitz, B. A. (2005). Dyslexia (specific reading disability). *Biological Psychiatry, 57*, 1301–1309.

Simos, P. G., Billingsley-Marshall, B., Sarkari, S., & Papanicolaou, A. C. (in press). Single-word reading: Perspectives from magnetic source imaging. In E. L. Grigorenko & A. Naples (Eds.), *Single-word reading*. Mahwah, NJ: Erlbaum.

Sing, C. F., & Reilly, S. L. (1993). Genetics of common diseases that aggregate, but do not segregate in families. In C. L. Harris (Ed.), *Genetics of cellular, individual family and population variability* (pp. 140–161). New York: Oxford University Press.

Smith, S. D., Kimberling, W. J., Pennington, B. F., & Lubs, H. A. (1983). Specific reading disability: Identification of an inherited form through linkage analyses. *Science, 219*, 1345–1347.

Snowling, M. J. (1996). Contemporary approaches to the teaching of reading. *Journal of Child Psychology and Psychiatry, 37*, 139–148.

Snowling, M. J., Bishop, D. V., & Stothard, S. E. (2000). Is preschool language impairment a risk factor for dyslexia in adolescence? *Journal of Child Psychology and Psychiatry, 41*, 587–600.

Snowling, M. J., Gallagher, A., & Frith, U. (2003). Family risk of dyslexia is continuous: Individual differences in the precursors of reading skill. *Child Development, 74*, 358–373.

Snyder, A. Z., Abdullaev, Y. G., Posner, M. I., & Raichle, M. E. (1995). Scalp electrical potentials reflect regional cerebral blood flow responses during processing of written words. *Proceedings of the National Academy of Sciences USA, 92*, 1689–1693.

Spearman, C. (1927). *The abilities of man*. New York: Macmillan.

Stein, J. (2001). The magnocellular theory of developmental dyslexia. *Dyslexia: The Journal of the British Dyslexia Association, 7*, 12–36.

Stevenson, J., Graham, P., Fredman, G., & McLoughlin, V. (1987). A twin study of genetic influences on reading and spelling ability and disability. *Journal of Child Psychology and Psychiatry, 28*, 229–247.

Tagamets, M. A., Novick, J. M., Chalmers, M. L., & Friedman, R. B. (2000). A parametric approach to orthographic processing in the brain: An fMRI study. *Journal of Cognitive Neuroscience, 12*, 281–297.

Taipale, M., Kaminen, N., Nopola-Hemmi, J., Haltia, T., Myllyluoma, B., Lyytinen, H., et al. (2003). A candidate gene for developmental dyslexia encodes a nuclear tetratricopeptide repeat domain protein dynamically regulated in brain. *Proceedings of the National Academy of Sciences USA, 20*, 11553–11558.

Tallal, P. (1980). Auditory temporal perception, phonics, and reading disabilities in children. *Brain and Language, 9*, 182–198.

Tallal, P., Miller, S., & Fitch, R. H. (1993). Neurobiological basis of speech: A case for the preeminence of temporal processing. *Annals of the New York Academy of Science, 682*, 27–47.

Thompson, G. (1994). Identifying complex disease genes: Progress and paradigms. *Nature Genetics, 8*, 108–110.

Thompson, G. H. (1939). *The factorial analysis of human ability.* London: University of London Press.

Thurstone, L. L. (1938). *Primary mental abilities.* Chicago: University of Chicago Press.

Turkeltaub, P. E., Eden, G. F., Jones, K. M., & Zeffiro, T. A. (2002). Meta-analysis of the functional neuroanatomy of single-word reading: Method and validation. *NeuroImage, 16,* 765–780.

Turkeltaub, P. E., Gareau, L., Flowers, D. L., Zeffiro, T. A., & Eden, G. F. (2003). Development of neural mechanisms for reading. *Nature Neuroscience, 6,* 767–773.

van Alphen, P., de Bree, E., Gerrits, E., de Jong, J., Wilsenach, C., & Wijnen, F. (2004). Early language development in children with a genetic risk of dyslexia. *Dyslexia: The Journal of the British Dyslexia Association, 10,* 265–288.

Varmus, H. (2002). Getting ready for gene-based medicine. *New England Journal of Medicine, 347,* 1526–1527.

Vellutino, F. R., Fletcher, J. M., Snowling, M. J., & Scanlon, D. M. (2004). Specific reading disability (dyslexia): What have we learned in the past four decades? *Journal of Child Psychology and Psychiatry and Allied Disciplines, 45,* 2–40.

Wagner, R. K., Torgesen, J. K., & Rashotte, C. A. (1994). Development of reading-related phonological processing abilities: New evidence of bidirectional causality from a latent variable longitudinal study. *Developmental Psychology, 30,* 73–87.

Wigg, K. G., Couto, J. M., Feng, Y., Anderson, B., Cate-Carter, T. D., Macciardi, F., et al. (2004). Support for EKN1 as the susceptibility locus for dyslexia on 15q21. *Molecular Psychiatry, 9,* 1111–1121.

Wijsman, E. M., Peterson, D., Leutenegger, A. L., Thomson, J. B., Goddard, K. A. B., Hsu, L., et al. (2000). Segregation analysis of phenotypic components of learning disabilities: I. Nonword memory and digit span. *American Journal of Human Genetics, 67,* 631–646.

Wolff, P. H., & Melngailis, I. (1994). Family patterns of developmental dyslexia. *American Journal of Medical Genetics (Neuropsychiatric Genetics), 54,* 122–131.

Ziegler, A., Konig, I. R., Deimel, W., Plume, E., Nothen, M. M., Propping, P., et al. (2005). Developmental dyslexia: Recurrence risk estimates from a German bi-center study using the single proband sib pair design. *Human Heredity, 59,* 136–143.

CHAPTER 6

Typical Reading Development and Developmental Dyslexia across Languages

Usha Goswami

The best predictor that we have of how well children will learn to read and write their language is their ability to detect and manipulate component sounds in words, called "phonological awareness." Furthermore, children who have specific problems in detecting and manipulating the speech sounds of language (phonology) are usually at risk for developmental dyslexia. The component sounds of language can be defined at a number of different linguistic levels, for example, syllables versus rhymes. Having a specific problem with phonology appears to be heritable (e.g., Fisher & DeFries, 2002; see also Grigorenko, Chapter 5, this volume) and can be measured long before reading tuition commences (e.g., Lundberg, Olofsson, & Wall, 1980; Schneider, Roth, & Ennemoser, 2000; see also Molfese et al., Chapter 8, this volume). However, there are systematic differences in the way that the orthographies of the world represent the sound patterns of the world's languages. Accordingly, there are systematic differences in the course of reading development and in the manifestation of developmental dyslexia (see Ziegler & Goswami, 2005). In some of the world's languages, developmental dyslexia was believed to be nonexistent (e.g., Makita, 1968, for Chinese). This hope has turned out to be misplaced. Developmental dyslexia has been found in all of the world's orthographies in which systematic studies have been done. Just as phonological awareness predicts reading acquisition across orthographies, an insensitivity to phonological structure is associated with developmental dyslexia across orthographies. This finding is not particularly surprising if it is remembered that the brain evolved for language, not for reading. The act of reading is the comprehension of speech written down. Hence, broadly speaking, biological unity for literacy would be expected across languages.

I argue here that data on literacy acquisition and dyslexia from different languages can be described theoretically by a "psycholinguistic grain-size" framework (see Goswami, Ziegler, Dalton, & Schneider, 2001, 2003; Ziegler & Goswami, 2005). According to this framework, the sequence of phonological development is essentially universal across languages. However, the ways in which sounds are mapped to letters (or other orthographic symbols) appears to be language-specific. In particular, solutions to the "mapping problem" of how sounds are related to symbols differ with orthographic consistency. When orthographies allow 1:1 mappings between symbols and sounds (e.g., as in Italian, a transparent or consistent orthography), children learn to read relatively quickly. When orthographies have a many:1 mapping between sound and symbol (*feedback* inconsistency, e.g., as in French, consider *pain/fin/hein*) or between symbol and sound (*feedforward* inconsistency, e.g., as in English, *cough/rough/bough*), children learn to read more slowly. French and English are examples of inconsistent (nontransparent) orthographies. Nevertheless, despite some language-specific differences in the strategies developed for reading, all children learn to read by creating mappings between sound and print. The idea that children can learn to read "visually," using rote visual memorization of all the printed words making up a language, has been shown to be characteristic of no language in the world.

In applying the psycholinguistic grain-size framework to developmental dyslexia, it is important to point out that this developmental disorder is quite different from the acquired dyslexias. This difference means that the theoretical frameworks that are useful in adult neuropsychology are unlikely to be of similar value in explaining development (e.g., Bishop, 1997; Goswami, 2003; Karmiloff-Smith, 1998). Adults with acquired dyslexias have usually suffered a neural insult, such as a stroke, which has affected the *developed* system. The developed system is the *end-state* of development. Analyses of this end-state may not be able to tell us anything about how the system evolved. In fact, most models of the acquired dyslexias are based on theoretical frameworks that assume modularity. Subtyping is popular, with characteristic patterns of deficit being observed following lesions in particular locations (e.g., a relatively pure problem with phonological processing, "phonological dyslexia," vs. a relatively pure problem with orthographic processing, "surface dyslexia"). Developmentally, a child cannot choose to learn to read either "phonologically" or "orthographically." There is no good evidence for subtyping in developmental dyslexia if stringent research designs are used (see Ziegler & Goswami, 2005). Rather, all developmental dyslexia appears to be phonological in origin. Children with developmental dyslexia have difficulties with sublexical phonology. They find it difficult to detect and manipulate units of sound at the subword level.

THE DEVELOPMENTAL TRAJECTORY OF PHONOLOGICAL AWARENESS ACROSS LANGUAGES

Phonological awareness is usually measured at three linguistic levels, which are hierarchically related. Children can become aware that (1) words can be broken down into *syllables* (e.g., two syllables in *window,* three syllables in *popsicle*); (2) syllables can be broken down into *onset-rime* units (to divide a syllable into onset and rime, divide at the vowel, as in *t-each* and *sp-eech*); and (3) onsets and rimes can be broken down into sequences of *phonemes*. Phonemes can be defined as the smallest speech sounds making up words, and for many languages phonemes correspond to the sounds made by alphabetic letters. Linguistically, phonemes are a relatively abstract concept and are defined in terms of sound substitutions that change meaning. For example, *pin* and *pit* differ in terms of their final phoneme, and *pin* and *pan* differ in terms of their medial phoneme. Children seem to learn about phonemes by learning about letters. Although letters are used to symbolize phonemes, the physical sounds corresponding to the same letter can be rather different. An example is the *p* in *pit, lap,* and *spoon.* As children learn the conventions of the spelling system of their language, they stop noticing these physical differences. To a prereading child, however, the sounds at the beginning of *chair* and *train* are more similar than the sounds at the beginning of *train* and *tip* (Read, 1986).

The development of phonological awareness appears to follow a similar trajectory across languages. Studies of preschoolers are particularly valuable, because phonological skills can be measured independently of literacy. For example, a 3-year-old can be asked to correct speech errors made by a hand puppet (*sie* for *pie*), to complete nursery rhymes ("Jack and Jill went up the—[hill]"), or to select the odd word out of a group of three rhyming words (oddity detection: cat, *pit*, fat; see Bradley & Bryant, 1983; Bryant, Bradley, Maclean, & Crosland, 1989; Chaney, 1992; Ho &

Bryant, 1997b). Individual differences in these different phonological awareness tasks are usually connected to individual differences in reading.

Cross-language studies reveal a language-invariant sequence in the development of phonological awareness. Children in all languages so far studied appear to become aware of "large" units of sound within words first. These units are the syllable, onset, and rime. The linguistic term *rime* is distinct from *rhyme* and is used because a multisyllabic word has many rimes. Although "mountain" and "captain" share the rime of the final syllable, they do not rhyme. A word such as *conversation* has four rimes (approximately corresponding to the sounds *on*, *er*, *ay*, *un*). The hierarchical structure of the syllable is shown in Figure 6.1.

Although studies of phonological awareness across languages reveal the universal emergence of large units first, the emergence of awareness of small units (phonemes) varies dramatically with language. Illiterate adults perform poorly in tasks requiring them to manipulate or detect single phonemes in all languages (e.g., Goswami & Bryant, 1990; Morais, Cary, Alegria, & Bertelson, 1979). However, children acquire phonemic awareness much faster in some languages than in others. Children learning transparent orthographies such as Turkish, Finnish, Greek, and Italian acquire phonemic awareness relatively quickly. Children learning nontransparent orthographies such as English, Danish, French, and Portuguese take much longer to acquire phonemic awareness. There seem to be two key factors that explain these cross-language differences. One is the phonological complexity of the spoken language; the other is the orthographic consistency of the written language.

Phonemic awareness usually emerges fairly rapidly in languages with consistent orthographies, and in languages that have a simple syllable structure (languages based on CV syllables are considered to have a simple structure, C = consonant, V = vowel). Most of the world's languages use a simple syllable structure. In these languages, the child has an advantage, because onset-rime units (which depend on dividing the syllable at the vowel, yielding C-V) and phonemes (which are also the C and the V) are equivalent. Consider Italian and Spanish as an example. Here, the onset-rime segmentation for the words *casa* and *mama* (a segmentation available

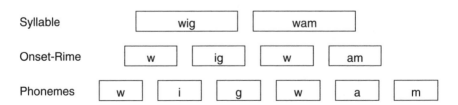

FIGURE 6.1. The hierarchical structure of the syllable.

prior to literacy) is /c/ /A/ /s/ /A/ and /m/ /A/ /m/ /A/. This is equivalent to segmenting these words into phonemes. For CVCV words, the onset-rime segmentation and the phonemic segmentation are equivalent. Now consider the fact that in both Spanish and Italian there is a 1:1 mapping between print and sound. One letter consistently maps to one phoneme. Many of these phonemes are already represented in the child's spoken lexicon of word forms, because they are also onsets and rimes (as in the examples of *casa* and *mama*). The extra advantage is obvious. Children who are learning to read consistent alphabetic orthographies such as Italian and Spanish can solve the "mapping problem" of mapping units of print (letters) to units of sound (phonemes) with relatively little effort. Most of the sounds that they need are already represented in the spoken lexicon via onset-rime segmentation. All of the letters that they meet will map onto only one of these sounds. The learning problem is simplified considerably.

The learning problem becomes more difficult if the spoken language has a more complex syllable structure. An example is German. German has some CV syllables, but it also has CVC syllables, CCVC syllables, and CVCC syllables (it even allows CCC clusters, as in *Pflaum* and *Strasse*). For most syllables in German, onset-rime segmentation will not be equivalent to phonemic segmentation. However, although the phonology is complex, the orthography is consistent. One letter maps to one and only one phoneme. This helps the German child to acquire phonemic awareness. Letters are a reliable clue to phonemes, and so despite the multiple consonant clusters, the German child is still at an advantage.

The child who is faced with the most difficult mapping problem is the child learning to read an orthographically inconsistent language that also has a complex syllable structure. Examples include English, French, Danish, and Portuguese. Like German, English allows CCC clusters (*string, sprain, split*). Some English syllables are CV (about 5%, think of *yoyo* and *cocoa*), but most are CVC, CCVC, or CVCC (see De Cara & Goswami, 2002). Hence, onset-rime segmentation is rarely equivalent to phonemic segmentation. English also has a relatively large number of monosyllables (around 4,000, whereas German has about 1,400 in comparison). In English, one letter may map to as many as five or more phonemes (e.g., the letter *a* maps to different vowel sounds in *cat, car, cake,* and *call*). Given this analysis, it is unsurprising to find that phonemic awareness develops relatively slowly in English-speaking children. The rate at which children learning to read different languages develop phonemic awareness can be measured by phoneme counting studies. A selection of studies carried out in different languages is summarized in Table 6.1.

What happens in nonalphabetic languages? The best-studied nonalphabetic language is Chinese. Chinese has a simple phonological structure with mainly CV syllables but includes some nasal codas (such as *n* and

TABLE 6.1. Data (% Correct) from Studies
Comparing Phoneme Counting in Different
Languages in Kindergarten or Early Grade 1

Language	% phonemes counted correctly
Greek[1]	98
Turkish[2]	94
Italian[3]	97
Norwegian[4]	83
German[5]	81
French[6]	73
English[7]	70
English[8]	71
English[9]	65

Note. 1 = Harris and Giannoulis (1999); 2 = Durgunoglu and
Oney (1999); 3 = Cossu, Shankweiler, Liberman, Katz, and Tola
(1988); 4 = Hoien, Lundberg, Stanovich, and Bjaalid (1995); 5 =
Wimmer, Landerl, Linortner, and Hummer (1991); 6 = Demont
and Gombert (1996); 7 = Liberman, Shankweiler, Fischer, and
Carter (1974); 8 = Tunmer and Nesdale (1985); 9 = Perfetti, Beck,
Bell, and Hughes (1987) and grade 2 children.

ng). The entire syllabary can be described using 22 onsets and 37 rimes (see
Siok & Fletcher, 2001). Studies suggest that Chinese preschoolers develop
good onset-rime level skills before entering school. For example, using a
Chinese version of the oddity task (cat, *pit*, fat) pioneered by Bradley and
Bryant (1983), Ho and Bryant (1997b) reported that Chinese 3-year-olds
attained high levels of performance (68% correct). Phonemic awareness
would seem unlikely to develop in Chinese-speaking children because they
are learning a character-based script. However, this is not the case. Chinese
has two instructional systems for teaching children the sounds of the characters, and both of these systems operate at an onset-rime level. They are
called Pinyin (used in mainland China), and Zhu-Yin-Fu-Hao (used in Taiwan). Pinyin uses the alphabet to represent the component sounds in syllables, whereas Zhuyin uses simple characters. Because most Chinese syllables have a CV structure, these instructional systems effectively teach
children correspondences for the phonemes in the syllables. Accordingly,
Chinese children growing up in Mainland China and in Taiwan perform
well in phonemic awareness tasks (Siok & Fletcher, 2001; Huang &
Hanley, 1994). However, Chinese children growing up in Hong Kong, who
learn the Chinese characters by rote and are not taught Pinyin or Zhuyin,
show very poor phonemic awareness (Huang & Hanley, 1994).

THE TRAJECTORY OF READING ACQUISITION ACROSS LANGUAGES

Grapheme–phoneme recoding skills develop in tandem with phonemic awareness. As might be expected, therefore, children learning to read different languages also develop grapheme–phoneme recoding skills at different rates. A comprehensive cross-language comparison of grapheme–phoneme recoding skills during the first year of acquisition was conducted by the European Concerted Action on Learning Disorders as a Barrier to Human Development. As part of this action, participating scientists from 14 European Community (EC) countries developed a matched set of items of simple real words and nonwords suitable for first-grade readers. The real and nonword items were then given to children from each country during their first year of reading instruction (see Seymour, Aro, & Erskine, 2003). Because children in different EC countries begin school at different ages, the children varied in age at the time of testing. However, they were equated for degree of reading instruction across orthography, because they were all tested at the same time point midway through their first year at school. The methods of reading instruction used by participating schools in the different countries could not be equated exactly; however, the schools were chosen so that all children were experiencing phoneme-level "phonics" teaching (including those children who were learning to read the more inconsistent orthographies). The data from this study for monosyllables are shown in Table 6.2.

The table is arranged so that the languages are listed from most to least orthographic consistency. This makes it easy to see that the children who were acquiring reading in the orthographically consistent EC languages (Greek, Finnish, German, Italian, Spanish) were those performing close to ceiling. This performance was true for both word and nonword reading. The children doing less well were those learning to read Danish (71% correct), Portuguese (73% correct), and French (79% correct). However, although grapheme–phoneme recoding skills were less accurate in these orthographies, the reduced levels of accuracy are in line with the reduced orthographic consistency of these languages. Danish is relatively inconsistent for reading (Elbro & Pallesen, 2002), whereas Portuguese and French are relatively inconsistent for spelling (Defior, Martos, & Cary, 2002; Ventura, Morais, Pattamadilok, & Kolinsky, 2004; Ziegler, Jacobs, & Stone, 1996). The children who were performing most poorly were those learning to read in English (34% correct). These children were retested a year later, following an extra year of phonics-based literacy instruction, and they still performed below children reading the other languages. However, this relatively poor performance would be predicted by

TABLE 6.2. Data (% Correct) from the COST A8 Study
of Grapheme–Phoneme Recoding Skills
for Monosyllables in 14 European Languages

Language	Familiar real words	Nonwords
Greek	98	97
Finnish	98	98
German	98	98
Austrian German	97	97
Italian	95	92
Spanish	95	93
Swedish	95	91
Dutch	95	90
Icelandic	94	91
Norwegian	92	93
French	79	88
Portuguese	73	76
Danish	71	63
Scottish English	34	41

Note. Data from Seymour, Aro, and Erskine (2003).

the bidirectional inconsistency of English (severe inconsistency in *both* reading and spelling; see Ziegler, Stone, & Jacobs, 1997). The English children face the most difficult learning problem. They are trying to learn correspondences for phonemes embedded in complex syllables, and the correspondences are not predictable (English does not follow a system of 1:1 mappings). On this analysis, it is not so surprising that the English children were lagging behind their European peers.

In order to be sure that differences between languages are due to the orthography rather than other factors, such as the particular words that the children had to read, it is necessary to run controlled experimental studies. A particularly helpful set of studies comparing English and German was carried out by Frith, Wimmer, and Landerl (1998). They studied nonword reading in German and English 7-, 8-, and 9-year-old children. The language comparison between German and English is ideal for matching items, because both languages have similar orthography and phonology. For example, words such as *ball, park,* and *hand* are identical in both languages. The difference is in the consistency of the spelling-to-sound correspondences. All three words in German have the same pronunciation for the grapheme *a*. However, this same grapheme has a *different* pronunciation in each word in English. If orthographic consistency affects the development of grapheme–phoneme recoding strategies, then English children at the same stage of reading development should be less efficient at recoding nonwords that include graphemes such as *a* compared to German children.

To test this idea, Frith and colleagues (1998) gave English and German children identical nonwords to read (such as *grall*). They found that the German children's nonword reading was close to ceiling after only 1 year of reading instruction. In contrast, the English children showed much lower reading accuracy. They did not approach ceiling levels of performance until they had been learning to read for at least 3 years. For nonwords such as *grall*, the 7-year-old English readers made errors in the region of 55%, compared to 15% for the German readers. In both language groups, performance improved with age, but differences between the languages were still strong at age 9. A significant difference in nonword reading was even found when the cross-language comparison was restricted to those German and English children whose word reading performance was 100% correct for analogous items (real words such as *ball*). The selected German children made only 8% errors with nonwords based on these real words (*grall-ball*), whereas the selected English-speaking children made 22% errors (for similar results in comparisons of English and German, see also Wimmer & Goswami, 1994; Wimmer & Hummer, 1990).

It might be objected that comparisons between English and German children cannot rule out cultural or social factors that might differ between the two countries, which in themselves might affect reading acquisition. One way around this objection is to design experimental comparisons of reading development in Welsh-speaking versus English-speaking children living in Wales. Welsh is a highly consistent orthography. In Wales, the same school districts include schools that teach in Welsh and schools that teach in English. The children attending these schools come from the same catchment areas and follow the same curricula (e.g., Hanley, Masterson, Spencer, & Evans, 2004; Spencer & Hanley, 2003; see also Ellis & Hooper, 2001). The only difference is the language of instruction (it is important to note that phonotactic complexity is similar in English and Welsh). Hanley and his colleagues have followed a group of Welsh-speaking children who were learning to read Welsh and a matched group of English-speaking children living in the same area of Wales who were learning to read English since they were 5 years old. By the age of 11, Hanley and his colleagues found that the groups of children were comparable in tests of single-word reading in their native languages and in nonword reading. However, in all previous comparisons the English children had performed more poorly than their Welsh peers, at each test point, demonstrating slower reading acquisition. The English children had also been slower to acquire phonemic awareness.

Clearly, therefore, grapheme–phoneme recoding skills develop more slowly in children learning to read English, and in large part this slow rate is due to the inconsistency of the orthography. However, although the English orthography is maximally inconsistent at the "small" grain size of the phoneme, it is less inconsistent at the larger grain size of the rime (Treiman, Mullennix, Bijeljac-Babic, & Richmond-Welty, 1995). Treiman and colleagues (1995) analyzed the spelling–sound correspondences of all the monosyllables of English at both the C-V-C level and also at the larger grain sizes of C-VC and CV-C. For English vowels, Treiman and her colleagues found that consistency in pronunciation across words was around 50%. For example, if a child met the vowel *a* in the word *cat* (or the like), the chances that the next word containing an *a* had the same grapheme–phoneme correspondence was 51%. In contrast, if the child noticed the spelling–sound correspondence for the entire rime, then consistency increased to 77%. Most words that share rime spellings have consistent pronunciations for the rime (e.g., *cat*, *hat*, *mat*), although not all of them (e.g., *ball*, *shall*). Average consistency is 77%, which is an improvement on the 51% yielded by a C-V-C analysis that treats the vowel as a unit independent of the coda (the final consonant phoneme is called the coda). Attaching the vowel to the onset phoneme did not improve consistency. The consistency of pronunciation for CV units (*cat*, *cab*, *car*) was only 52%.

These analyses of orthographic consistency make it likely that English children need to develop phonological recoding strategies at more than one grain size in order to become competent readers. They need to develop efficient grapheme–phoneme recoding strategies, but they also need to develop "rhyme analogy" strategies to take advantage of spelling–sound consistency at the large-unit level of the rime. Children learning to read English do indeed use rhyme analogy strategies (making connections between spelling patterns in analogous words such as *beak* and *peak*), and this use has been shown by a variety of experimental techniques, including making analogies from clue words (Goswami, 1986, 1988), reading pseudo-homophones (Goswami et al., 2001), and comparing the decoding of large-unit versus small-unit nonwords (Goswami et al., 2003). Brown and Deavers (1999) have suggested that children learning to read in English adopt "flexible unit size" strategies. Nevertheless, it is important to point out that there are more orthographic units to learn when the grain size is big than when the grain size is small. For example, in order to decode the most frequent 3,000 monosyllabic English words at the level of the rime, a child needs to learn mappings between approximately 600 different orthographic patterns and 400 phonological rimes. In addition, English-speaking children need to develop whole-word recognition strategies to supplement rhyme analogies and grapheme–phoneme recoding. Some spelling patterns in English are unique (e.g., *choir*, *people*). These patterns must be learned holistically, using "look and say" methods.

Finally, the role of visual skills in learning to read logographic orthographies should be mentioned. Logographies such as Chinese and Japanese usually depend on visually distinctive symbols that are created from the same basic elements (e.g., horizontal strokes versus vertical strokes). Chinese characters are quite visually complex and therefore require fine-grained visual analysis and storage. Surprisingly, perhaps, individual differences in visual processing only make a difference to learning during the first year of reading acquisition (e.g., Siok & Fletcher, 2001). It is phonological awareness rather than visual processing skills that predicts reading development in Chinese. This finding has been replicated with a wide range of visual tasks. For example, individual differences in the ability to recall abstract designs over short periods of time, to discriminate visual forms, to detect the odd design out of three abstract spatial designs presented in different orientations, and to learn visual paired associates are not related to reading acquisition in Chinese (Ho, 1997; Ho & Bryant 1997a; Huang & Hanley, 1994, 1997).

DEVELOPMENTAL DYSLEXIA IN CHILDREN ACROSS LANGUAGES

If we now turn to consider dyslexia, we find analogous cross-language differences in the manifestation (but not in the incidence) of developmental reading problems. In all languages so far studied, children with developmental dyslexia show deficits in phonological awareness. They are poor at performing tasks such as the oddity task and phoneme counting, they have difficulties with short-term (phonological) memory, and they are significantly slower in producing highly familiar words under timed conditions (e.g., in rapidly naming colors, called rapid automatized naming, or RAN). The deficit in phonological awareness can be measured at the linguistic levels of syllable, onset-rime, and phoneme, as would be predicted by the psycholinguistic grain-size framework. However, whereas in inconsistent orthographies such as English, developmental dyslexia can be diagnosed on the basis of reduced *accuracy* in phonological awareness tasks, in consistent orthographies developmental dyslexia is usually diagnosed on the basis of reduced *speed*. Dyslexic children who learn to read consistent orthographies can use spelling information to help them succeed in phonological tasks. For example, they can visualize the spelling pattern of a word and count its phonemes (because there is a 1:1 correspondence between graphemes and phonemes). However, they tend to do this extremely slowly.

Diagnosis of developmental dyslexia in most languages follows the OECD (Organisation for Economic Co-operation and Development) definition. This definition states that developmental dyslexia is a specific problem with reading and spelling that cannot be accounted for by low intelligence, poor educational opportunities, or obvious sensory or neurological damage. In consistent orthographies, this specific problem manifests in extremely effortful decoding and inaccurate spelling. Dyslexic children learning to read languages such as Italian, Spanish, and German can recode both words and nonwords accurately, but they do this so slowly that they are functionally dyslexic compared to their peers. Furthermore, their reduced phonological memory means that by the time they have decoded all the words in a sentence, they may have forgotten the beginning of the sentence, and so meaning may be lost. However, the hallmark of developmental dyslexia in these languages is unexpectedly poor spelling. Because orthographies that are consistent for reading are frequently inconsistent for spelling (i.e., there are many possible orthographic patterns that can be used to represent a particular sound), it is spelling rather than reading that reveals inaccurate performance.

In contrast, developmental dyslexia in inconsistent orthographies is usually obvious because of the inaccurate and effortful reading of the child. Children who lack phonological sensitivity find it very difficult to acquire grapheme–phoneme recoding skills in these orthographies, because graphemes are not a consistent guide to phonemes. Furthermore, it is difficult for these children to use orthographic knowledge to improve the quality of their phonological representations. Children learning to read in inconsistent orthographies cannot use spelling information to succeed on phonological tasks, or at least cannot use spelling information as a consistent guide to accurate performance. For example, the words *pitch* and *rich* contain the same number of phonemes, but this is not obvious from their spellings (see Ehri & Wilce, 1980). Hence performance in phonological awareness tasks continues to be inaccurate as well as slow. Dyslexic children in nonalphabetic languages experience similar difficulties in acquiring logographies and syllabaries. Reduced phonological sensitivity makes it difficult to acquire print–sound relationships even when these are at the whole-word (i.e., character) level. Studies in Chinese show that dyslexic children have the same problems with phonological processing that characterize dyslexic children in English. As in consistent orthographies, however, the most striking manifestation of their dyslexia is in writing rather than in reading. Chinese children with developmental dyslexia can recode characters to sound accurately, but when they need to select the correct character to represent a sound, they have striking difficulties.

Before giving examples of studies in individual languages conducted within the psycholinguistic grain-size framework, the importance of stringent subject matching should be mentioned. Obviously, because dyslexia occurs in children of wide cognitive ability, cognitive skills should be equivalent across the children with dyslexia and comparison children. Because phonological abilities in dyslexic children are necessarily affected by reading experience, however, it is important to compare dyslexic children to younger children who are reading at the same level (a "reading-level" or "RL-match" design). This control group should be used in addition to children matched for chronological age (or CA). Children who are the same age as the dyslexic children will obviously be much better readers. However, if the phonological or reading subskills of the dyslexic children are inferior even to those of the *younger* children who can read the same number of words, then any deficits found are likely to be fundamental rather than a simple consequence of poorer reading experience. In prereaders, only CA match controls can be used, because an RL match is impossible to achieve. A limitation of studying individuals with developmental dyslexia when they are adults is that only CA controls can be used here, too. Usually, if adult readers can be found who have reading skills comparable to those with dyslexia (i.e., relatively poor reading skills), these adults also have cognitive deficits that preclude an I.Q. match.

THE DEVELOPMENTAL TRAJECTORY
OF PHONOLOGICAL AWARENESS IN DYSLEXIA

Studies across languages using stringent experimental designs have shown that dyslexic children have phonological deficits. A number of studies in English using the RL match design have reported syllable- and onset-rime-level deficits, as well, of course, as the ubiquitous phoneme-level difficulties (e.g., Bowey, Cain, & Ryan, 1992; Bradley & Bryant, 1978; Bruck, 1992; Swan & Goswami, 1997). For example, Bradley and Bryant (1978) reported that English 10-year-olds with dyslexia were significantly poorer in the oddity task than both 10-year-old CA controls and 7-year-old RL controls. Using a phoneme version of the oddity task, Bowey and colleagues (1992) reported a similar result for Australian 9-year-olds. The children with dyslexia were significantly poorer at recognizing shared phonemes than *both* CA and RL controls. In fact, children and adults with dyslexia in nontransparent languages such as English never seem to develop accurate phoneme awareness skills (e.g., Bruck, 1992). In Bruck's (1992) study, she asked children with dyslexia ages 8–15 years and RL and CA controls to count the phonemes in two- to four-phoneme nonwords such as *tisk* and *leem*. The children with dyslexia performed correctly in 47% of trials, as compared to 72% of trials for the RL-matched children and 77% of trials for the CA-matched children. When Bruck then compared adults with dyslexia to third-grade normally progressing readers, she found that the children were significantly better than the adults with dyslexia at both phoneme counting and phoneme deletion. The phoneme deficit in dyslexia in inconsistent orthographies is therefore extremely pervasive.

In contrast, the phoneme deficit in dyslexia in consistent orthographies is only observable in terms of accuracy at the very beginning of reading acquisition. Porpodas (1999) studied Greek first graders with serious literacy difficulties and found significant differences in phoneme awareness between children with dyslexia and control children. The children with dyslexia scored 88% correct in a phoneme segmentation task, as compared to 100% correct for CA controls; and 78% correct in a phoneme deletion task, as compared to 98% correct for the CA controls (note that the participating children were beginning readers and hence an RL control group could not be generated). The Greek first graders with literacy difficulties had been selected out of an initial cohort of 564 children and were at least two standard deviations below the controls in spelling accuracy and at least 1 standard deviation below the controls in decoding time.

Wimmer (1993) studied 10-year-old German children with dyslexia using a phoneme substitution task. In this task, the children had to substitute a consistent phoneme such as /i/ (e.g., "*Mama ist krank*" became "*Mimi ist krink*"). Wimmer found that the children with dyslexia made correct substitutions on 86% of trials. Younger RL control children also made correct substitutions on 86% of trials. The CA control children made correct substitutions on 95% of trials, a significant difference. However, it is important to note that the children with dyslexia had been learning to read a consistent orthography for about 4 years. When Wimmer (1996) retrospectively examined the performance of the German children with dyslexia on a phoneme awareness task in grade 1, before they were diagnosed as dyslexic, he found large differences in comparison to CA controls. The to-be-dyslexic children scored on average 22% correct in the phoneme reversal task used, compared to an average of 69% correct for the control children. Wimmer concluded that German children with dyslexia exhibit the same difficulties in phonemic segmentation exhibited by older English children with dyslexia, but only in the earliest phase of learning to read. Greek children with dyslexia appear to be similar.

Longitudinal studies of children who are at risk for reading difficulties are rare but provide extremely valuable evidence concerning entry-level phonological skills. Such studies also reveal phonological deficits at the rhyme and syllable level in children learning to read consistent orthographies. For example, Schneider, Roth, and Ennemoser (2000) studied a large group of 208 at-risk German children when they were in kindergarten. They found that the at-risk children performed significantly more poorly than control children on tasks of rhyme production, rhyme matching, and syllable segmentation. The control children were German kindergartners in the same nurseries who were not thought to be at risk of later reading difficulties. In a Dutch longitudinal study, similar results were found. Those children who were later diagnosed with dyslexia showed poorer rhyme awareness than their controls when tested in kindergarten (De Jong & van der Leij, 2003). Longitudinal studies of prereading children at risk for reading difficulties in English have also reported poorer syllable and onset-rime awareness compared to controls (Carroll & Snowling, 2003).

Studies of children with dyslexia who are learning to read non-alphabetic orthographies are rare. Nevertheless, available data suggest that these children, too, display phonological deficits at the levels of syllable, rhyme, and phoneme. For example, Ho, Law, and Ng (1998) showed that Chinese children with dyslexia ages 8–9 years were significantly poorer than *both* CA and RL controls in rhyme awareness and phonological memory tasks. Kobayashi, Kato, Haynes, Macaruso, and Hook (2003) reported that Japanese children with developmental dyslexia displayed difficulties in tasks such as syllable deletion, syllable reversal, nonword repetition, and rapid automatized naming, the same type of tasks that distinguish children with dyslexia in other languages. In a study on dyslexia in Korea, 11-year-old children with dyslexia scored only 37% correct in an oddity task in which the deviating element was the second phoneme of the first syllable (e.g., *mo-ki, bo-ki, ko-ki, sa-ki*). This score was in comparison to 83% correct for CA controls (Kim & Davis, 2004). In all world languages so far studied, therefore, children with developmental dyslexia have difficulties in recognizing and manipulating phonological units at all linguistic levels. However, learning to read a consistent alphabetic orthography can help to improve the accuracy of phonological representations in some languages. Nevertheless, children who are dyslexic in these languages still display a phonological deficit in terms of the speed of their phonological processing skills.

THE TRAJECTORY OF READING ACQUISITION IN DYSLEXIA

As noted earlier, grapheme–phoneme recoding skills develop in tandem with phonemic awareness, so it might be expected that the development of phonological recoding skills in children with dyslexia would be impaired. This is indeed the case. As with typical development, however, there are important cross-language differences. Although the impaired development of phonological recoding skills is a hallmark of developmental dyslexia across languages, being most often measured in terms of nonword reading skills, in languages with consistent alphabetic orthographies children can eventually achieve quite accurate performance. The problem is that even though children learning to read languages such as Greek, German, and Spanish can recode nonwords to sound accurately, they do so extremely slowly. This pace makes them functionally dyslexic in comparison to their peers.

The nonword reading deficit in consistent alphabetic orthographies is most marked in younger children with dyslexia. When children are studied at the beginning of the acquisition process, clear deficits in accuracy as well as in speed are apparent. For example, when Wimmer (1996) compared the nonword reading accuracy of German children in kindergarten after discovering (via a longitudinal study) which of them were destined to be dyslexic, he found that 7 out of 12 children who later became dyslexic read less than 60% of simple nonwords such as *Mana* (Mama) and *Aufo* (Auto) accurately. In comparison, beginning readers who did not subsequently become dyslexic showed an average performance rate of 96% correct with these simple nonwords. Three years later, when the children with dyslexia were 10, Wimmer compared them to younger RL-matched children who could read the same number of real words. The nonword reading deficit had apparently disappeared (Wimmer, 1993). In terms of accuracy, the German dyslexic children could recode as many nonwords to sound as their younger controls. However, they showed a marked phonological recoding deficit in terms of reading *speed*. It took the German children with dyslexia on average twice as long as the younger children to recode the nonwords to sound. Similar findings have been reported by Porpodas (1999) for Greek and by López and Jiminez González (2000) for Spanish.

In contrast, studies of children with dyslexia who are learning to read English suggest that accuracy deficits in nonword reading are very persistent. A review paper of published studies showed that error rates were typically rather high, between 40 and 60% (Rack, Snowling, & Olson, 1992). Most studies find that children with dyslexia continue to be less accurate in nonword reading than younger RL controls. For example, Landerl, Wimmer, and Frith (1997) gave 12-year-old English children with dyslexia and 8-year-old RL control children nonwords to read that were one, two, or three syllables in length. The one- and two-syllable nonwords were constructed by changing the onsets of real words (e.g., *ball–grall, butter–sutter*). The three-syllable nonwords were constructed by syllable substitution (*semater, chacustre*), and consequently made greater demands on grapheme–phoneme recoding procedures. Overall the English children with dyslexia found the nonword reading task significantly more difficult than the RL controls (scoring 48% correct compared to 65% correct). For the three-syllable nonwords, the English children with dyslexia scored at 30% correct.

Again, if we search for comparable developmental studies in non-alphabetic orthographies, the database is sparse. Kim and Davis (2004) reported that children with dyslexia in Korea read 72% of nonwords correctly compared to 100% for CA controls. In Hebrew, Breznitz (1997) found that third graders with dyslexia were inferior in a nonword reading task compared to children in first grade (RL controls), who were matched to the dyslexic group for word recognition accuracy and reading comprehension. Phonological problems in nonalphabetic scripts are even more marked in writing. In most world orthographies, sound-to-spelling relations are many-to-one, and this is particularly true for Chinese Kanji (note that Japanese children also need to learn around 1,000 Kanji). There may be as many as eight choices of Kanji to represent one sound. This finding mirrors findings in transparent alphabetic orthographies (German, Greek), where children with dyslexia typically become able to decode quite accurately (albeit, extremely slowly) but never become fluent writers.

BIOLOGICAL UNITY:
THE BRAIN BASIS OF DEVELOPMENTAL DYSLEXIA

According to the cross-language analysis developed above, developmental dyslexia in all of the world's languages should have the same underlying neural causation. Children with developmental dyslexia in all languages so far studied systematically show the same characteristic phonological deficit. Children with developmental dyslexia have difficulties with phonological tasks measuring syllable, rhyme, and phoneme awareness; they have difficulties with tasks measuring phonological memory; and they have difficulties with "rapid automatized naming" tasks. These are the three hallmark areas of a phonological difficulty. This analysis predicts that at the neural level, similar deficits in brain activity should be found, whether the child is dyslexic in English, French, German, or Chinese. The core difficulty for children with dyslexia is a linguistic (phonological) one, and language is represented in the same neural areas whether the language is English or Chinese.

Work by Turkeltaub and colleagues has shown that three distinct neural areas are involved in these different aspects of phonological processing in children (Turkeltaub, Gareau, Flowers, Zeffiro, & Eden, 2003). Phonological working memory appears to depend on neural activity in the left intraparietal sulcus (as in adults); phonological awareness, on a network of areas centered on the left posterior superior temporal sulcus (also the primary area recruited by young children at the beginning of reading development); and RAN on a different, bilateral network, including right posterior superior temporal gyrus, right middle temporal gyrus, and left ventral inferior frontal gyrus. Although studies with children learning to read other languages have yet to be done, in studies of adults with developmental dyslexia across languages, the most consistent findings concern underactivation in left temporoparietal and left occipitotemporal cortices (Eden et al., 2004; Paulesu et al., 2001). This finding has led researchers such as Paulesu to propose that a common neurological network underpins dyslexia across languages, despite some superficial behavioral differences across countries (which can be ascribed to differences in orthographic consistency).

Nevertheless, there is currently some debate about whether "biological unity" should be expected for literacy, which is a culturally acquired skill rather than a natural adaptation of the brain. For example, in a recent fMRI study of eight Chinese children with developmental dyslexia, it was claimed that neural imaging data showed increased activity in brain regions responsible for *visuospatial analysis* rather than phonological analysis (Siok, Perfetti, Jin, & Tan, 2004). The children with developmental dyslexia in this study showed reduced activity in the left middle frontal gyrus, an area involved in visuospatial analysis, but apparently did not show reduced activity in left temporoparietal regions.

Clearly, accurate visuospatial analysis is mandatory in acquiring a character-based system. However, if individual differences in visuospatial memory do not predict individual differences in typical reading development in Chinese (as discussed earlier), then why should a deficit in visuospatial analysis be the cause of a difficulty in reading acquisition in Chinese? This difference may be a product of the impaired reading development of the children being studied rather than a clue to the cause of their reading difficulties. In fact, the eight children with dyslexia studied by Siok and colleagues (2004) did have a phonological deficit. This was evident in their poorer performance on the behavioral task, which was a homophone judgment task. In this task, the participants had to silently read two characters and decide whether they were pronounced in the same way or not. The children with dyslexia were significantly worse at recognizing homophones than the controls, and they also took significantly longer to make homophone decisions. Furthermore, no comparisons with RL-matched controls were reported. The atypical imaging profile reported (i.e., reduced activation in left middle frontal gyrus, an area associated with the representation and working memory of visuospatial and verbal information) may have been the profile to be expected for the character reading level achieved by the children. Without longitudinal data and reading level controls, we cannot tell whether or not there is biological unity at the neural level in dyslexia.

CONCLUSION

Across all languages so far studied, there is a fundamental and causal relationship between a child's phonological awareness and his or her acquisition of reading and spelling skills. There is an apparently universal sequence of phonological development, from awareness of large units (syllables, onsets, rimes) to awareness of small units (phonemes). Alongside this apparently universal sequence of phonological development, variations in the phonological complexity of languages and variations in the consistency with which phonology is represented in orthography generate cross-language differences in reading acquisition and in the manifestation of dyslexia. The nature of these cross-language differences can be predicted a priori by considering the availability and consistency of phonological and orthographic units at different grain sizes.

The probable biological unity for literacy at the neural level suggests that the teaching of reading should follow a similar approach across cultures, beginning with direct instruction in how print is linked to sound, followed by building fluency through repeated practice of decoding. Similarly, remedial programs for children with dyslexia are likely to need the same components across orthographies, focusing on developing phonological skills and on linking phonology to orthography. Given the underactivation of key areas for reading in remediated adults with dyslexia, it seems likely that the development of fluency will continue to be problematic, even for children with dyslexia who are learning to read transparent orthographies. However, the dearth of imaging studies across languages means that systematic cross-language comparisons of neurocognitive trajectories during literacy development are needed before strong recommendations for the classroom can be made.

REFERENCES

Bishop D. V. M. (1997). Cognitive neuropsychology and developmental disorders: Uncomfortable bedfellows. *Quarterly Journal of Experimental Psychology, 50A,* 899–923.

Bowey, J. A., Cain, M. T., & Ryan, S. M. (1992). A reading-level design study of phonological skills underlying fourth grade children's word reading difficulties. *Child Development, 63,* 999–1011.

Bradley, L., & Bryant, P. E. (1978). Difficulties in auditory organization as a possible cause of reading backwardness. *Nature, 271,* 746–747.

Bradley, L., & Bryant, P. E. (1983). Categorising sounds and learning to read: A causal connection. *Nature, 310,* 419–424.

Breznitz, Z. (1997). Enhancing the reading of dyslexic children by reading acceleration and auditory masking. *Journal of Educational Psychology, 89*(1), 103–113.

Brown, G. D. A., & Deavers, R. P. (1999). Units of analysis in nonword reading: Evidence from children and adults. *Journal of Experimental Child Psychology, 73,* 208–242.

Bruck, M. (1992). Persistence of dyslexics' phonological awareness deficits. *Developmental Psychology, 28,* 874–886.

Bryant, P., Bradley, L., Maclean, M., & Crosland, J. (1989). Nursery rhymes, phonological skills and reading. *Journal of Child Language, 16,* 407–428.

Carroll, J. M., & Snowling, M. J. (2003). Language and phonological skills in children at high risk of reading difficulties. *Journal of Child Psychology and Psychiatry, 45,* 631–640.

Chaney, C. (1992). Language development, metalinguistic skills, and print awareness in 3–year-old children. *Journal of Applied Psycholinguistics, 13,* 485–514.

Cossu, G., Shankweiler, D., Liberman, I. Y., Katz, L., & Tola, G. (1988). Awareness of phonological segments and reading ability in Italian children. *Applied Psycholinguistics, 9,* 1–16.

De Cara, B., & Goswami, U. (2002). Similarity relations among spoken words: The special status of rimes in English. *Behavior Research Methods, Instruments and Computers, 34*(3), 416–423.

Defior, S., Martos, S., & Cary, L. (2002). Differences in reading acquisition development in two shallow orthographies: Portuguese and Spanish. *Applied Psycholinguistics, 23,* 135–148.

De Jong, P. F., & van der Leij, A. (2003). Developmental changes in the manifestation of a phonological deficit in dyslexic children learning to read a regular orthography. *Journal of Educational Psychology, 95,* 22–40.

Demont, E., & Gombert, J. E. (1996). Phonological awareness as a predictor of recoding skills and syntactic awareness as a predictor of comprehension skills. *British Journal of Educational Psychology, 66,* 315–332.

Durgunoglu, A. Y., & Oney, B. (1999). A cross-linguistic comparison of phonological awareness and word recognition. *Reading and Writing, 11,* 281–299.

Eden, G. F., Jones, K. M., Cappell, K., Gareau, L., Wood, F. B., Zeffiro, T. A., et al. (2004). Neural changes following remediation in adult developmental dyslexia. *Neuron, 44,* 411–422.

Ehri, L. C., & Wilce, L. S. (1980). The influence of orthography on readers' conceptualisation of the phonemic structure of words. *Applied Psycholinguistics, 1,* 371–385.

Elbro, C., & Pallesen, B. R. (2002). The quality of phonological representations: A causal link? In L. Verhoeven, C. Elbro, & P. Reitsma (Eds.), *Precursors of functional literacy* (Vol. 11, pp. 17–32). Amsterdam: Benjamins.

Ellis, N. C., & Hooper, A. M. (2001). Why learning to read is easier in Welsh than in English: Orthographic transparency effects evinced with frequency-matched tests. *Applied Psycholinguistics, 22,* 571–599.

Fisher, S. E., & DeFries, J. C. (2002). Developmental dyslexia: Genetic dissection of a complex cognitive trait. *Nature Reviews: Neuroscience, 3,* 767–780.

Frith, U., Wimmer, H., & Landerl, K. (1998). Differences in phonological recoding in German- and English-speaking children. *Scientific Studies of Reading, 2,* 31–54.

Goswami, U. (1986). Children's use of analogy in learning to read: A developmental study. *Journal of Experimental Child Psychology, 42,* 73–83.

Goswami, U. (1988). Orthographic analogies and reading development. *Quarterly Journal of Experimental Psychology, 40A,* 239–268.

Goswami, U. (2003). Why theories about developmental dyslexia require developmental designs. *Trends in Cognitive Sciences, 7,* 534–540.

Goswami, U., & Bryant, P. E. (1990). *Phonological skills and learning to read.* Hillsdale, NJ: Erlbaum.

Goswami, U., Ziegler, J., Dalton, L., & Schneider, W. (2001). Pseudohomophone effects and phonological recoding procedures in reading development in English and German. *Journal of Memory and Language, 45,* 648–664.

Goswami, U., Ziegler, J., Dalton, L., & Schneider, W. (2003). Nonword reading across orthographies: How flexible is the choice of reading units? *Journal of Applied Psycholinguistics, 24,* 235–247.

Hanley, J. R., Masterson, J., Spencer, L. H., & Evans, D. (2004). How long do the advantages of learning a transparent orthography last? An investigation of the reading skills and incidence of dyslexia in Welsh children at 10 years of age. *Quarterly Journal of Experimental Psychology, 57*(8), 1393–1410.

Harris, M., & Giannoulis, V. (1999). Learning to read and spell in Greek: The importance of letter knowledge and morphological awareness. In M. Harris & G. Hatano (Eds.), *Learning to read and write: A cross-linguistic perspective* (pp. 51–70). Cambridge, UK: Cambridge University Press.

Ho, C. S.-H. (1997). The importance of phonological awareness and verbal short-term memory to children's success in learning to read Chinese. *Psychologia, 40*(4), 211–219.

Ho, C. S.-H., & Bryant, P. (1997a). Development of phonological awareness of Chinese children in Hong Kong. *Journal of Psycholinguistic Research, 26,* 109–126.

Ho, C. S.-H., & Bryant, P. (1997b). Phonological skills are important in learning to read in Chinese. *Developmental Psychology, 33,* 946–951.

Ho, C. S.-H., Law, T. P.-S., & Ng, P. M. (1998). The phonological deficit hypothesis in Chinese developmental dyslexia. *Reading and Writing, 32,* 276–289.

Hoien, T., Lundberg, L., Stanovich, K. E., & Bjaalid, I. K. (1995). Components of phonological awareness. *Reading and Writing, 7,* 171–188.

Huang, H. S., & Hanley, J. R. (1994). Phonological awareness and visual skills in learning to read Chinese and English. *Cognition, 54,* 73–98.

Huang, H. S., & Hanley, J. R. (1997). A longitudinal study of phonological awareness, visual skills, and Chinese reading acquisition among first-graders in Taiwan. *International Journal of Behavioral Development, 20,* 249–268.

Karmiloff-Smith, A. (1998). Development itself is the key to understanding developmental disorders. *Trends in Cognitive Sciences, 2,* 389–398.

Kim, J., & Davis, C. (2004). Characteristics of poor readers of Korean Hangul: Auditory, visual and phonological processing. *Reading and Writing, 17*(1–2), 153–185.

Kobayashi M., Kato J., Haynes, C. W., Macaruso, P., & Hook, P. (2003). Cognitive linguistic factors in Japanese children's reading. *Japanese Journal of Learning Disabilities, 12,* 240–247.

Landerl, K., Wimmer, H., & Frith, U. (1997). The impact of orthographic consistency on dyslexia: A German–English comparison. *Cognition, 63,* 315–334.

Liberman, I. Y., Shankweiler, D., Fischer, F. W., & Carter, B. (1974). Explicit syllable and phoneme segmentation in the young child. *Journal of Experimental Child Psychology, 18,* 201–212.

López, M. R., & González, J. E. J. (2000). IQ vs phonological recoding skill in explaining differences between poor readers and normal readers in word recognition: Evidence from a naming task. *Reading and Writing, 12,* 129–142.

Lundberg, I., Olofsson A., & Wall, S. (1980). Reading and spelling skills in the first school years predicted from phonemic awareness skills in kindergarten. *Scandinavian Journal of Psychology, 21,* 159–173.

Makita, M. (1968). The rarity of reading disability in Japanese children. *American Journal of Orthopsychiatry, 38,* 599–614.

Morais, J., Cary, L., Alegria, J., & Bertelson, P. (1979). Does awareness of speech as a sequence of phones arise spontaneously? *Cognition, 7,* 323–331.

Paulesu, E. (2001). Dyslexia: Cultural diversity and biological unity. *Science, 291,* 2163–2167.

Perfetti, C. A., Beck, I., Bell, L., & Hughes, C. (1987). Phonemic knowledge and learning to read are reciprocal: A longitudinal study of first grade children. *Merrill–Palmer Quarterly, 33,* 283–319.

Porpodas, C. D. (1999). Patterns of phonological and memory processing in beginning readers and spellers of Greek. *Journal of Learning Disabilities, 32,* 406–416.

Rack, J. P., Snowling, M. J., & Olson, R. (1992). The nonword reading deficit in developmental dyslexia: A review. *Reading Research Quarterly, 27,* 29–53.

Read, C. (1986). *Children's creative spelling.* London: Routledge.

Schneider W., Roth E., & Ennemoser M. (2000). Training phonological skills and letter knowledge in children at risk for dyslexia: A comparison of three kindergarten intervention programs. *Journal of Educational Psychology, 92,* 284–295.

Seymour, P. H., Aro, M., & Erskine, J. M. (2003). Foundation literacy acquisition in European orthographies. *British Journal of Psychology, 94,* 143–174.

Siok, W. T., & Fletcher, P. (2001). The role of phonological awareness and visual–orthographic skills in Chinese reading acquisition. *Developmental Psychology, 37,* 886–899.

Siok, W. T., Perfetti, C. A., Jin, Z., & Tan, L. H. (2004). Biological abnormality of impaired reading is constrained by culture. *Nature, 431,* 71–76.

Spencer, L. H., & Hanley, J. R. (2003). Effects of orthographic transparency on reading and phoneme awareness in children learning to read in Wales. *British Journal of Psychology, 94*(1), 1–28.

Swan, D., & Goswami, U. (1997). Phonological awareness deficits in development dyslexia and the phonological representations hypothesis. *Journal of Experimental Child Psychology, 66,* 18–41.

Treiman, R., Mullennix, J., Bijeljac-Babic, R., & Richmond-Welty, E. D. (1995). The special role of rimes in the description, use, and acquisition of English orthography. *Journal of Experimental Psychology: General, 124,* 107–136.

Tunmer, W. E., & Nesdale, A. R. (1985). Phonemic segmentation skill and beginning reading. *Journal of Educational Psychology, 77,* 417–527.

Turkeltaub, P. E., Gareau, L., Flowers, D. L., Zeffiro, T. A., & Eden, G. F. (2003). Development of neural mechanisms for reading. *Nature Neuroscience, 6,* 767–773.

Ventura, P., Morais, J., Pattamadilok, C., & Kolinsky, R. (2004). The locus of the orthographic consistency effect in auditory word recognition. *Language and Cognitive Processes, 19*(1), 57–95.

Wimmer, H. (1993). Characteristics of developmental dyslexia in a regular writing system. *Applied Psycholinguistics, 14,* 1–33.

Wimmer, H. (1996). The nonword reading deficit in developmental dyslexia: Evidence from children learning to read German. *Journal of Experimental Child Psychology, 61,* 80–90.

Wimmer, H., & Goswami, U. (1994). The influence of orthographic consistency on reading development: Word recognition in English and German children. *Cognition, 51*(1), 91–103.

Wimmer, H., & Hummer, P. (1990). How German speaking first graders read and spell: Doubts on the importance of the logographic stage. *Applied Psycholinguistics, 11,* 349–368.

Wimmer, H., Landerl, K., Linortner, R., & Hummer, P. (1991). The relationship of phonemic awareness to reading acquisition: More consequence than precondition but still important. *Cognition, 40,* 219–249.

Ziegler, J. C., & Goswami, U. (2005). Reading acquisition, developmental dyslexia, and skilled reading across languages: a psycholinguistic grain size theory. *Psychological Bulletin, 131*(1), 3–29.

Ziegler, J. C., Jacobs, A. M., & Stone, G. O. (1996). Statistical analysis of the bidirectional inconsistency of spelling and sound in French. *Behavior Research Methods, Instruments, and Computers, 28,* 504–515.

Ziegler, J. C., Stone, G. O., & Jacobs, A. M. (1997). What's the pronunciation for __OUGH and the spelling for /u/? A database for computing feedforward and feedback inconsistency in English. *Behavior Research Methods, Instruments, and Computers, 29,* 600–618.

CHAPTER 7

Neurocognitive Correlates of Developmental Verbal and Orofacial Dyspraxia

Frederique Liegeois
Angela Morgan
Faraneh Vargha-Khadem

Relatively little is known about the neural mechanisms through which verbal communication is achieved. Speech requires input from four main operational levels for every spoken word: (1) choosing and accessing a word that is semantically and syntactically correct, (2) retrieving the phonological or sound structure of the word, (3) encoding or syllabifying the sounds of the word in context, and (4) planning and producing the phonetic or articulatory gestures (Levelt, 1999). This complicated process, culminating in fluent and articulate speech, occurs at the rate of two to three words per second, in the context of a very low error rate. The spontaneity and accuracy with which speech is produced, even in very young children, has led to the proposal that this unique human attribute has a strong neurogenetic basis (Chomsky, 1959; Lenneberg, 1964). In support of this proposal, evidence has accumulated over the past two decades indicating that some forms of speech and language disorder are inherited (e.g., Bishop, North, & Donlan, 1996; Hurst, Baraitser, Auger, Graham, & Norell, 1990; Lewis, 1992; Scheffer, 2000; Tallal, Townsend, Curtiss, & Wulfeck, 1991;

Vargha-Khadem, Watkins, Alcock, Fletcher, & Passingham, 1995; Vargha-Khadem et al., 1998). One form of speech and language disorder that shows strong heritability is "verbal dyspraxia" (i.e., a motor–speech disorder), best exemplified in studies of the unique KE family (Alcock, Passingham, Watkins, & Vargha-Khadem, 2000a, 2000b; Hurst et al., 1990; Vargha-Khadem et al., 1995, 1998; Vargha-Khadem, Gadian, Copp, & Mishkin, 2005; Watkins, Dronkers, & Vargha-Khadem, 2002).

Half of the members of the large three-generational KE family present with a severe speech and language disorder, which is transmitted as an autosomal-dominant monogenic trait (Hurst et al., 1990; Pembrey, 1992) and encoded by the *FOXP2* gene (Lai, Fisher, Hurst, Vargha-Khadem, & Monaco, 2001). The core deficit in the affected members is a severe and chronic developmental verbal and orofacial dyspraxia (DVOFD) that seriously interferes with the rapid selection, sequencing, and execution of sounds that culminates in the production of articulate and intelligible speech. In addition, the affected KE members suffer from a plethora of expressive and receptive language problems and have difficulties with aspects of reading, writing, and nonverbal intellectual abilities as well as with perception and execution of rhythms (Alcock et al., 2000a; Vargha-Khadem et al., 1995, 1998; Watkins, Dronkers, & Vargha-Khadem, 2002a). It is not yet clear whether each of these language, cognitive, and rhythm impairments constitute independent secondary deficits or result directly from the core deficits of verbal and orofacial dyspraxia.

The neural correlates of DVOFD in the affected KE members have been identified through a series of structural and functional magnetic resonance imaging (fMRI) investigations (Belton, Salmond, Watkins, Vargha-Khadem, & Gadian, 2003; Liegeois et al., 2003; Watkins et al., 2002). The structural studies have revealed relatively reduced gray matter bilaterally, compared to that in controls, in the cerebellum, neostriatum, and both dorsomedial premotor and inferior frontal areas, as well as relatively increased gray matter bilaterally in the superior temporal and angular gyri, among other regions. The ontogenetic processes giving rise to this pattern of abnormality are still unknown, but the anatomical abnormalities documented in adulthood provide a clear neuropathological basis for the behavioral phenotype, particularly the speech dyspraxia. The structural evidence is complemented by functional neuroimaging studies during covert and overt speech, which show relative underactivation, compared to that in controls, in some of the structurally abnormal motor-related areas, and relative overactivation in some of the structurally abnormal posterior cortical areas.

By reviewing the speech and language, cognitive, and brain imaging findings on DVOFD resulting from the *FOXP2* mutation, the first aim of this chapter is to compare the phenotype of the affected KE members with that reported for developmental verbal dyspraxia (DVD) and with adult-onset aphasia, which is often comorbid with an acquired verbal dyspraxia (AVD). The second aim is to provide plausible hypotheses about the abnormal neural systems and mechanisms that may underlie the phenotype of DVOFD in the affected KE members.

DVOFD IN THE AFFECTED KE MEMBERS COMPARED WITH DVD

Morley, Court, and Miller (1954) were the first to describe DVD, noting a similar pattern of disordered speech characteristics in children compared to adults with aphasia and AVD. Despite the disorder being reported more than 50 years ago, the diagnosis and identification of the underlying causes have proven problematic (Shriberg, Aram, & Kwiatkowski, 1997). Moreover, it has been difficult to quantify the separate components of verbal dyspraxia because lexical, phonological, and articulation deficits co-occur and are commonly assessed simultaneously during clinical evaluation (Maassen, 2002). However, a consensus has emerged among clinicians regarding key characteristics of DVD and AVD, including the presence of articulatory struggle (groping), particularly at the beginning of words; substitution errors; markedly inconsistent production on repetitions of the same word; increased phoneme and syllable deletions; increased vowel/diphthong errors; and prosodic disturbance (Austin & Shriberg, 1996; Forrest, 2003).

    To date, there have been no reports of a direct comparison between the key diagnostic characteristics of individuals with DVD and KE members with DVOFD. However, studies of affected KE members have revealed markedly similar phenotypic characteristics to those displayed by children with DVD, including articulatory groping (Morgan, Liegeois, Vogel, Connelly, & Vargha-Khadem, 2005), substitution errors (Fee, 1995), increased phoneme and syllable deletions (Fee, 1995), increased vowel/diphthong errors (Ciocca, van Fletcher, Vargha-Khadem, & Belton, 2004), restricted knowledge of prosodic rules (Piggott & Kessler-Robb, 1999), and token-to-token variability (Fee, 1995; Morgan et al., 2005). In addition, other key features of chronic speech impairment commonly noted in, but not unique to, children with DVD have also been noted in the KE family, including markedly delayed acquisition of phonemes and inconsistent use of phonemes already present in their sound repertoire (Fee, 1995). Impairment on the diadochokinesis (DDK) task (e.g., repeating *pata* as quickly and clearly as possible) has also been advocated as a potential diagnostic marker for DVD (Thoonen, Maassen, Gabreels, & Schreuder, 1999); affected members of the KE family demonstrate poor skills on DDK tasks with respect to both consistency and accuracy of word or nonword repetitions (Belton et al., 2003; Belton, Gadian, & Vargha-Khadem, 2004).

In addition to verbal dyspraxia, the affected KE members also present with an orofacial dyspraxia. This is an impairment in the execution of voluntary nonspeech oral movements, with automatic or involuntary oral movements remaining relatively intact. In principle, the diagnosis of orofacial dyspraxia should be made independently of verbal or speech dyspraxia (Ozanne, 1995). In practice, however, this diagnostic distinction is difficult to make because verbal and orofacial dyspraxia are often comorbid in children with DVD (Dewey, Roy, Square-Storer, & Hayden, 1988; Milloy, 1991; Stackhouse, 1992). Moreover, it is possible that the limits of orofacial control are best revealed during verbal praxis and not during nonspeech orofacial movements, which have less precision and range of motor demand. Since the comorbidity of verbal and orofacial dyspraxia has not been experimentally investigated in children with DVD, it is not clear whether a dissociation between these two aspects of oromotor function exists in this population. In the absence of such evidence, it is difficult to determine whether any differences between the diagnostic characteristics of DVOFD and DVD are due to the confound of features in the former condition.

DVOFD IN AFFECTED KE MEMBERS COMPARED WITH AVD

A major difference between developmental and acquired verbal dyspraxia is that the primary diagnosis in the latter condition is usually one of aphasia, with the verbal dyspraxia presenting as a comorbid feature. The absence of aphasia in association with a neurodevelopmental disorder or a frank unilateral lesion sustained early in life is not surprising, given that during infancy and childhood enhanced brain plasticity and reorganizational capacity will ensure the preservation of speech and language function at a basic level (Vargha-Khadem, Isaacs, & Muter, 1994; Vargha-Khadem et al., 1997; Vargha-Khadem & Mishkin, 1997). Such is not the case with acquired adult-onset aphasia, in which speech and language function can be *selectively* and chronically impaired after a left-sided brain lesion, often resulting in aphasic subtypes (e.g., Broca's aphasia, anomia, conduction aphasia) and comorbid features (e.g., dysarthria, verbal dyspraxia). Whereas with DVD a major underlying problem is presumed to be inefficient movement coordination of the orovocal system, with AVD secondary to an aphasic syndrome there is controversy about whether the verbal dyspraxia arises from a language impairment or from a motor programming and execution problem.

Frequently denoted as apraxia of speech, AVD is clinically described as a motor programming disorder resulting from a cerebral lesion, typically to Broca's area, and primarily manifested as an articulatory impairment (Darley, 1982, p. 10). Disturbed prosody is a common secondary feature of the disorder (Murdoch, 1990). Very few cases of "pure" AVD in the absence of aphasia are reported in the literature (Fox, Kasner, Chatterjee, & Chalela, 2001; Mendez, 2004; Pellat et al., 1991; Rapin & Allen, 1988). Pure AVD is reportedly a disorder that affects speech disproportionately to language (Halpern, Darley, & Brown, 1973). Adult patients with a pure form of the disorder demonstrate speech that is significantly impaired in comparison to the modalities of listening, reading, and writing (Murdoch, 1990). In contrast, patients with a primary diagnosis of aphasia with or without coexisting apraxia of speech demonstrate a profile wherein auditory, visual, and spoken modalities are more equally affected.

Given that the diagnostic criteria for DVD are based on AVD, it is not surprising to note that the error patterns are almost identical in the two disorders. The main features of AVD are visible and audible groping, variable production of repeated words, and increased articulatory error with increasing complexity or word length of the articulatory exercise (see Croot, 2002; Peach, 2004, for a review). As noted previously, affected members of the KE family demonstrate all of these features and are therefore comparable to patients with AVD with regard to speech production at a clinical level.

To date, there are two reports directly comparing the speech and language and limb and orofacial praxis of the affected KE members with two different groups of adult-onset aphasic patients, some of whom also demonstrate AVD. Watkins, Dronkers, and Vargha-Khadem (2002) compared the performance of affected KE members ($n = 13$) to a group of adults with left-hemispheric stroke and expressive aphasia ($n = 11$) and unaffected family members ($n = 12$) on measures of receptive vocabulary (lexical decision) and receptive grammar, word and nonword repetition, naming to confrontation, verbal fluency, expressive inflectional and derivational morphology, past tense production, nonword reading and spelling, and nonverbal intelligence. Only six of the patients with expressive aphasia presented with comorbid verbal apraxia, but this was also accompanied by dysarthria and/ or anomia, or conduction disorder.

Results indicated that affected KE members and the patients with expressive aphasia were equally impaired relative to the unaffected KE members on receptive grammar, naming accuracy, expressive morphology, past tense production, and nonword reading and spelling (Watkins, Dronkers, & Vargha-Khadem, 2002). On the measure of word and nonword repetition, an interesting dissociation emerged between the two speech- and language-disordered groups. Whereas both the affected members and the patients with aphasia were equally impaired relative to the unaffected members on the measure of nonword repetition (particularly nonwords with complex articulation patterns and those with increased number of syllables), the aphasic patients performed significantly better than the affected KE members on word repetition. The advantage of the aphasic group on word repetition is presumably attributable to the normal articulation patterns of words that had been acquired premorbidly. For the affected KE members, there was no difference between the accuracy of repetitions for words compared to nonwords, suggesting that semantic representation of real words did not aid repetition accuracy.

In contrast to the disadvantage shown on word repetition, the affected KE group showed a significant advantage compared to the aphasic group on all three tests of semantic, phonemic, and written fluency, though they were impaired on each measure relative to the unaffected members. This advantage is presumably due to the developmental nature of the speech and language disorder, which guards against chronic and persistent aphasic symptoms—characteristics of adult-onset nonfluent aphasia.

Although DVOFD appears to spare fluency in the affected members, it adversely affects the development of nonverbal intellectual functions. Thus, relative to both the unaffected and aphasic groups, the affected group had a significantly reduced nonverbal (i.e., Performance) intelligence quotient. This finding suggests that DVOFD extends beyond the speech and language domain to influence nonverbal intellectual functions, in contrast to adult-onset expressive aphasia, which spares these functions but affects speech and language functions *selectively*. As already noted, however, the deficit in nonverbal intelligence in DVOFD may be a separate deficit.

As in children diagnosed with DVD, limb and orofacial dyspraxia may co-occur in AVD (Kimura & Watson, 1989; Mateer, 1978; Mateer & Kimura, 1977; Square, Roy, & Martin, 1997). A comparison of affected KE members with two groups of patients with adult-onset expressive aphasia (one with nonfluent aphasia, speech difficulties, and problems with oral movements; Alcock et al., 2000b; Watkins, Dronkers, & Vargha-Khadem, 2002) showed that neither DVOFD nor expressive aphasia interferes with limb praxis. Such is not the case with orofacial praxis, which is significantly impaired in relation to controls in both KE members with DVOFD and patients with adult-onset aphasia. Although both the KE and aphasic groups were able to perform simple single oromotor movements, they experienced difficulties with complex single movements (involving two or more articulators) and sequenced oral movements (Alcock et al., 2000b; Watkins, Dronkers, & Vargha-Khadem, 2002).

These results suggest that the DVOFD in the affected KE members—and possibly the adult-onset expressive aphasia, which in some cases is also associated with verbal dyspraxia—may arise, at least in part, from a lower-level deficit in orofacial praxis. The integrity of this aspect of oromotor control appears to be critical for articulate speech (Vargha-Khadem et al., 2005).

THE NEURAL BASIS OF DVOFD IN AFFECTED KE MEMBERS

To date, the neural basis of DVD, and indeed the more general form of language disorder known as specific language impairment (SLI), has remained unknown. Investigations using imaging techniques to detect subtle brain pathology (see below) have yet to be reported in these populations. Although family and twin studies of children with DVD (Lewis et al., 2004) or SLI have provided strong evidence in support of a genetic origin (Bishop, North, & Donlan, 1995), the relationship between the phenotype of these developmental disorders of speech and language and their neural substrates is unclear. Such is not the case with the affected KE members, in whom the gene responsible for the DVOFD has been identified and the relationship of this phenotype to an underlying neural network has been studied through a series of MRI studies.

Neurodevelopmental disorders (e.g., dyslexia, dyscalculia, SLI) without comorbid neurological impairments (e.g., frank motor, visual, auditory, or other sensory deficits) are not associated with obvious anatomical brain abnormalities as indicated by routine MRI studies. In this respect, DVOFD is not an exception. However, systematic examination of MRI datasets using quantitative techniques (e.g., voxel-based morphometry—VBM [Ashburner & Friston 2000]; volumetric measurements of regions of interest [Van Paesschen, Revesz, Duncan, Kling, & Connelly, 1997]; T2 relaxometry [Jackson, Connelly, Duncan, Grunewald, & Gadian, 1993]; or magnetic resonance spectroscopy—1HMRS [Gadian et al., 1996]) can be extremely valuable in revealing subtle neurodevelopmentally based pathology that may not be identifiable using visual inspection alone. Correlations can then be examined between any subtle pathology thus found and the behavioral and/or cognitive indices of the disorder (i.e., the phenotype in question) in order to seek a direct link between brain abnormality and consequent dysfunction. Such structural MRI techniques have been applied successfully in patient groups to study brain abnormalities underlying conditions such as dyscalculia (Isaacs, Edmonds, Lucas, & Gadian, 2001), autism and Asperger syndrome (Courshesne, Townsend, & Saitoh, 1994; Salmond et al., 2005), and amnesia (Gadian et al., 2000; Vargha-Khadem et al., 2003). Subsequent studies using fMRI can then address specific questions about the sites associated with impaired functions and their relationship to both the structural and behavioral abnormalities.

Brain–behavior relationships indicated in this way are particularly informative in identifying the neural systems that may be implicated in a specific neurodevelopmental disorder and in providing hypotheses about aberrant neural mechanisms.

BILATERAL PATHOLOGY AFFECTING THE NEURAL SUBSTRATES OF SPEECH AND LANGUAGE

Despite the fact that the disorder in the affected KE members is developmental in origin, it has failed to resolve throughout childhood and adolescence, a time when brain plasticity and reorganizational capacity are hypothesized to be at a maximum. Individual affected members have received intensive speech and language therapy throughout their school years and have attended speech and language units to ameliorate their articulation and expressive language disorder. Despite these interventions, the disorder has persisted into adulthood. Against this background, the main aim of the brain imaging studies was to identify which brain regions, likely to be part of the circuitry that produces coherent and intelligible speech, have failed to develop properly. Before considering the findings, the issues of age at injury and laterality of function need to be considered relative to two hypotheses about the KE phenotype.

It is well established that in adulthood, injury to the left hemisphere alone is sufficient to produce a chronic and severe aphasia. In childhood, however, examination of various groups of patients with focal injuries indicates that damage to either hemisphere alone is insufficient to produce aphasia (Bates et al., 2001; Teuber, 1975; Vargha-Khadem & Polkey, 1992; Vargha-Khadem, Isaacs, Watkins, & Mishkin, 2000; for an illustrative case, see Vargha-Khadem et al., 1997). Indeed, it is apparently because damage to the perisylvian regions of both hemispheres is so rare that cases of congenital aphasia are also extremely rare.

One such unusual case is the patient Adam (Vargha-Khadem, Watters, & O'Gorman, 1985), who had chronic aphasia after apparently limited bifrontal lesions that were incurred perinatally. Adam's lesion on the left side encompassed Broca's area entirely. His lesion on the right side was located somewhat more dorsally, yet it was apparently close enough to the region homologous to Broca's area to result in virtual mutism. Although he was not diagnosed until age 6, at which time his lesions were discovered, he did receive intensive and extended speech and language therapy thereafter. Yet, up to 4 years later, Adam still had not developed intelligible speech. This case revealed that focal brain damage in or near Broca's area must be bilateral in order to produce a chronic aphasic-like symptom in children who have suffered these pathologies early in life.

TWO HYPOTHESES ABOUT PATHOPHYSIOLOGY IN THE KE PHENOTYPE

Based on the findings with Adam (Vargha-Khadem et al., 1985) and also from a large number of individual cases and patient groups with unilateral focal lesions, including hemidecortication (Bates et al., 2001; Vargha-Khadem, Isaacs, Papaleloudi, Polkey, & Wilson, 1991; Vargha-Khadem & Polkey, 1992; Vargha-Khadem et al., 1997, 2000), two hypotheses were proposed about the brain pathology that might have given rise to the KE family phenotype. First, in the affected family members, the brain pathology was predicted to be bilateral because of the neurodevelopmental origin of the disorder. Second, the brain regions affected were predicted to include one or more components of the motor system, because one of the core deficits of the phenotype is an orofacial dyspraxia. Thus, the two hypotheses called for bilaterality and involvement of the motor system.

STRUCTURAL BRAIN ABNORMALITIES

Two of the quantitative MRI techniques referred to above, voxel-based morphometry (VBM) and volumetric measurement of specific structures, were used to examine the MRI datasets of the affected KE members in relation to the unaffected family members and normal controls. The first technique, VBM, provides a quantitative measure of gray matter density in voxels across the entire brain and allows for comparison of differences between groups. This technique can also be restricted to detect bilateral abnormalities—that is, those found in homotopic regions of the left and right hemispheres (Salmond, Ashburner, Vargha-Khadem, Gadian, & Friston, 2000). Through the application of this method, abnormal levels of gray matter density in the affected members of the KE family, with respect to both unaffected members and controls, were identified (Belton et al., 2003). The second technique involved volumetric measurements of specific structures that were found to be abnormal in the VBM analyses and/or were considered important in relation to the two hypotheses outlined above (Watkins et al., 2002).

The results of the VBM analyses showed that both motor- and language-related systems are affected bilaterally by the *FOXP2* mutation. Reduced gray matter density was found in the head of the caudate nucleus, the dorsal inferior frontal gyrus, the precentral gyrus (primary motor cortex), temporal pole, and the ventral cerebellum (lobule VIIB and VIIIB; for anatomical reference, see Schmahmann et al., 1999), whereas more gray matter was found in the posterior superior temporal gyrus and the angular gyrus. These findings were consistent with gene expression studies in mice and human embryos (see Vargha-Khadem et al., 2005, for a review), which confirmed that in all species *FOXP2* was expressed in the cerebellum and basal ganglia. A volumetric analysis also revealed that the caudate nucleus was significantly reduced in the affected members of the KE family relative to both controls and unaffected members (Vargha-Khadem et al., 1998; Watkins et al., 2002). Altogether, morphological studies suggest that both cerebellar- and striatal-cortical networks have been disrupted by the *FOXP2* mutation. How this neural phenotype relates to the behavioral phenotype is examined in the next section in conjunction with results from functional imaging studies and from studies of patients with lesions to these regions.

FUNCTIONAL BRAIN ABNORMALITIES

A series of fMRI studies of the KE family provided further evidence that the structural abnormalities were indeed associated with functional abnormalities in language and motor-related circuits (Liegeois et al., 2003). The first experiment examined the pattern of brain activation during *covert* speech in five affected KE members, five unaffected members, and ten controls. When performing a task involving the silent generation of a verb to a noun (e.g., *BREAD-cut*), the affected members of the KE family showed under-activation (i.e., significantly lowered blood flow) in the putamen, the posterior part of Broca's area (BA; pars opercularis, BA 44), as well as in the precentral gyrus (primary motor cortex) and the supramarginal gyrus (Liegeois et al., 2003). Overall, activation in the affected members was atypical and more posterior and diffuse than in the unaffected and control groups, suggesting functional abnormalities even when the execution of motor–speech sequences was not required.

In the second experiment, the family members (five unaffected and five affected) were asked to perform an *overt* (i.e., aloud) verb generation task and a word repetition task to explore functional abnormalities related to internally generated as compared to externally cued words. Significant underactivation was found in the putamen and the inferior frontal gyrus (Brodmann's area 45, anterior part of BA) during the overt verb generation task, with underactivation in Brodmann's area 45 being detected during word repetition as well. Results of this study suggest that the putamen was underactive during internally generated mental search for words, whereas the inferior frontal gyrus was underactive when words were either covertly or overtly generated. Such a pattern of underactivation is consistent with a functionally abnormal striatocortical circuit.

NEURAL MECHANISMS DISRUPTED IN DVOFD

The phenotype described in the affected KE members may arise from the disruption of one or more putative neural circuits subserving motor planning, timing, procedural learning, and/or phonological processing (Vargha-Khadem et al., 2005). Based on the available data, it is not clear whether disruption of any one or more of these neural circuits can fully account for the phenotype of verbal and orofacial dyspraxia in the KE family. Nevertheless, it is informative to review the reported findings in patients with neurological disorders resulting in speech and language disturbances akin to those in the affected KE members and the results of neuroimaging studies of normal individuals with a view to understanding the role of each of these components.

Disruption of Neural Networks Involved in Motor Planning

As described earlier, the phenotype of the KE family is characterized as a verbal and orofacial dyspraxia. Traditionally, a motor–speech impairment of this type has been viewed as a disorder of planning and coordination of sequences of orofacial movements involved in speech. The finding that the affected KE members show underactivation of the posterior part of BA (pars opercularis), the primary motor cortex, and the putamen during covert verb generation is consistent with the disruption of the circuit responsible for motor planning.

The role of the basal ganglia in the planning of motor sequences has long been suspected, based on dyspraxic features associated with neostriatal infarcts in adults. For instance, an adult with bilateral abnormality of the basal ganglia due to hypoxemia was reported to suffer from speech and language deficits, with particular difficulties sequencing articulatory gestures (Pickett, Kuniholm, Protopapas, Friedman, & Lieberman, 1998), and another person with infarct to the lentiform nucleus showed transient signs of speech apraxia (Warren, Smith, Denson, & Waddy, 2000). Involvement of BA in verbal praxis is evident from the study of adults with left-hemispheric stroke (Watkins, Dronkers, & Vargha-Khadem, 2002) and has been the subject of several lesion analyses. A recent study of 80 adults with left-hemispheric stroke (Hillis et al., 2004) indicated that apraxia of speech was associated with a lesion in the posterior part of the inferior frontal gyrus (BA 44) and not in the anterior insular cortex, as previously suggested (Dronkers, 1996), consistent with the hypothesis that the posterior part of BA is involved in speech planning. An adult with multiple sclerosis and verbal dyspraxia showed MRI abnormality in a region subjacent to Brodmann's area 44/45 (Jaffe, Glabus, Kelley, & Minager, 2003). Interestingly, normalization of speech was observed when tissue inflammation in that region was reduced. The strong interconnectivity between the basal ganglia and the inferior frontal gyrus is reflected in the finding that sustained cortical hypoperfusion (lowered blood flow) in the inferior frontal gyrus, although not visible on structural imaging, may be at the root of the speech and language impairments observed after subcortical stroke (Nadeau & Crosson, 1997).

At least two cases of children with chronic and severe speech and articulation difficulties (i.e., apraxia of speech) associated with bilateral damage to BA and its homologue on the right side, and direct or indirect damage to the basal ganglia, have been described in the literature. The first case, Adam, described earlier (Vargha-Khadem et al., 1985), remained mute as a consequence of perinatal bilateral prefrontal lesions. The second case was that of a young boy with bilateral damage to the head of the caudate nuclei (Tallal, Jernigan, & Trauner, 1994). This patient presented with delayed speech acquisition, language and articulation deficits, and difficulties producing verbal as well as nonverbal motor sequences. This case raises the question of the role of the basal ganglia in the early acquisition of speech–motor sequences that may be crucial for the subsequent normal development of intelligible speech.

Although there is evidence of ventral cerebellar abnormality in the affected KE members on morphometric analyses (Watkins et al., 2002), and gene expression studies in both human embryo and mouse implicate this structure as an early site of *Foxp2* expression, it is not possible to determine, on the basis of available data, whether any motor planning deficits in the KE phenotype are specifically attributable to abnormality in the inferior frontal cerebellar loop (Vargha-Khadem et al., 2005). Similarly, there is no convincing evidence from studies of patients with lesions of the cerebellum to suggest a direct link between pathology in this structure and presence of verbal dyspraxia. For example, cerebellar tumors in children (e.g., van Mourik, Catsman-Berrevoets, Yousef-Bak, Paquier, & van Dongen, 1998) and adults (Kent, 2000) typically result in ataxic dysarthria, but no reported dyspraxic features. Nevertheless, a recent neuroimaging study has concluded that the preparation of movements is carried out by a network that includes the left supplementary motor area, the left anterior insula, the left dorsolateral prefrontal cortex (including BA), and the right superior cerebellum (Riecker et al., 2005).

Disruption of Neural Networks Involved in the Timing of Motor Execution

As discussed previously, the results of a study by Alcock and colleagues (2000b) suggested that a deficit in timing might underlie the phenotype of verbal and orofacial dyspraxia in the affected KE members. Although timing was a component of the task used in this study, there were other factors, such as cross-modal transfer or intramodal perception of the stimuli, that could have interacted with a timing deficit.

Numerous researchers have argued that the cerebellum is involved in fine-tuning the timing of movement sequences (see Ivry & Spencer, 2004, for a review). Identification of the role of the cerebellum in timing and movement execution comes mainly from the observation of patients with lesions to the cerebellum who suffer from hypermetria, in which movements are erratic, oscillatory, and hardly reach the targets (see "cerebellar motor syndrome" in Schmahmann, 2004). Timing is, however, also implicated in neurodegenerative diseases affecting the basal ganglia, such as in the dysarthria associated with Huntington disease (Ackermann & Hertrich, 1994; Hertrich & Ackermann, 1994). Some authors have argued that patients with Huntington disease or those with Parkinson disease are not impaired at the level of planning motor sequences but have an underlying problem with timing (Ludlow, Connor, & Bassich, 1987). Developmental stuttering is another speech disorder that originates in early childhood and persists into adulthood and is marked by timing problems. There is increasing evidence that the basal ganglia circuits are implicated in developmental stuttering, although the nature of the disorder remains controversial (see Alm, 2004, for a review).

There is now increasing evidence from the neuroimaging literature that both cerebellar and striatal networks are involved in the timing of motor execution (e.g., Rao et al., 1997). In the domain of speech, a study of normal adults, in which activation during covert (i.e., silent) repetition of the syllable /ta/ at different rates was examined, has reported greater basal ganglia activation during slow repetition rates, but greater cerebellar activation during the fastest rate, suggesting different roles played by cerebellar and striatal loops in the control and timing of movement sequences (Wildgruber, Ackermann, & Grodd, 2001). In a recent review, it was similarly suggested that both striatal and cerebellar loops contribute to the timing of speech movements (Schirmer, 2004). However, it should be noted that acquired damage to the cerebellum or the basal ganglia in adults does not result in verbal dyspraxia but rather in different subtypes of dysarthria.

Disruption of Neural Networks Involved in Procedural Learning

A third possible explanation of the KE phenotype is that the disorder is not caused by a *planning* or *execution* deficit, per se, but by a *learning* deficit. It is well established, on the basis of research with nonhuman primates, that an important neural network implicated in the learning of habits and rule-based information is the procedural memory system (Mishkin, Malamut, & Bachavalier, 1984; Squire & Knowlton, 2000; Squire, Knowlton, & Musen, 1993). Procedural learning is implicit, and acquisition of the particular habit or skill builds up gradually during multiple trials. The neural substrate for procedural learning involves the frontal/basal ganglia loop, with the caudate nucleus and the putamen playing critical roles in the learning of new skills.

Recently, it has been proposed that disruption of this network during development can underlie some aspects of cognitive, language, and grammatical deficits that are commonly found in children with SLI (Ullman, 2004; Ullman & Pierpont, 2005). A procedural learning deficit of this type could conceivably affect a wide array of implicit processes that contribute to cognitive learning and retrieval.

Neuroimaging studies using positron emission tomography (PET) and fMRI in healthy adults have revealed that the learning of a new task modifies activation in cortical areas, such as the primary motor cortex, but also in interconnected regions such as the neostriatum and the cerebellum (Hazeltine, Grafton, & Ivry, 1997; Karni et al., 1995). In a review of the neural basis of learning skilled motor acts, Ungerleider, Doyon, and Karni (2002) concluded that changes in the primary motor cortex occurred slowly and over the course of weeks, whereas changes in the cerebellum and the putamen were more rapid and dynamic over the course of days.

For example, a study involving the learning of sequences of key presses concluded that the cerebellum is involved during the process of automatization, whereas the putamen is involved during both learning and retrieval (Jenkins, Brooks, Nixon, Frackowiak, & Passingham, 1994). Another study examining implicit sequence learning in healthy adults reported that despite interindividual variability in the side and site (caudate or putamen) of basal ganglia activation, the "best learners" were the ones who showed greatest putamen activation (Rauch et al., 1997). In addition, there was a positive correlation between activation in the putamen and the gain in reaction time associated with learning. Similarly, learning-related changes in the putamen and in the left motor cortex and supplementary motor area have been observed in a PET study involving an implicit serial reaction time task (Hazeltine et al., 1997). Changes in fMRI activation from cerebellar- to striatal-cortical networks have also been detected with extended practice during a motor sequence learning task (Doyon et al., 2002). Altogether, data from functional imaging studies suggest that the corticostriatal and corticocerebellar systems are involved at different stages of skill acquisition (for a review, see Doyon, Penhune, & Ungerleider, 2003). The cerebellum appears to be active during the fast learning (Doyon et al., 2002) or automatization phase (Jenkins et al., 1994), but its involvement decreases with practice. In contrast, the striatum is more active when asymptotic performance has been reached relative to the beginning of the acquisition process (Doyon et al., 2002), as well as during retrieval (Jenkins et al., 1994).

To date, direct measurement of procedural learning ability has not been reported in the affected KE family members. It is noteworthy, however, that retrieval of previously learned words during repetition is as restricted as the repetition of nonwords, suggesting that semantic representations associated with known words do not aid retrieval of previously learned utterance patterns. Whether the neostriatal pathology in the affected KE members interferes with procedural learning, particularly the acquisition of articulation patterns of words, and whether this restriction leads in turn to deficient retrieval remains to be determined (Vargha-Khadem et al., 2005).

Disruption of the Neural Networks Involved in Phonological Processing

Functional imaging studies of healthy adults have identified a neural network involved in phonological processing. In view of the longstanding problems with literacy in the affected KE members, particularly the reading and writing of nonwords (Watkins, Dronkers, & Vargha-Khadem, 2002), it is possible that abnormality in this neural network is the underlying cause of the speech and language disorder. In healthy adults, the fMRI paradigm involving covert and overt generation of verbs has been shown to activate semantic processing areas of the left hemisphere, in addition to BA and the frontostriatal articulatory loop (Liegeois et al., 2003). In the affected KE members, however, abnormal underactivation was found in the two regions typically associated with phonological processing, namely, the supramarginal gyrus (Xu et al., 2001) and the inferior frontal gyrus (Siok, Jin, Fletcher, & Tan, 2003). Although the possibility cannot be readily dismissed that a phonological processing impairment lies at the root of the disorder in the KE family, a more parsimonious account is that phonological impairment is a by-product of atypical motor learning or sequencing, and that this ultimately leads to disrupted development of phonological representations. Even if deficient phonological representation is not at the root of the disorder in the KE family, the comorbidity of oromotor and literacy deficits in the affected members and in those with DVD and/or SLI cannot be ignored. It is now well established that the development of adequate phonological representations is a prerequisite for the development of good literacy skills (e.g., Muter, Hulme, Snowling, & Stevenson, 2004; see also Molfese et al., Chapter 8; Grigorenko, Chapter 5; and Goswami, Chapter 6, this volume).

SUMMARY

In the first section of this chapter, the major aim was to determine whether the phenotype of two neurodevelopmental disorders of speech and language—namely, DVOFD, resulting from the *FOXP2* mutation, and DVD of unknown etiology—was distinct. On the basis of the available evidence, it was not possible to provide a differential diagnosis between the two disorders. The clinical symptoms are very similar, and both quantitative measures of motor–speech deficits and classification of speech dyspraxia and/or dysarthria are required before any similarities or differences can be reliably identified.

A secondary aim of the first section was to compare the two developmental disorders of speech and language with acquired verbal dyspraxia associated with aphasia in adults. Here the problem was that only some aphasic patients have accompanying speech dyspraxia, and as a result, the comparison of the phenotype was confounded by the presence of other comorbid speech- and language-related problems. Nevertheless, direct comparison of the language and cognitive profiles of DVOFD, associated with the *FOXP2* mutation, with AVD did show striking similarities in the core deficits characteristic of speech dyspraxia, but also differences across measures of fluency.

In the second part of the chapter, the neural substrate associated with the *FOXP2* mutation in the KE family was considered. Here the aim was to account for neural mechanisms that could have been disrupted as a result of the genetic mutation, thus leading to the phenotype of verbal and orofacial dyspraxia. Overall, it is concluded that fluent and intelligible speech is the product of multiple sensory and cognitive processes that are subserved by similarly complex and interacting neural systems, and that dysfluent and unintelligible speech may be the product of atypical development in one or more of these systems. Many of these processes function in parallel, and dissection of the relevant components, both at the behavioral and the neural level, awaits future research.

REFERENCES

Ackermann, H., & Hertrich, I. (1994). Speech rate and rhythm in cerebellar dysarthria: An acoustic analysis of syllabic timing. *Folia Phoniatrica et Logopaedica, 46*, 70–78.

Alcock, K. J., Passingham, R. E., Watkins, K. E., & Vargha-Khadem, F. (2000a). Oral dyspraxia in inherited speech and language impairment and acquired dysphasia. *Brain and Language, 75*(1), 17–33.

Alcock, K. J., Passingham, R. E., Watkins, K., & Vargha-Khadem, F. (2000b). Pitch and timing abilities in inherited speech and language impairment. *Brain and Language, 75*(1), 34–46.

Alm, P. A. (2004). Stuttering and the basal ganglia circuits: A critical review of possible relations. *Journal of Communication Disorders, 37*, 325–369.

Ashburner, J., & Friston, K. J. (2000). Voxel-based morphometry: The methods. *NeuroImage, 11*, 805–821.

Austin, D., & Shriberg, L. D. (1996). *Lifespan reference data for ten measures of articulation competence using the Speech Disorders Classification System (SDCS)* (Tech. Rep. No. 3). Madison: University of Wisconsin, Waisman Center, Phonology Project.

Bates, E., Reilly, J., Wulfeck, B., Dronkers, N., Opie, M., Fenson, J., et al. (2001). Differential effects of unilateral lesions on language production in children and adults. *Brain and Language, 79*, 223–265.

Belton, E., Gadian, D. E., & Vargha-Khadem, F. (2004). *The KE family: A severe motoric deficit to speech* [Abstract]. Washington, DC: Society for Neuroscience.

Belton, E., Salmond, C. H., Watkins, K. E., Vargha-Khadem, F., & Gadian, D. G. (2003). Bilateral brain abnormalities associated with dominantly inherited verbal and orofacial dyspraxia. *Human Brain Mapping, 18*(3), 194–200.

Bishop, D. V., North, T., & Donlan, C. (1995). Genetic basis of specific language impairment: Evidence from a twin study. *Developmental Medicine and Child Neurology, 37*, 56–71.

Bishop, D. V., North, T., & Donlan, C. (1996). Nonword repetition as a behavioural marker for inherited language impairment: Evidence from a twin study. *Journal of Child Psychology and Psychiatry, 37*(4), 391–403.

Chomsky, N. (1959). Review of *Verbal Behaviour*, by B. F. Skinner. *Language, 35,* 26–58.

Ciocca, V., Yan, T., Fletcher, O., Vargha-Khadem, F., & Belton, E. (2004). *Diphthong and vowel production errors in speakers with genetic speech and language disorder* (Publication No. 93295). Layfayette, LA: ICPLA.

Courshesne, E., Townsend, J., & Saitoh, O. (1994). The brain in infantile autism: Posterior fossa structures are abnormal. *Neurology, 44,* 214–223.

Croot, K. (2002). Diagnosis of AOS: Definition and criteria. *Seminars in Speech and Language, 23*(4), 267–280.

Darley, F. L. (1982). *Aphasia.* Philadelphia: Saunders.

Dewey, D., Roy, E. A., Square-Storer, P. A., & Hayden, D. (1988). Limb and oral praxic abilities of children with verbal sequencing deficits. *Developmental Medicine and Child Neurology, 30*(6), 743–751.

Doyon, J., Penhune, V., & Ungerleider, L. G. (2003). Distinct contribution of the cortico–striatal and cortico–cerebellar systems to motor skill learning. *Neuropsychologia, 41,* 252–262.

Doyon, J., Song, A. W., Karni, A., Lalonde, F., Adams, M. M., & Ungerleider, L. G. (2002). Experience-dependent changes in cerebeller contributions to motor sequence learning. *Proceedings of the National Academy of Sciences USA, 99,* 1017–1022.

Dronkers, N. F. (1996). A new brain region for coordinating speech articulation. *Nature, 384,* 159–161.

Fee, E. J. (1995). The phonological system of a specifically language-impaired population. *Clinical Linguistics and Phonetics, 9,* 189–209.

Forrest, K. (2003). Diagnostic criteria of developmental apraxia of speech used by clinical speech-language pathologists. *American Journal of Speech Language Pathology, 12*(3), 376–380.

Fox, R. J., Kasner, S. E., Chatterjee, A., & Chalela, J. A. (2001). Aphemia: An isolated disorder of articulation. *Clinical Neurology and Neurosurgery, 103,* 123–126.

Gadian, D. G., Aicardi, J., Watkins, K. E., Porter, D. A., Mishkin, M., & Vargha-Khadem, F. (2000). Developmental amnesia associated with early hypoxic-ischaemic injury. *Brain, 123,* 499–507.

Gadian, D. G., Isaacs, E. B., Cross, J. H., Connelly, A., Jackson, G. D., King, M.D., et al. (1996). Lateralization of brain function in childhood revealed by magnetic resonance spectroscopy. *Neurology, 46,* 974–977.

Halpern, H., Darley, F. L., & Brown, J. R. (1973). Differential language and neurologic characteristics in cerebral involvement. *Journal of Speech and Hearing Disorders, 38*(2), 162–173.

Hazeltine, E., Grafton, S. T., & Ivry, R. (1997). Attention and stimulus characteristics determine the locus of motor-sequence encoding: A PET study. *Brain, 120*(1), 123–140.

Hertrich, I., & Ackermann, H. (1994). Acoustic analysis of speech timing in Huntington's disease. *Brain and Language, 47,* 182–196.

Hillis, A. E., Work, M., Barker, P. B., Jacobs, M. A., Breese, E. L., & Maurer, K.

(2004). Re-examining the brain regions crucial for orchestrating speech articulation. *Brain, 127,* 1479–1487.

Hurst, J. A., Baraitser, M., Auger, E., Graham, F., & Norell, S. (1990). An extended family with a dominantly inherited speech disorder. *Developmental Medicine and Child Neurology, 32,* 352–355.

Isaacs, E. B., Edmonds, C. J., Lucas, A., & Gadian, D. G. (2001). Calculation difficulties in children of very low birthweight: A neural correlate. *Brain, 124*(9), 1701–1707.

Ivry, R. B., & Spencer, R. M. (2004). The neuronal representation of time. *Current Opinion in Neurobiology, 14,* 225–232.

Jackson, G. D., Connelly, A., Duncan, J. S., Grunewald, R. A., & Gadian, D. G. (1993). Detection of hippocampal pathology in intractable partial epilepsy: Increased sensitivity with quantitative magnetic resonance T2 relaxometry. *Neurology, 43,* 1793–1799.

Jaffe, S. L., Glabus, M. F., Kelley, R. E., & Minager, A. (2003). Acute verbal dyspraxia, a rare presentation in multiple sclerosis: A case report with MRI localization. *Multiple Sclerosis, 9,* 630–632.

Jenkins, I. H., Brooks, D. J., Nixon, P. D., Frackowiak, R. S., & Passingham, R. E. (1994). Motor sequence learning: A study with positron emission tomography. *Journal of Neuroscience, 14,* 3775–3790.

Karni, A., Meyer, G., Jezzard, P., Adams, M. M., Turner, R., & Ungerleider, L. G. (1995). Functional MRI evidence for adult motor cortex plasticity during motor skill learning. *Nature, 377,* 155–158.

Kent, R. D. (2000). Research on speech motor control and its disorders: A review and prospective. *Journal of Communication Disorders, 33,* 391–427.

Kimura, D., & Watson, N. (1989). The relation between oral movement control and speech. *Brain and Language, 37*(4), 565–590.

Lai, C. S., Fisher, S. E, Hurst, J. A., Vargha-Khadem, F., & Monaco, A. P. (2001). A forkhead-domain gene is mutated in a severe speech and language disorder. *Nature, 413,* 519–523.

Lenneberg, E. H. (1964). Speech as a motor skill with special reference to nonaphasic disorders. *Monographs of the Society for Research in Child Development, 29,* 115–127.

Lewis, B. A. (1992). Pedigree analysis of children with phonology disorders. *Journal of Learning Disabilities, 25*(9), 586–597.

Lewis, B. A., Freebairn, L. A., Hansen, A., Gerry-Taylor, H., Iyengar, S., & Shriberg, L. D. (2004). Family pedigrees of children with suspected childhood apraxia of speech. *Journal of Communication Disorders, 37*(3), 157–175.

Levelt, W. J. (1999). Models of word production. *Trends in Cognitive Sciences, 3*(6), 223–232.

Liegeois, F., Baldeweg, T., Connelly, A., Gadian, D. G., Mishkin, M., & Vargha-Khadem, F. (2003). Language fMRI abnormalities associated with *FOXP2* gene mutation. *Nature Neuroscience, 6*(11), 1230–1237.

Ludlow, C. L., Connor, N. P., & Bassich, C. J. (1987). Speech timing in Parkinson's and Huntington's disease. *Brain and Language, 32,* 195–214.

Maassen, B. (2002). Issues contrasting adult acquired versus developmental apraxia of speech. *Seminars in Speech and Language, 23*(4), 257–266.

Mateer, C. (1978). Impairments of nonverbal oral movements after left hemisphere damage: A follow-up analysis of errors. *Brain and Language, 6*(3), 334–341.

Mateer, C., & Kimura, D. (1977). Impairment of nonverbal oral movements in aphasia. *Brain and Language, 4*(2), 262–276.

Mendez, M. F. (2004). Aphemia-like syndrome from a right supplementary motor area lesion. *Clinical Neurology and Neurosurgery, 106*(4), 337–339.

Milloy, N. R. (1991). *Breakdown of speech: Causes and remediation.* London: Chapman & Hall.

Mishkin, M., Malamut, B., & Bachevalier, J. (1984). Memories and habits: Two neural systems. In G. Lynch, J. L. McGaugh, & N. W. Weinburger (Eds.), *Neurobiology of human learning and memory* (pp. 65–87). New York: Guilford Press.

Morgan, A., Liegeois, F., Vogel, A., Connelly, A., & Vargha-Khadem, F. (2005). *Electropalatography findings and functional brain abnormalities associated with an inherited speech disorder.* Paper presented at the Fourth International Electropalatography symposium, Queen Margaret University College, Edinburgh, UK.

Morley, M., Court, D., & Miller, H. (1954). Developmental dysarthria. *British Medical Journal, 2,* 8–10.

Murdoch, B. E. (1990). *Acquired speech and language disorders: Neuroanatomical and functional neurological approach.* London: Chapman & Hall.

Muter, V., Hulme, C., Snowling, M. J., & Stevenson, J. (2004). Phonemes, rimes, vocabulary, and grammatical skills as foundations of early reading development: Evidence from a longitudinal study. *Developmental Psychology, 40,* 665–681.

Nadeau, S. E., & Crosson, B. (1997). Subcortical aphasia. *Brain and Language, 58,* 355–402.

Ozanne, A. E. (1995). The search for developmental verbal dyspraxia. In B. Dodd (Ed.), *Differential diagnosis of children with speech disorder* (pp. 91–109). San Diego, CA: Singular.

Peach, R. K. (2004). Acquired apraxia of speech: Features, accounts, and treatment. *Topics in Stroke Rehabilitation, 11*(1), 49–58.

Pellat, J., Gentil, M., Lyard, G., Vila, A., Tarel, V., Moreau, O., et al. (1991). Aphemia after a penetrating brain wound: A case study. *Brain and Language, 40*(4), 459–70.

Pembrey, M. (1992). Genetics and language disorders. In P. Fletcher & D. Hall (Eds.), *Specific speech and language disorders in children: Correlates, characteristics, outcomes* (pp. 51–62). London: Whurr.

Pickett, E. R., Kuniholm, E., Protopapas, A., Friedman, J., & Lieberman, P. (1998). Selective speech motor, syntax and cognitive deficits associated with bilateral damage to the putamen and the head of the caudate nucleus: A case study. *Neuropsychologia, 36,* 173–188.

Piggott, G. L, & Kessler-Robb, M. (1999). Prosodic features of familial language impairment: Constraints on stress assignment. *Folia Phoniatrica et Logopaedica, 51*(1–2), 55–69.

Rao, S. M., Harrington, D. L., Haaland, K. Y., Bobholz, J. A., Cox, R. W., & Binder, J. R. (1997). Distributed neural systems underlying the timing of movements. *Journal of Neuroscience, 17,* 5528–5535.

Rapin, I., & Allen, D. A. (1988). Syndromes in developmental dysphasia and adult aphasia. *Research Publications—Association for Research in Nervous and Mental Disease, 66,* 57–75.

Rauch, S. L., Whalen, P. J., Savage, C. R., Curran, T., Kendrick, A., Brown, H. D., et al. (1997). Striatal recruitment during an implicit sequence learning task as measured by functional magnetic resonance imaging. *Human Brain Mapping, 5,* 124–132.

Riecker, A., Mathiak, K., Wildgruber, D., Erb, M., Hertrich, I., Grodd, W., et al. (2005). fMRI reveals two distinct cerebral networks subserving speech motor control. *Neurology, 64,* 700–706.

Salmond, C. H., Ashburner, J., Connelly, A., Friston, K. J., Gadian, D. G., & Vargha-Khadem, F. (2005). The role of the medial temporal lobe in autistic spectrum disorders. *European Journal of Neuroscience, 22*(3), 764–772.

Salmond, C. H., Ashburner, J., Vargha-Khadem, F., Gadian, D. G., & Friston, K. J. (2000). Detecting bilateral abnormalities with voxel-based morphometry. *Human Brain Mapping, 11,* 223–232.

Scheffer, I. E. (2000). Autosomal dominant rolandic epilepsy with speech dyspraxia. *Epileptic Disorders, 2*(Suppl. 1), S19–S22.

Schirmer, A. (2004). Timing speech: A review of lesion and neuroimaging findings. *Brain Research: Cognitive Brain Research, 21,* 269–287.

Schmahmann, J. D. (2004). Disorders of the cerebellum: Ataxia, dysmetria of thought, and the cerebellar cognitive affective syndrome. *Journal of Neuropsychiatry and Clinical Neuroscience, 16,* 367–378.

Schmahmann, J. D., Doyon, J., McDonald, D., Holmes, C., Lavoie, K., Hurwitz, A. S., et al. (1999). Three-dimensional MRI atlas of the human cerebellum in proportional stereotaxic space. *NeuroImage, 10,* 233–260.

Shriberg, L. D., Aram, D. M, & Kwiatkowski, J. (1997). Developmental apraxia of speech: I. Descriptive and theoretical perspectives. *Journal of Speech, Language, and Hearing Research, 40*(2), 273–285.

Siok, W. T., Jin, Z., Fletcher, P., & Tan, L. H. (2003). Distinct brain regions associated with syllable and phoneme. *Human Brain Mapping, 18,* 201–207.

Square, P. A, Roy, E. A., & Martin, R. E. (1997). Apraxia of speech: Another form of praxis disruption. In L. A. Gonzales-Rothi & K. M. Heilman (Eds.), *Apraxia: The neuropsychology of action* (pp. 173–206). Hillsdale, NJ: Erlbaum.

Squire, L. R., & Knowlton, B. J. (2000). The medial temporal lobe, the hippocampus, and the memory systems of the brain. In M. S. Gazzaniga (Ed.), *The new cognitive neurosciences* (pp. 765–780). Cambridge, MA: MIT Press.

Squire, L. R., Knowlton, B., & Musen, G. (1993). The structure and organization of memory. *Annual Review of Psychology, 44,* 453–495.

Stackhouse, J. (1992). Developmental verbal dyspraxia: 1. A review and critique. *European Journal of Disorders of Communication, 27*(1), 19–34.

Tallal, P., Jernigan, T. L., & Trauner, D. (1994). Developmental bilateral damage to the head of the caudate nuclei: Implications for speech–language pathology. *Journal of Medical Speech–Language Pathology, 2,* 23–28.

Tallal, P., Townsend, J., Curtiss, S., & Wulfeck B. (1991). Phenotypic profiles of language-impaired children based on genetic/family history. *Brain and Language, 41*(1), 81–95.

Teuber, H. L. (1975). Recovery of function after brain injury in man. In R. Porter & D. W. Fitzsimons (Eds.), *Outcome of severe damage to the central nervous system: CIBA Foundation Symposium 34* (pp. 159–190). Amsterdam: Elsevier.

Thoonen, G., Maassen, B., Gabreels, F., & Schreuder, R. (1999). Validity of maximum performance tasks to diagnose motor speech disorders in children. *Clinical Linguistics and Phonetics, 13*(1), 1–23.

Ungerleider, L. G., Doyon, J., & Karni, A. (2002). Imaging brain plasticity during motor skill learning. *Neurobiology of Learning and Memory, 78,* 553–564.

Ullman, M. T. (2004). Contributions of memory circuits to language: The declarative/procedural model. *Cognition, 92,* 231–270.

Ullman, M. T., & Pierpont, E. I. (2005). Specific language impairment is not specific to language: The procedural deficit hypothesis. *Cortex, 41,* 399–433.

van Mourik, M., Catsman-Berrevoets, C. E., Yousef-Bak, E., Paquier, P. F., & van Dongen, H. R. (1998). Dysarthria in children with cerebellar or brainstem tumors. *Pediatric Neurology, 18,* 411–414.

Van Paesschen, W., Revesz, T., Duncan, J. S., Kling, M. D., & Connelly, A. (1997). Quantitative neuropathology and quantitative magnetic resonance imaging of the hippocampus in temporal lobe epilepsy. *Annals of Neurology, 42,* 756–766.

Vargha-Khadem, F., Carr, L. J., Isaacs, E., Brett, E., Adams, C., & Mishkin, M. (1997). Onset of speech after left hemispherectomy in a nine-year-old boy. *Brain, 120*(1), 159–182.

Vargha-Khadem, F., Gadian, D. G., Copp, A., & Mishkin, M. (2005). *FOXP2* and the neuroanatomy of speech and language. *Nature Reviews: Neurosciences, 6,* 131–138.

Vargha-Khadem, F., Isaacs, E., & Muter, V. (1994). A review of cognitive outcome after unilateral lesions sustained during childhood. *Journal of Child Neurology, 9*(Suppl. 2), 67–73.

Vargha-Khadem, F., Isaacs, E., Papaleloudi, H., Polkey, C., & Wilson, J. (1991). Development of language in six hemispherectomized patients. *Brain, 114,* 463–495.

Vargha-Khadem, F., Isaacs, E., Watkins, K., & Mishkin, M. (2000). Ontogenetic specialization of hemispheric function. In J. M. Oxbury, C. E. Polkey, & M. Duchowney (Eds.), *Intractable focal epilepsy: Medical and surgical treatment* (pp. 405–418). London: Harcourt.

Vargha-Khadem, F., & Mishkin, M. (1997). Speech and language outcome after hemispherectomy in childhood. In I. Tuxhorn, H. Holthausen, & H. E.

Boenigk (Eds.), *Paediatric epilepsy syndromes and their surgical treatment* (pp. 774–784). London: Libbey.

Vargha-Khadem, F., & Polkey, C. (1992). A review of cognitive outcome after hemidecortication in humans. In D. Rose & D. Johnson (Eds.), *Recovery from brain damage: Reflections and directions* (pp. 32–48). New York: Plenum Press.

Vargha-Khadem, F., Salmond, C. H., Watkins, K. E., Price, C. E., Ashburner, J., Alcock, K. J., et al. (2003). Developmental amnesia: Effect of age at injury. *Proceedings of the National Academy of Sciences USA, 100,* 10055–10060.

Vargha-Khadem, F., Watkins, K., Alcock, K., Fletcher, P., & Passingham, R. (1995). Praxic and nonverbal cognitive deficits in a large family with a genetically transmitted speech and language disorder. *Proceedings of the National Academy of Sciences USA, 92*(3), 930–933.

Vargha-Khadem, F., Watkins, K. E., Price, C. J., Ashburner, J., Alcock, K. J., Connelly, A., et al. (1998). Neural basis of an inherited speech and language disorder. *Proceedings of the National Academy of Sciences USA, 95*(21), 12695–12700.

Vargha-Khadem, F., Watters, G., & O'Gorman, A. (1985). Development of speech and language following bilateral frontal lesions. *Brain and Language, 25,* 167–183.

Warren, J. D., Smith, H. B., Denson, L. A., & Waddy, H. M. (2000). Expressive language disorder after infarction of left lentiform nucleus. *Journal of Clinical Neuroscience, 7,* 456–458.

Watkins, K. E., Dronkers, N. F., & Vargha-Khadem, F. (2002). Behavioural analysis of an inherited speech and language disorder: Comparison with acquired aphasia. *Brain, 125*(3), 452–464.

Watkins, K. E., Vargha-Khadem, F., Ashburner, J., Passingham, R. E., Connelly, A., Friston K. J., et al. (2002). MRI analysis of an inherited speech and language disorder: Structural brain abnormalities. *Brain, 125*(3), 465–478.

Wildgruber, D., Ackermann, H., & Grodd, W. (2001). Differential contributions of motor cortex, basal ganglia, and cerebellum to speech motor control: Effects of syllable repetition rate evaluated by fMRI. *NeuroImage, 13,* 101–109.

Xu, B., Grafman, J., Gaillard, W. D., Ishii, K., Vega-Bermudez, F., Pietrini, P., et al. (2001). Conjoint and extended neural networks for the computation of speech code: The neural basis of selective impairment in reading words and pseudowords. *Cerebral Cortex, 11,* 267–277.

Neurotypical　　　　Autism

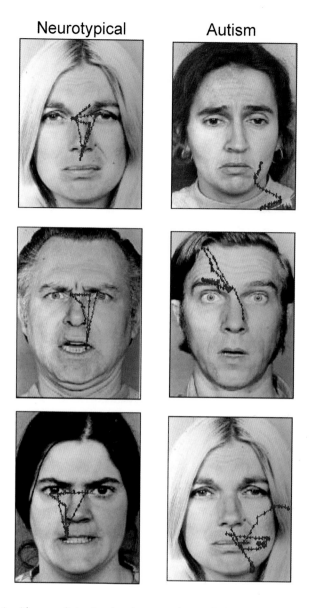

PLATE 3.1. Abnormalities in visual scanpaths made by individuals with autism (right column) relative to neurologically normal individuals (left column). Among other deficits in social perception and social cognition, individuals with autism exhibit abnormal scanpaths when viewing faces, typically spending little time on the core features of the face, particularly the eyes. This deficit is comparable to that shown by a patient with bilateral lesions of the amygdala, implicating this structure for functioning in face scanning and processing of information from core facial features, especially the eyes. The cross marks and lines together indicate the subject's point of regard over time during the presentation of the face. Reproduced with kind permission of Springer Science and Business Media from Pelphrey, K. A., Sasson, N. J., Reznick, J. S., Paul, G., Goldman, B. D., & Piven, J. (2002). Visual scanning of faces in autism. *Journal of Autism and Developmental Disorders, 32*(4), 249–261.

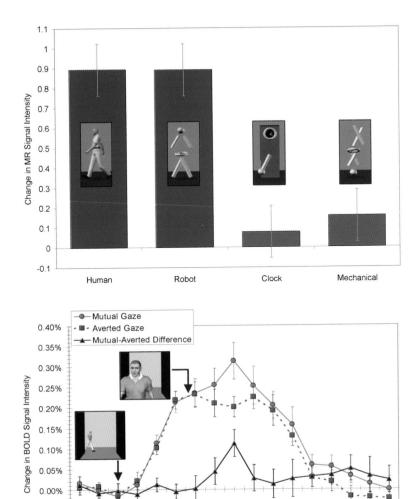

PLATE 3.2. *Top panel*: Measurements of the peak amplitudes from all voxels in the right hemisphere superior temporal sulcus for each of four conditions: walking human, walking robot, ticking grandfather clock, and moving mechanical assembly. Adapted with permission from Pelphrey, K. A., Mitchell, T. V., McKeown, M. J., Goldstein, J., Allison, T., & McCarthy, G. (2003). Brain activity evoked by the perception of human walking: Controlling for meaningful coherent motion. *Journal of Neuroscience*, 23(17), 6819–6825. *Bottom panel*: The time courses of average BOLD signal changes from the activated right superior temporal sulcus voxels in response to mutual and averted gaze movements made by a man walking down a hallway. The mutual and averted gaze conditions are plotted along with a difference waveform of mutual-averted gaze. Adapted with permission from Pelphrey, K. A., Viola, R. J., & McCarthy, G. (2004). When strangers pass: Processing of mutual and averted social gaze in the superior temporal sulcus. *Psychological Science*, 15(9), 598–603.

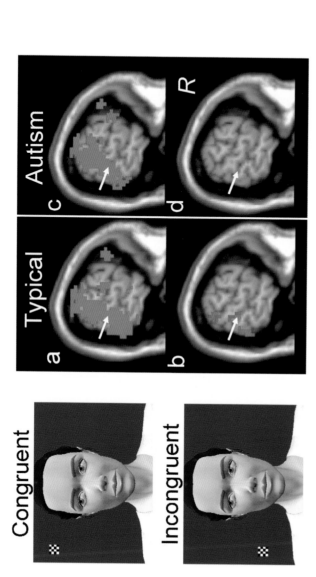

PLATE 3.3. *Left panel:* A small checkerboard appeared and flickered in the woman's field of view for 5 seconds. In two conditions, she either shifted her gaze toward (congruent with viewer expectations) or away from (incongruent) the checkerboard after a delay of 1 or 3 seconds. *Right panel:* Incongruent trials evoked greater superior temporal sulcus activity than did congruent trials in the typically developing individuals (see panel sections *a* and *b*). Although the same brain regions were activated in the individuals with autism, these subjects did not differentiate between the congruent and incongruent trials (see panel sections *c* and *d*), indicating that the activity was not modulated by the context of the perceived gaze shifts. Adapted with permission from Pelphrey, K. A., Morris, J., & McCarthy, G. (2005). Neural basis of eye gaze processing deficits in autism. *Brain, 128*(5), 1038–1048.

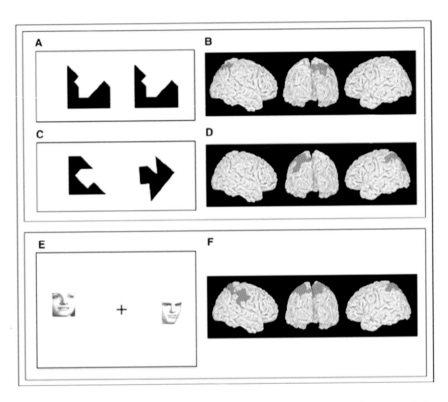

PLATE 4.1. Stimuli and significant group differences in activation between adults with WS and controls in three fMRI tasks. (*A*) Example of stimuli for matching task. (*B*) Significant hypoactivation in WS compared to controls in the match-versus-baseline contrast (matching task). (*C*) Example of square completion stimuli. (*D*) Significant hypoactivation in WS compared to controls in the construction-versus-match contrast (square completion task). (*E*) Example of object-versus-location-task stimuli. Both face (shown) and house stimuli were used. (*F*) Significant hypoactivation in WS compared to controls in the location > object contrast (location-versus-object task). All activation difference maps are significant at $p < .05$ cluster level corrected for multiple comparisons (voxel threshold, $p < .001$). Reproduced with permission from Elsevier from Meyer-Lindenberg, A., Kohn, P., Mervis, C. B., Kippenhan, J. S., Olsen, R. K., Morris, C. A., et al. (2004). Neural basis of genetically determined visuospatial construction deficit in Williams syndrome. *Neuron, 43*, 623–631.

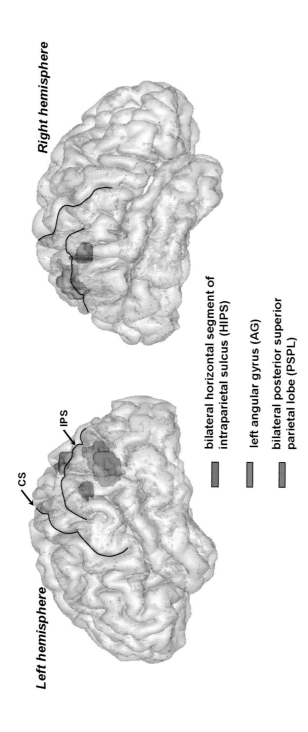

Right hemisphere

Left hemisphere

CS

IPS

bilateral horizontal segment of
intraparietal sulcus (HIPS)

left angular gyrus (AG)

bilateral posterior superior
parietal lobe (PSPL)

PLATE 9.1. Three-dimensional representation of parietal regions activated in numerical tasks (see text for details). For better visualization, the clusters show all parietal voxels activated in at least 40% of studies in a given group. Adapted with permission from Dehaene, S., Piazza, M., Pinel, P., & Cohen, L. (2003). Three parietal circuits for number processing. *Cognitive Neuropsychology, 20,* 487–506, http://www.psypress.co.uk/journals.asp.

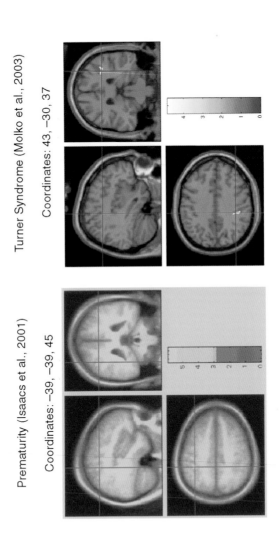

Prematurity (Isaacs et al., 2001)

Coordinates: −39, −39, 45

Turner Syndrome (Molko et al., 2003)

Coordinates: 43, −30, 37

PLATE 9.2. *Left:* Reduced gray matter density in the intraparietal sulcus in dyscalculia, in children born prematurely; reproduced with permission from Oxford University Press from Isaacs, E. B., Edmonds, C. J., Lucas, A., & Gadian, D. G. (2001). Calculation difficulties in children of very low birthweight: A neural correlate. *Brain, 124*(9), 1701–1707). *Right:* Women with Turner syndrome; reproduced with permission from Elsevier from Dehaene, S., Molko, N., Cohen, L., & Wilson, A. J. (2004). Arithmetic and the brain. *Current Opinion in Neurobiology, 14*(2), 218–224.

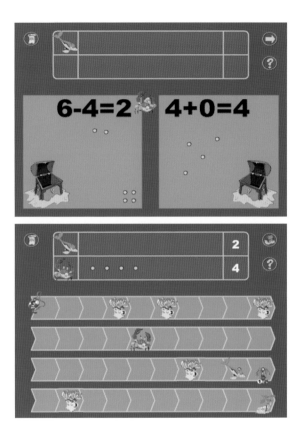

PLATE 9.3. Screenshots from "The Number Race," remediation software for dyscalculia in the form of an adaptive game (produced in our laboratory by Anna Wilson). The child plays the character of the dolphin and has to choose the larger of two numerosities before his or her competitor (the crab) arrives at the key and steals this many pieces of gold. Here we see a high difficulty level, with addition and subtraction required before numerical comparison is performed. The child then wins the same amount of squares on a game board, where he or she must avoid landing on anemone hazards. Once the child arrives at the end of the board, he or she wins a "reward" fish to add to his or her collection. Winning enough of these rewards unlocks access to the next character.

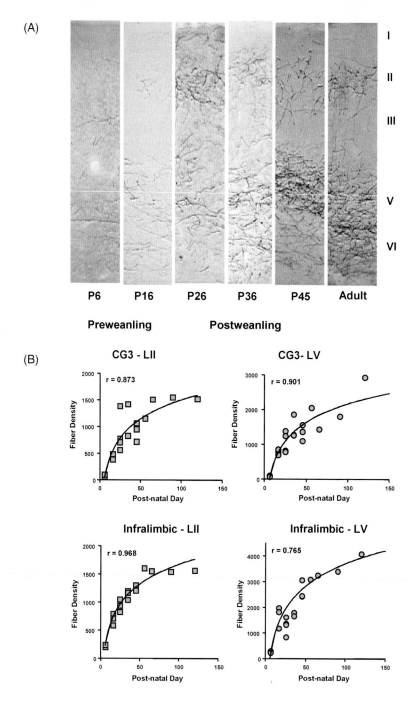

PLATE 13.1. Postnatal development of amygdalocingulate connections. (*A*) A set of photomicrographs showing a progressive increase in the density of labeled fibers originating in the basolateral amygdala. (*B*) A set of graphs showing a curvilinear increase in the numerical density of amygdalocortical projections between the preweaning and early adult periods in the rat brain.

CHAPTER 8

Relation between Early Measures of Brain Responses to Language Stimuli and Childhood Performance on Language and Language-Related Tasks

Dennis L. Molfese
Victoria J. Molfese
Peter J. Molfese

For decades, researchers interested in language development have focused their efforts on investigations of the development of phonology, syntax, semantics, and morphology (e.g., Reese & Lipsitt, 1970). Research interest in language development was ignited in part by Chomsky's (1957) work on the syntactic structures of language and research evidence of a biological basis for human language learning (e.g., Lenneberg, 1967). This work challenged the then prevailing view that language development relied heavily on modeling and reinforcement for word meaning (semantics) and grammar (syntax). Thus began the historical "scientific revolution" in language research (Fraser, Bellugi, & Brown, 1963; Jenkins & Palermo, 1964). The theoretical (Chomsky & Halle, 1968) and empirical research on phonological development (Templin, 1957) and the study of speech perception (Liberman, Cooper, Shankweiler, & Studdert-Kennedy, 1967) attracted the attention of a number of investigators interested in language and phonological development in infancy (Eimas, Siqueland, Jusczyk, & Vigorito,

1971). Interest in phonology has continued into the present time and, indeed, flourished as investigators have begun to expand their research to language-related skills, such as reading, whose development relies on phonological skills.

Phonological skills refer to the abilities to perceive and understand the speech sounds that make up words. The discrimination of speech sounds and the skills needed to identify words from both individual sounds and sound combinations are involved in phonological processing. Phonological skills occur at many levels, including phonological awareness (detecting the individual sounds that comprise words), phonological retrieval (the ability to access and use the sounds and names of words), and phonological memory (the ability to code phonological information such as a string of words or nonwords into memory). Children learn to use phonological skills to learn and identify words that they hear as well as to sound out or decode written words; that is, phonological skills are used to write words as well as for the oral production of words. For children with language disorders or reading disabilities, detecting phonological information and using phonological skills may be difficult and inaccurate (Aram & Kamhi, 1982; Bishop, 1997; Camarata, 1995; Fletcher, Foorman, Shaywitz, & Shaywitz, 1999; see also Goswami, Chapter 6, this volume). The renewed interest in phonology as an important aspect of language skill has resulted in greater interest in learning about how phonological skills play a role in the typical and atypical development of language and reading skills.

This chapter reviews research on the perception of speech sounds during infancy and how phonological skills are linked to the later development of language and reading skills. We focus specifically on studies using electrophysiological and behavioral assessment techniques to study the brain's role in speech perception. The evidence for brain and behavior relations in measures of speech perception and the development of language and reading skills is discussed from theoretical and empirical perspectives.

PHONOLOGICAL PROCESSING AND LANGUAGE SKILLS

The belief that there could be an early biologically related influence on the acquisition of language can be traced to a number of research findings. Lenneberg (1967) argued that a biological substrate subserves language abilities and that evidence for this substrate could be seen at a number of levels in humans. For example, human beings are physically structured to produce speech sounds via the anatomical characteristics of the human vocal tract, and to hear these speech sounds via specific auditory processing

mechanisms, with the pinna of the ear structured to favor acoustic information in the range of frequencies known to carry much of the speech code.
Such biological factors were found to have homologues in nonhuman
mammals as well. For example, Kuhl and Miller (1975) found that chin-
chillas discriminate some speech cues, such as voicing cues, along dimen-
sions that are similar to the discrimination shown by humans. Morse and
Showdon (1975) and Kuhl and Padden (1983) reported a somewhat similar effect with rhesus monkeys. Studies by Morse, Molfese, Laughlin,
Linnville, and Wetzel (1987) and Molfese and colleagues (1986) also
reported that the electrophysiological responses of infant rhesus monkeys
had similarities to those reported in studies of humans. Together these findings indicated that several different mammalian species discriminate speech
sounds in a fashion comparable to humans—findings that support the
notion of a biological substrate for speech perception.

At a neurological level, Lenneberg linked brain organization to the
development of language skills. For Lenneberg, lateralization of brain functions was a biological indicator of language acquisition (Lenneberg, 1967).
Although research evidence supported his general view that there are specific biological underpinnings that facilitate language development, investigators challenged his views that brain lateralization occurred after language
acquisition. Molfese (1972) and Molfese, Freeman, and Palermo (1975)
reported the first evidence of brain lateralization in early infancy, before
the beginning of language. In these and later publications, Molfese reported
that electrophysiological responses of full-term and preterm newborn
infants as well as 2-month-old infants indicate that the left and right hemispheres respond differently to specific speech cues (Molfese & Molfese,
1983). Other researchers reported that damage to the left hemisphere in the
first year of life had detrimental effects on the acquisition of syntactic skills
in childhood (Dennis & Whitaker, 1976). Thus this research showed that
before language production skills were evident, lateralized regions in the
brains of young children were already differentially responsive to the
speech and language environment.

Whereas early research employed different behavioral paradigms to
study the discrimination of different auditory stimuli, later research began
to examine more systematically the perception of the auditory dimensions
of speech sounds and to involve measures of brain processing. This
research was greatly facilitated by the use of event-related potential (ERP)
techniques that use scalp electrodes to detect electrical activity generated by
neurons in the brain. These brain responses, in turn, can be related to
behavioral measures as a way to identify reliable commonalities that would
be useful for understanding how brain mechanisms correspond to behavior, such as the discrimination of different speech-sound contrasts.

The ERP is a synchronized portion of the ongoing electroencephalo-gram (EEG) and reflects changes in brain activity over time during stimu-lus processing (Molfese, Molfese, & Pratt, in press; Rockstroh, Elbert, Birbaumer, & Lutzenberger, 1982). Changes in brain activity are reflected in the amplitude (in microvolts [µV] or height of the wave at different tem-poral points) and latency (time lapsed in milliseconds [ms] measured from the onset of the stimulus) of regions of the ERP waveform. Based on brain electrophysiology and statistical analyses, specific peaks within the ERP waveform are identified and examined to determine if they are systemati-cally related to independent variables under study, such as voice-onset time (VOT) of an auditory stimulus. The ERP differs from the more traditional EEG measure because it reflects a portion of the ongoing EEG activity that is time-locked to the onset of a specific external event, such as the presenta-tion of a speech sound, or the onset of an internal event, such as a cognitive process (e.g., detecting semantic differences between words such as tennis *ball* versus Cinderella's *ball*; Molfese, Papanicolaou, Hess, & Molfese, 1979). This time-locked feature is the real strength of the ERP measure because it enables researchers to track the processing of stimulus events across time. The temporal event-related specificity of the ERP technique represents a major advantage over the traditional EEG measures as well as other techniques such as fMRI and MRI (Cacioppo, Tassinary, & Berntson, 2000; Papanicolaou, 1998).

ERP responses allow researchers to examine direct correlations be-tween rapid changes in brain responses from different electrode regions that may originate from different brain areas and behaviors that reflect processing across the very short time periods that are involved. As re-searchers began to examine more specific dimensions of auditory stimuli, they noted variations in ERP components (waveform peak amplitudes and latencies) that occurred in response to changes in stimulus dimen-sions in adults (Molfese, 1978, 1980) as well as in infants and children (Dehaene-Lambertz & Peña, 2001; Dehaene-Lambertz, Peña, Christophe, & Landrieu, 2004; Cheour, Alho, et al., 1998; Cheour, Ceponiene, et al, 1998; Cheour et al., 2002; Martynova, Kirjavainen, & Cheour, 2003; Molfese, 1978, 1980, 1989; Molfese & Hess, 1978). As researchers pur-sued these investigations, some sought ways to investigate whether a link could be identified between the ability to discriminate auditory stimuli, as evidenced by changes in the ERP, and concurrent or later developing cogni-tive skills, particularly in infants (Molfese & Molfese, 1985). This interest in developmental changes in brain responses and the meaning of the changes in terms of predicting later outcomes opened what has become a robust area of research. Investigation of the relations between early mea-sures of brain responsiveness and language development has been particu-larly popular.

THE USE OF ERPs TO PREDICT LANGUAGE

Among the earliest studies attempting to relate measures of brain responsiveness to later behavioral measures are a series of studies using visual ERPs with infants and children, recorded in response to a simple flash of light. An early peak in the brain wave (with the latency of the first negative component occurring at approximately 146 ms after the onset of the light flash) was found that correlated with several behavioral measures. For example, Butler and Engel (1969) reported correlations between the visual ERP latencies obtained from neonates and later measures of intelligence obtained in infancy. In this study, a sample of 433 children was obtained from the Collaborative Project on Cerebral Palsy, Mental Retardation, and Other Neurological and Sensory Disorders of Infancy and Childhood. Performance scores on the Bayley Scales of Infant Development at 8 months were obtained and used as the criterion measures. Although the correlations between the behavioral measures and visual ERP latencies were significant, the effects were moderate (r's ranged from .23 to .33) and accounted for only small amounts of variance. Correlations between gestational age and Bayley scores were similar in magnitude, although the correlations between birth weight and Bayley scores were somewhat smaller. Although photic latency was found to contribute to the correlations with Bayley developmental scores independently of gestational age and birthweight, the amount of variance accounted for by photic latency alone was little better than that accounted for by gestational age alone. In a follow-up to this study, Jensen and Engel (1971) subsequently reported correlations between neonatal photic latencies and developmental scores (i.e., age of walking) at 1 year of age. In that study visual ERP responses were obtained from 1,074 neonates. When the ERP latencies were divided into three regions (short, middle, and long), it was found that infants with short photic latencies were the first to walk.

Unfortunately, researchers reported less success when attempting to extend prediction beyond the first year of life and into early childhood. Engel and Fay (1972) investigated the relationship between visual ERPs recorded in 852 neonates and later performance on tests of articulation obtained at 3 years of age and on the Stanford–Binet Intelligence Test obtained at 4 years of age. These researchers reported that infants with faster visual ERP latencies (less than 146 ms) performed better at 3 years of age on an initial and final consonant articulation task than did slow reactors. Visual ERP latencies, however, were not predictive of differences in performance on the Stanford–Binet at 4 years. The authors concluded that although visual ERP latency may be predictive of motor development, such as that involved in articulation, it is not predictive of symbolic/intellectual development. Engel and Henderson (1973) and Henderson and Engel

(1974) conducted subsequent studies with somewhat older children. These studies failed to find a relationship between five peaks identified in the visual ERPs of neonates and scores on the Wechsler Intelligence Scale for Children—Revised (WISC-R) subtests and the Bender-Gestalt test obtained when the children (*n* = 122) were 7–8 years of age. The authors concluded that the latencies of neonatal visual ERP responses in neurologically normal children are not related to later intelligence test performance. Henderson and Engel reached a similar conclusion in their follow-up study, in which they assessed whether neonatal visual ERPs could be used to predict total WISC-R intelligence and subtest scores, sensorimotor, perceptuomotor, and achievement test scores at 7 years of age. The visual ERP latency data from the 809 infants participating in the study did not significantly correlate with any of the performance scores.

Studies conducted during the late 1960s and the 1970s reported some early links between visual ERP measures and subsequent motor, cognitive–motor, or language-related abilities during the first year of life. However, when longer-term predictions were attempted, researchers failed to find reliable correlations. Although such findings dampened hopes of identifying factors in infancy that could be used to identify children's status on developmental outcome measures, a series of longitudinal studies was begun in the late 1970s that offered new evidence that early predictive factors could be reliably identified from brain and behavior measures (Molfese, 2000; Molfese & Molfese, 1985; Molfese & Searock, 1986). In retrospect, it appears that the differences in success between the earlier and later studies were due to changes in research methodology and data analyses. For example, Molfese and his associates focused their analyses on the entire evoked potential waveform (a time period of approximately 700 ms), thus expanding the portion of the brain responses that was analyzed. Analyzing a longer portion of the waveform enabled statistical techniques to be applied to more data in an effort to identify whether brain responses recorded in infancy were systematically related to behaviors measured at later ages. The frequency range of the ERPs analyzed was also expanded to include frequencies below 2 Hz because frequencies in this range are characteristic of the evoked potentials of young infants. The inclusion of lower-frequency signals through a change in the filtering of the brain responses enabled an enhanced and more comprehensive brain response to be examined.

Later studies also used language-related stimuli, such as speech sounds, as the evoking stimuli rather than the light flashes used by the researchers cited above. The relation of light flashes to the types of cognitive processing reflected in language skills and in the various cognitive skills tapped by intelligence tests is not known. However, data are available indicating that speech perception abilities are specifically related to language skill and that

the verbal skills of young children play an important part in their performance on intelligence tests (Molfese, Yaple, Helwig, Harris, & Connell,
1992). Because predictors of successful performance are generally better if
they measure factors more directly related to the predicted skills, the inclusion of more language-relevant materials as the evoking stimuli in later
studies increased the likelihood of predicting later language-related skills.
These methodological changes yielded more successful results from predictive studies designed to link early speech perception skills with later language and language-related cognitive skills, such as reading.

Molfese and colleagues (1975) were the first to report evidence of
functional laterality to speech sounds in young infants. This early work is
significant because theoreticians previously had speculated that the absence
of hemispheric or lateralized differences in the brain indicated that the child
was at risk for certain cognitive or language disabilities (Travis, 1931).
Three decades later, Lenneberg (1967) argued that lateralization is a biological sign of language and that the presence of hemispheric differences,
per se, is predictive of language development. In sharp contrast to this view,
Molfese and colleagues reported that lateralized brain responding is present
in very early infancy, even before language skills become evident. This finding was subsequently replicated and supported by results obtained by other
investigators using a variety of different methodologies. A decade later,
Molfese and Molfese (1985) argued that lateralization, per se, was not an
effective predictor of later language development. Rather, they argued, and
reported evidence to support, the contention that predictions concerning
language performance are effective only when specific speech perception
processing capacities are lateralized.

In their study, Molfese and Molfese (1985) recorded ERPs from 16
infants, in response to different consonant and vowel sounds and using
electrodes placed over the left and right temporal scalp areas (traditionally
identified as T3 and T4 in the 10–20 electrode placement system; Jasper,
1958). These electrodes were referenced to linked ears, and ERPs were
recorded with a bandpass set to 0.1–30 Hz. ERPs were recorded at birth
and again at 6-month intervals until the child's third birthday. Information
was also obtained about prenatal and perinatal events, intelligence, language, socioeconomic status (SES), and child-centered activities in the
home. In this study, six speech stimuli (/bi/, /bae/, /bau/, /gi/, /gae/, /gau/)
and six nonspeech 1-Hz bandwidth sine-wave stimuli, which mimicked the
frequency changes of the speech stimuli, comprised the stimulus set. Analyses indicated that ERPs recorded at birth identified children who performed
better or worse on language tasks by 3 years of age. Two ERP components
discriminated between these two groups of children. The first component
was an initial large negative peak (N230) over left-hemispheric electrodes,
which reliably discriminated children whose scores on the Verbal Index

from the McCarthy Scales of Children's Abilities (McCarthy, 1972) were above 50 (the high group) from those with lower scores (i.e., the low group). Unlike the high group, the low group displayed no lateralized N230 component reflecting discrimination for either the speech or the nonspeech sounds. A second component of the ERP, a late negative peak (N664), also discriminated high from low groups This second component occurred at 664 ms over both hemispheres and therefoee reflected bilateral activity. This component discriminated speech from nonspeech stimuli in the high group only and discriminated specific consonant sounds only when consonants were combined with certain vowels. Thus, both lateralized and bilateral components in the neonatal ERP responses discriminated between the two groups of infants, based on differences between speech and nonspeech sounds. This finding shows that the ERPs reflected a sensitivity to language-related cues rather than brain responsivity to any auditory stimulus.

In subsequent analyses of these data, Molfese and Molfese (1986) investigated the generalizability of the ERP components that predicted language measures. A stepwise multiple regression model used the Peabody Picture Vocabulary Test (PPVT; Dunn, 1965) and McCarthy Verbal Index scores obtained at 3 years of age as the dependent variables. The ERP waveform components obtained at birth that best discriminated the different speech sounds in previous research served as the independent variables. This model accounted for 78% of the total variance in predicting McCarthy Verbal Index scores using the brain responses, whereas 69% of the variance was accounted for in predicting PPVT scores. Clearly, a strong relation exists between early ERP discrimination of speech sounds and later language skills. Interestingly, the inclusion of perinatal measures and Brazelton (1973) scores improved the amount of variance by less than 3%, reinforcing the notion that the brain responses at this early stage of development were more potent than other neonatal status measures in predicting later developmental outcomes, at least in the healthy children who participated in the research.

Molfese (1989) replicated these findings using a different sample of infants, different electrode placements, and different statistical approaches. In that study, ERPs were recorded at birth from frontal, temporal, and parietal scalp areas over the left and right hemispheres of 30 infants, in response to the speech syllables /bi/ and /gi/ and their nonspeech analogues. The infants were brought back at their birthdates for behavioral testing on a variety of cognitive measures, including the McCarthy Scales of Children's Abilities. Discriminant function analyses used the ERP regions identified by Molfese and Molfese (1985) to classify each of the 720 averaged ERPs obtained from the infants into one of two groups (that resembled the low or high language performers of Molfese & Molfese, 1985).

Classification accuracy was significantly above chance, accounting for 68.6% of the children in the high group and 69.7% of those in the low group.

In a study with older infants, Molfese and Searock (1986) extended the predictive relationship between early ERP activity and emerging language skills at 3 years of age to include the discrimination of vowel sounds. ERPs that reflected greater discrimination between vowel sounds at 1 year of age characterized infants who performed better on language tasks at 3 years. Thus, ERPs at birth as well as at 1 year successfully predicted language performance at 3 years. This replication, as well as the other replications reported above, is noteworthy because it indicates the stability of specific regions in the brain waves across different samples of infants measured at different ages. Overall, these data across studies clearly indicate that ERPs in infancy can be used to accurately predict future language skills.

More recently, Molfese and Molfese (1997) found that the relationship between neonatal ERPs and later language performance measures continues into the preschool years. ERPs were recorded from 71 full-term infants in response to nine consonant–vowel syllables that combined each of three initial consonants, b, d, g, with one of three following vowels, a, i, u. Electrode sites and recording procedures were identical to Molfese (1989). Children were retested at 5 years of age using the Stanford–Binet Intelligence Test. These 71 children were divided into two groups based on their Stanford–Binet verbal scores: 62 children with verbal intelligence scores above 100 (high group) and 9 children with verbal intelligence scores less than 100 (the break point of 100 was based on the standardized norms for this test, in which the average score is 100). No differences were noted between groups on prenatal, perinatal, or SES measures. A discriminant function analysis, in which experimental variables were used to differentiate participant groups, correctly classified 8 of 9 children belonging to the low group (88.9%) along with 60 of 62 children (96.8%) belonging to the high group. Thus, analyses indicated a high level of accuracy in using neonatal ERPs recorded in response to speech-sound stimuli to classify children's language performance, as measured by the standard Stanford–Binet verbal scale, at 5 years of age.

WHY IS SPEECH PERCEPTION PREDICTIVE OF LANGUAGE DEVELOPMENT?

Molfese and Molfese (1997) hypothesized that the findings described above reflected underlying perceptual mechanisms upon which aspects of later developing and emerging verbal and cognitive processes are based. Both behavioral and electrophysiological studies indicate that some phonological skills, important for analyzing patterns in speech sounds, are present at or near birth (e.g., discriminating differences in speech sounds based on place of articulation), and other skills (e.g., discriminating differences in speech sounds based on VOT) develop during infancy. Young infants discriminate between speech sounds that contain phonetic contrasts characteristic of their language environments and also appear to be sensitive to phonetic contrasts that are characteristic of other languages (Eilers, Wilson, & Moore, 1977; Eimas et al., 1971; Molfese, 2000; Molfese & Molfese, 1979a, 1979b). This sensitivity changes in later infancy toward increased attention to phonetic contrasts unique to the infant's language environment, a change that appears to facilitate language acquisition.

Further development of phonological skills is evident in the abilities of preschool children to segment spoken monosyllabic words into onset sounds and rimes or rhymes, and thus to play nursery rhyme games (Vellutino & Scanlon, 1987; see also Goswami, Chapter 6, this volume). Children later learn to use phonological skills to segment polysyllabic words into syllables as they approach kindergarten age and monosyllabic words into phonemes at around first grade (Liberman et al., 1967). For most children, fundamental perceptual abilities enable them to use phonological skills to discriminate stimuli within the environment in quite similar ways and to use these phonological skills to develop language and language-related abilities.

For other children, however, their perceptual processes may not respond to environmental elements in the same way. This differential response could indicate future difficulties, given that there is already evidence that phonological skills play a role in some types of disorders evident in language and reading. For example, Kraus and colleagues (1996) tested 90 control children and 91 children with learning disabilities between 6 and 15 years of age. The latter group was diagnosed clinically with learning disabilities, attention-deficit disorders, or both. All children had intelligence test scores greater than 85, but the two groups differed on measures of listening comprehension, visual processing speed, reading, spelling, and auditory memory for words. Both groups discriminated small temporal differences (5 ms) between speech stimuli such as /ba/ versus /wa/, but group differences were found for stimuli such as /ba/ versus /ga/. Kraus et al. found that children who differed in language-related skills also generated different ERP responses to these speech sounds. Other researchers have reported comparable results using a behavioral paradigm. Breier and colleagues (2001) engaged children 7–15 years of age in a behavioral task involving the labeling of speech and nonspeech sounds. Participants were characterized by dyslexia, attention-deficit/hyperactivity disorder (ADHD), comorbidity for both dyslexia and ADHD, or absence of any impairment.

Children with dyslexia were poorer at labeling speech as well as nonspeech sounds and performed at a lower level on measures of phonological processing compared to the other groups.

A link between early speech-sound discrimination skills and later language and reading skills has also been reported in studies of children at risk for dyslexia because of family history (see also Grigorenko, Chapter 5, this volume). In one set of studies, ERP responses to consonant–vowel speech sounds were obtained in the neonatal period from a longitudinal sample of Finnish infants with familial risk for dyslexia. In these studies, brain responses were recorded to standard and deviant stimuli to reflect speech discrimination. Leppanen, Pihko, Eklund, and Lyytinen (1999) and Pihko and colleagues (1999) found, in an examination of difference waves (comparing responses to the standard and deviant stimuli), that neonates at risk for dyslexia had significantly smaller amplitudes over the left hemisphere (between 590 and 625 ms and between 715 and 755 ms) as compared to neonates who were not at risk. These group differences in responsivity had not changed when the infants were retested at 6 months of age. A subsequent study of the same sample of infants used the neonatal ERP responses to predict later language and verbal memory skills when the children were preschool-age (Guttorm et al., 2003). Distinctive hemispheric differences in the ERPs to speech sounds at birth were identified that were predictive of receptive vocabulary skills at 2.5 and 3.5 years of age and of verbal memory skills at 5 years of age in children who were not at risk. These relations between ERP responses and later language and verbal memory skills were not found in the group of infants at familial risk for dyslexia. Despite using different paradigms across studies to investigate speech-sound discrimination, these findings are supportive of the hypothesis that early differences in the brain's processing of speech sounds predict later variations in language abilities.

BRAIN RESPONSES TO SPEECH SOUNDS AND READING SKILLS

It is not clear why some children develop the phonological processing skills needed to decode words and show normal reading skills, whereas others do not develop these skills or develop them to a lesser extent and have problems with reading. Fowler (1991) argued that a minimum level of language and cognitive development is necessary for the beginning of reading abilities. Early cognitive skills, such as (1) short-term memory for words, digits, and other verbally coded material; (2) specific early language skills (including utterance length and receptive and expressive vocabulary); and (3) rapid serial naming skills (reciting the names of object, letter, digit, and color stimuli from rows of pictures) have all been found to be successful discriminators of children with good reading skills compared to those with poor reading skills (Catts, 1989; Fowler, 1991; Gathercole, Willis, Emslie, & Baddeley, 1991; Sawyer, 1992; Scarborough, 1990; Scarborough & Dobrich, 1990; Silva, McGee, & Williams, 1984). It is also clear that cognitive development is necessary but not sufficient for reading success because level of intelligence, per se, is not a good determinant of either successful or poor reading (Siegel, 1989, 1992; Stanovich, 1988).

Other researchers point to the influence of language experiences, such as rhyming and word-sound game activities (the reading activities that characterize some homes) as well as other aspects of the child's environment, as key factors in fostering language and the development of the emergent literacy skills needed for word-level reading skills (Bradley & Bryant, 1983, 1985; Lonigan, Anthony, Bloomfield, Dyer, & Samwel, 1999; Share, Jorm, Maclean, Matthews, & Waterman, 1983). Some researchers also have argued that general auditory processing skills are important for the normal development of reading skills. For example, Tallal and colleagues (1996) proposed that children with reading disabilities have difficulty processing complex auditory tones when they are presented in quick succession but not when they are presented at slower rates. Although some researchers have provided support for this view in research on adults with and without reading disabilities (Hari & Renvall, 2001), other researchers argue that processing difficulties for children with dyslexia are due to speech-related processing problems rather than to general auditory processing problems (Mody, Studdert-Kennedy, & Brady, 1997). Indeed, an increasing number of researchers argue that specific deficits in phonological processing skills and in other specific language skills generally characterize children with dyslexia (Catts, 1996; Fletcher et al., 1999; see also Goswami, Chapter 6, this volume).

We have examined the relation between speech perception and reading skills across several longitudinal studies. Molfese (2000) reported the results from a longitudinal study in which neonatal ERPs were examined to determine if these responses could be used to predict reading skills of the children at 8 years of age. In that study, auditory ERPs were recorded from the left and right hemispheres at frontal, temporal, and parietal scalp regions of 48 participants during the neonatal period to speech stimuli /bi/ and /gi/ and to nonspeech homologues of these sounds. All participants were subsequently tested within 2 weeks of their 8-year birthdates, using a variety of language, reading, and general cognitive skills measures. By 8 years of age, performance on the reading and intelligence assessments allowed the children to be divided into three groups: 17 children were classified as dyslexic based on average intelligence scores and below-average reading skills, 7 children were classified as poor readers based on low intelligence scores and low reading skills, and 24 children were classified as controls who were matched to the other children on the basis of intelligence scores and reading scores. In a prospective analysis, neonatal ERP measures were examined to identify the peak latencies and amplitudes from the ERP regions earlier identified by Molfese and Molfese (1985). These peak latency and amplitude measures were the dependent measures in a discriminant function analysis used to classify the children's reading performance at 8 years. The results showed that two infant ERP components were strongly correlated with reading scores at 8 years (see Figure 8.1). These components included a measure of the peak latency recorded over the right temporal region elicited in response to the speech syllable /gi/ and the latency of a left-hemispheric frontal peak to the same syllable. Interestingly, this right temporal response had been identified in a previous study (Molfese & Molfese, 1997) as predictive of the language performance of children at 5 years of age.

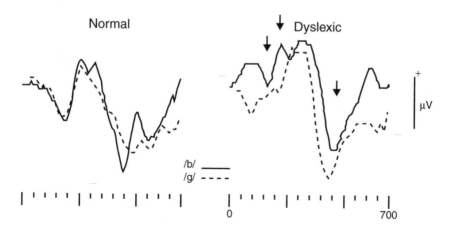

FIGURE 8.1. Auditory evoked potentials averaged across frontal, temporal, and parietal electrode sites and elicited in response to /b/ (solid line) and /g/ (dashed line) initial consonant–vowel speech syllables recorded from 24 newborn infants who, by 8 years of age, exhibited normal reading skills, and 24 infants whose reading skills were significantly impaired (1.5 *SD* below the mean for the Wide Range Achievement Test–3 [WRAT-3]) at 8 years. The arrows indicate points of maximal ERP differences between the two groups for both speech sounds. The initial large negativity at approximately 220 ms was larger in the infants who were likely to develop normal reading skills, whereas the following positive peak (~260 ms) was smaller in the group with dyslexia, and the late negative peak (~475 ms) was larger. Duration is 700 ms from stimulus onset. Voltage is positive up with calibration at 2.5 µV.

As a follow-up to the study published in 2000, Molfese, Molfese, and Modglin (2001) investigated two approaches to using ERP and behavioral measures to predict reading skills at 8 years of age. Data were used from 96 children participating in the longitudinal research and included ERP responses to speech stimuli obtained when the children were born as well as measures obtained at 3 years of age on language, short-term memory, and child-centered activities in the home related to language and reading skills. The purpose was to determine the effectiveness of these measures for discriminating between children based on reading group membership compared to the effectiveness of using these measures to predict reading scores as a continuum of abilities. In general, the same variables were found to influence the results whether they were used to discriminate reading groups or to predict a continuum of reading scores, but there were large differences in the amount of variance accounted for. More variance was accounted for in the discriminant function analyses (65–69%, depending on the model tested) than in the regression analyses (15–19%, depending on which variables were included in the model tested). Importantly, regardless of the model tested or the type of analysis used, the ERP measures accounted for more variance than the language, memory, or home environment measures. Furthermore, growth curve analyses of ERP measures obtained from 3 through 7 years of age for these two groups of children show evidence of biologically based differences in the perception and processing of auditory information (Andrews Espy, Molfese, Molfese, & Modglin, 2004). These ERP responses (illustrated in Figure 8.2) reflect group differences in reading proficiencies of the children at 8 years of age.

CONCLUSIONS

Much has been learned from studies of the brain and speech perception skills over the past three decades. Across our studies as well as those of other researchers, ERP responses recorded to speech sound stimuli at birth, as well as at later ages, are highly predictive of subsequent language and reading performance in the preschool and early elementary periods. Such findings open the possibility that ERPs and behavioral assessment techniques can be used together for the early identification of children at risk for language and reading disabilities. If accurate, early identification can occur during the infancy and early preschool periods, it should be possible to begin interventions much earlier than is currently attempted. Such early interventions, if they targeted key underlying phonological skills, could potentially lead to the mitigation or even elimination of some types of later emerging cognitive disabilities. Early identification allows time to re-

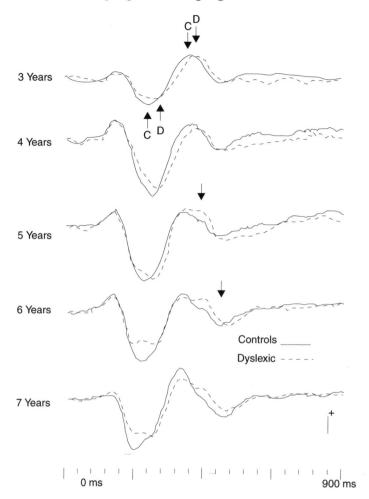

FIGURE 8.2. Auditory evoked potentials averaged across frontal, temporal, and parietal electrode sites to speech syllables recorded from 24 children at 3 through 7 years of age who, by 8 years, exhibited normal reading skills (solid line), and 24 children whose reading skills were significantly impaired (dotted line) at 8 years. Amplitude variations continue to occur between the groups after birth and into the early elementary school years. Duration is 900 ms from onset. Voltage is positive up with calibration at 2.5 µV.

mediate potential deficits in the development of perceptual skills and, when coupled with the early plasticity that neurocognitive systems appear to possess, could provide exciting breakthroughs in the treatment of disabilities. At this point it appears that particularly effective interventions are those emphasizing phonological skills, such as segmentation and blending of phonemes, combined with training in alphabetic skills (letter names and letter sounds); such approaches have been used with kindergarten children and have shown positive effects on reading skills (Ball & Blachman, 1991; Bradley & Bryant 1985; Oudeans, 2003). The development of effective interventions for remediating early language and reading disabilities needs to interface with brain and behavioral assessment techniques previously found to have high levels of accuracy in identifying young children with risk characteristics. Subsequent studies must then include both early identification and early intervention components to determine if this approach is effective in improving the language and reading performance of at-risk children.

ACKNOWLEDGMENTS

This work was supported in part by grants from the National Institute of Child Health and Human Development (No. R01-HD17860) and the U.S. Department of Education (Nos. R215K000023, R215R990011).

REFERENCES

Andrews Espy, K., Molfese, D., Molfese, V., & Modglin, A. (2004). Development of auditory event-related potentials in young children and relations to word-level reading abilities at age 8 years. *Annals of Dyslexia, 54*, 9–38.

Aram, D., & Kamhi, A. (1982). Perspectives on the relationship between phonological and language disorders. *Seminars in Speech, Language and Hearing, 3*, 3–22.

Ball, E. W., & Blachman, B. A. (1991). Does phoneme awareness training in kindergarten make a difference in early word recognition and developmental spelling? *Reading Research Quarterly, 26*, 49–66.

Bishop, D. (1997). *Uncommon understanding: Development and disorders of language comprehension in children.* Hove, UK: Psychology Press.

Bradley, L., & Bryant, P. (1983). Categorizing sounds and learning to read: A causal connection. *Nature, 30*, 419–421.

Bradley, L., & Bryant, P. (1985). *Rhyme and reason in reading and spelling.* Ann Arbor: University of Michigan Press.

Brazelton, T. (1973). Neonatal Behavioral Assessment Scale. *Clinics in Developmental Medicine, 50.* London: Heinemann.

Breier, J., Gray, L., Fletcher, J., Diehl, R., Klaas, P., Foorman, B., et al. (2001). Perception of voice and tone onset time continua in children with dyslexia with and without attention deficit/hyperactivity disorder. *Journal of Experimental Child Psychology, 80,* 245–270.

Butler, B., & Engel, R. (1969). Mental and motor scores at 8 months in relation to neonatal photic responses. *Developmental Medicine and Child Neurology, 11,* 77–82.

Cacioppo, J., Tassinary, L., & Berntson, G. (Eds.). (2000). *Handbook of psychophysiology.* Cambridge, UK: Cambridge University Press.

Camarata, S. (1995). A rationale for naturalistic speech intelligibility intervention. In M. E. Fey, J. Windsor, & S. F. Warren (Eds.), *Language intervention: Preschool through the elementary years* (pp. 63–84). Baltimore: Brookes.

Catts, H. W. (1989). Phonological processing deficits and reading disabilities. In A. Kamhi & H. Catts (Eds.), *Reading disabilities: A developmental language perspective* (pp. 101–132). Boston: Allyn & Bacon.

Catts, H. W. (1996). Defining dyslexia as a developmental language disorder: An expanded view. *Topics in Language Disorders, 16*(2), 14–29.

Cheour, M., Alho, K., Ceponiene, R., Reinikainen, K., Sainio, ´ K., Pohjavuori, M., et al. (1998). Maturation of mismatch negativity in infants. *International Journal of Psychophysiology, 29,* 217–226.

Cheour, M., Ceponiene, R., Lehtokoski, A., Luuk, A., Allik, J., Alho, K., et al. (1998). Development of language-specific phoneme representations in the infant brain. *Nature Neuroscience, 1,* 351–353.

Cheour, M., Martynova, O., Naatanen, R., Erkkola, R., Sillanpaa, M., Kero, P., et al. (2002). Speech sounds learned by sleeping newborns. *Nature, 415,* 599–600.

Chomsky, N. (1957). *Syntactic structures.* The Hague: Mouton.

Chomsky, N., & Halle, M. (1968). *The sound pattern of English.* New York: Harper & Row.

Dehaene-Lambertz, G., & Peña, M. (2001). Electrophysiological evidence for automatic phonetic processing in neonates. *NeuroReport, 12,* 3155–3158.

Dehaene-Lambertz, G., Peña, M., Christophe, A., & Landrieu, P. (2004). Phoneme perception in a neonate with a left sylvian infarct. *Brain and Language, 88,* 26–38.

Dennis, M., & Whitaker, H. (1976). Language acquisition following hemidecortication: Linguistic superiority of the left over the right hemisphere. *Brain and Language, 3,* 404–433.

Dunn, L. (1965). *Peabody Picture Vocabulary Test.* Circle Pines, MN: American Guidance Service.

Eilers, R., Wilson, W., & Moore, J. (1977). Developmental changes in speech discrimination in infants. *Journal of Speech and Hearing Research, 20,* 766–780.

Eimas, P. D., Siqueland, E., Jusczyk, P., & Vigorito, J. (1971). Speech perception in infants. *Science, 171,* 303–306.

Engel, R., & Fay, W. (1972). Visual evoked responses at birth, verbal scores at three years, and IQ at four years. *Developmental Medicine and Child Neurology, 14,* 283–289.

Engel, R., & Henderson, N. (1973). Visual evoked responses and IQ scores at school age. *Developmental Medicine and Child Neurology, 15,* 136–145.

Fletcher, J. M., Foorman, B. R., Shaywitz, S. E., & Shaywitz, S. A. (1999). Conceptual and methodological issues in dyslexia research: A lesson for developmental disorders. In H. Tager-Flusberg (Ed.), *Neurodevelopmental disorders* (pp. 271–305). Hillsdale, NJ: Erlbaum.

Fowler, A. E. (1991). How early phonological development might set the stage for phoneme awareness. In S. A. Brady & D. P. Shankweiler (Eds.), *Phonological processes in literacy: A tribute to Isabelle Y. Liberman* (pp. 97–118). Hillsdale, NJ: Erlbaum.

Fraser, C., Bellugi, U., & Brown, R. (1963). Control of grammar in imitation, comprehension, and production. *Journal of Verbal Learning and Verbal Behavior, 2,* 121–135.

Gathercole, S. E., Willis, C., Emslie, H., & Baddeley, A .D. (1991). The influences of number of syllables and wordlikeness on children's repetition of nonwords. *Applied Psycholinguistics, 12,* 349–367.

Guttorm, T. K., Leppänen, P. H. T., Eklund, K. M., Poikkeus, A.-M., Lyytinen, P., & Lyytinen, H. (2003). *Brain responses to changes in vowel duration measured at birth predict later language skills in children with familial risk for dyslexia.* Manuscript submitted for publication.

Hari, R., & Renvall, H. (2001). Impaired processing of rapid stimulus sequences in dyslexia. *Trends in Cognitive Science, 5,* 525–532.

Henderson, N., & Engel, R. (1974). Neonatal visual evoked potentials as predictors of psychoeducational testing at age sever. *Developmental Psychology, 10,* 269–276.

Jasper, H. (1958). The ten–twenty system of the International Federation of Societies for Electroencephalography: Appendix to report of the committee on methods of clinical examination in electroencephalography. *Journal of Electroencephalography and Clinical Neurophysiology, 10,* 371–375.

Jenkins, J., & Palermo, D. (1964). Mediation processes and the acquisition of linguistic structure. In U. Bellugi & R. Brown (Eds.), *The acquisition of language* (pp. 141–169). *Monograph of the Society for Research in Child Development, 29.*

Jensen, D. R., & Engel, R. (1971). Statistical procedures for relating dichotomous responses to maturation and EEG measurements. *Electroencephalography and Clinical Neurophysiology, 30,* 437–443.

Kraus, N., McGee, T. J., Carrell, T. D., Zecker, S. G., Nicol, T. G., & Koch, D. B. (1996). Auditory neurophysiologic responses and discrimination deficits in children with learning problems. *Science, 273,* 971–973.

Kuhl, P. K., & Miller, J. D. (1975). Speech perception by the chinchilla: Voiced–voiceless distinction in alveolar plosive consonants. *Science, 190,* 69–72.

Kuhl, P. K., & Padden, D. M. (1983). Enhanced discriminability at the phonetic boundaries for the place feature in macaques. *Journal of the Acoustical Society of America, 73,* 1003–1010.

Lenneberg, E. (1967). *Biological foundations of language.* New York: Wiley.

Leppanen, P., Pihko, E., Eklund, K., & Lyytinen, H. (1999). Cortical responses of infants with and without a genetic risk for dyslexia: II. Group effects. *NeuroReport, 10*, 969–973.

Liberman, A. M., Cooper, F. S., Shankweiler, D., & Studdert-Kennedy, M. (1967). Perception of the speech code. *Psychological Review, 74*, 431–461.

Lonigan, C. J., Anthony, J. L., Bloomfield, B. G., Dyer, S. M., & Samwel, C. S. (1999). Effects of two shared-reading interventions on emergent literacy skills of at-risk preschoolers. *Journal of Early Intervention, 22*, 306–322.

Martynova, O., Kirjavainen, J., & Cheour, M. (2003). Mismatch negativity and late discriminative negativity in sleeping human newborns. *Neuroscience Letters, 340*, 75–78.

McCarthy, D. (1972). *Manual for the McCarthy Scales of Children's Abilities.* New York: Psychological Corporation.

Mody, M., Studdert-Kennedy, M., & Brady, S. (1997). Speech perception deficits in poor readers: Auditory processing or phonological coding? *Journal of Experimental Child Psychology, 64*, 199–231.

Molfese, D. L. (1972). *Cerebral asymmetry in infants, children and adults: Auditory evoked responses to speech and music stimuli.* Unpublished doctoral dissertation, Pennsylvania State University, University Park.

Molfese, D. L. (1978). Neuroelectrical correlates of categorical speech perception in adults. *Brain and Language, 5*, 25–35.

Molfese, D. L. (1980). Hemispheric specialization for temporal information: Implications for the perception of voicing cues during speech perception. *Brain and Language, 11*, 285–299.

Molfese, D. L. (1989). The use of auditory evoked responses recorded from newborns to predict later language skills. In N. Paul (Ed.), *Research in infant assessment* (Vol. 25, No. 6, pp. 47–62). White Plains, NY: March of Dimes.

Molfese, D. L. (2000). Predicting dyslexia at 8 years using neonatal brain responses. *Brain and Language, 72*, 238–245.

Molfese, D. L., Freeman, R., & Palermo, D. (1975). The ontogeny of lateralization for speech and nonspeech stimuli. *Brain and Language, 2*, 356–368.

Molfese, D. L., & Hess, T. M. (1978). Speech perception in nursery school age children: Sex and hemispheric differences. *Journal of Experimental Child Psychology, 26*, 71–84.

Molfese, D. L., Laughlin, N. K., Morse, P. A., Linnville, S., Wetzel, F., & Erwin, R. (1986). Neuroelectrical correlates of categorical perception for place of articulation in normal and lead-treated rhesus macaques. *Journal of Clinical and Experimental Neuropsychology, 8*, 680–696.

Molfese, D. L., & Molfese, V. J. (1979a). Hemisphere and stimulus differences as reflected in the cortical responses of newborn infants to speech stimuli. *Developmental Psychology, 15*, 505–511.

Molfese, D. L., & Molfese, V. J. (1979b). Infant speech perception: Learned or innate? In H. Whitaker & H. Whitaker (Eds.), *Advances in neurolinguistics* (Vol. 4, pp. 225–240). New York: Academic Press.

Molfese, D. L., & Molfese, V. J. (1983). Development of symmetrical and asymmetrical hemisphere responses to speech sounds: Electrophysiological correlates. In E. Lasky & J. Katz (Eds.), *Central auditory processing disorders:*

Problems of speech, language and learning (pp. 69–89). Baltimore: University Park Press.

Molfese, D. L., & Molfese, V. J. (1985). Electrophysiological indices of auditory discrimination in newborn infants: The bases for predicting later language development. *Infant Behavior and Development, 8,* 197–211.

Molfese, D. L., & Molfese, V. J. (1986). Psychophysical indices of early cognitive processes and their relationship to language. In J. E. Obrzut & G. W. Hynd (Eds.), *Child neuropsychology: Vol. 1. Theory and research* (pp. 95–115). New York: Academic Press.

Molfese, D. L., & Molfese, V. J. (1997). Discrimination of language skills at five years of age using event related potentials recorded at birth. *Developmental Neuropsychology, 13,* 135–156.

Molfese, D. L., Molfese, V. J., & Pratt, N. L. (in press). The use of event-related evoked potentials to predict developmental outcomes. In M. de Haan (Ed.), *Infant EEG and event-related potentials.* Hove, UK: Psychology Press.

Molfese, D. L., Papanicolaou, A., Hess, T. S., & Molfese, V. (1979). Neuro-electrical correlates of semantic processes. In H. Begleiter (Ed.), *Evoked brain potentials and behavior.* New York: Plenum Press.

Molfese, D. L., & Searock, K. (1986). The use of auditory evoked responses at one year of age to predict language skills at 3 years. *Australian Journal of Communication Disorders, 14,* 35–46.

Molfese, V. J., Molfese, D. L., & Modglin, A. (2001). Newborn and preschool predictors of second grade reading scores: An evaluation of categorical and continuous scores. *Journal of Learning Disabilities, 34,* 545–554.

Molfese, V. J., Yaple, K., Helwig, S., Harris, L., & Connell, S. (1992). Stanford–Binet Intelligence Scale (4th ed.): Factor structure and verbal subscale scores for three year olds. *Journal of Psychoeducational Assessment, 10,* 47–58.

Morse, P. A., Molfese D. L., Laughlin, N. K., Linnville, S., & Wetzel, W. F. (1987). Categorical perception for voicing contrasts in normal and lead-treated rhesus monkeys: Electrophysiological indices. *Brain and Language, 30,* 63–80.

Morse, P. A., & Snowdon, C. (1975). An investigation of categorical speech discrimination by rhesus monkeys. *Perception and Psychophysics 17,* 9–16.

Oudeans, M. (2003). Integration of letter–sound correspondences and phonological awareness skills of blending and segmenting: A pilot study examining the effects of instructional sequence on word reading for kindergarten children with low phonological awareness. *Learning Disabilities Quarterly, 26,* 258–280.

Papanicolaou, A. C. (1998). *Fundamentals of functional brain imaging: A guide to the methods and their applications to psychology and behavioral neurosciences.* Netherlands: Swets & Zeitlinger.

Pihko, E., Leppanen, P. H., Eklund, K. M., Cheour, M., Guttorm, T. K., & Lyytinen, H. (1999). Cortical responses of infants with and without a genetic risk for dyslexia: I. Age effects. *NeuroReport, 10,* 901–905.

Reese, H., & Lipsitt, L. (1970). *Experimental child psychology* (pp. 425–477). New York: Academic Press.

Rockstroh, B., Elbert, T., Birbaumer, N., & Lutzenberger, W. (1982). *Slow brain potentials and behavior.* Baltimore: Urban-Schwarzenberg.

Sawyer, D. (1992). Language abilities, reading acquisition, and developmental dyslexia: A discussion of hypothetical and observed relationships. *Journal of Learning Disabilities, 25,* 82–95.

Scarborough, H. (1990). Very early language deficits in dyslexic children. *Child Development, 61,* 1728–1743.

Scarborough, H., & Dobrich, W. (1990). Development of children with early language delay. *Journal of Speech and Hearing Research, 33,* 70–83.

Share, D., Jorm, A., Maclean, R., Matthews, R., & Waterman, B. (1983). Early reading achievement, oral language ability, and a child's home background. *Australian Psychologist, 18,* 75–87.

Siegel, L. (1989). IQ is irrelevant to the definition of learning disabilities. *Journal of Learning Disabilities, 22,* 469–486.

Siegel, L. (1992). Dyslexia v. poor readers. Is there a difference? *Journal of Learning Disabilities, 25,* 618–629.

Silva, P., McGee, R., & Williams, S. (1984). A seven year follow-up study of the cognitive development of children who experienced common perinatal problems. *Australian Pediatric Journal, 20,* 23–28.

Stanovich, K. (1988). Explaining the differences between dyslexic and the garden-variety poor reader: The phonological core variable difference model. *Journal of Learning Disabilities, 21,* 590–604.

Tallal, P., Miller, S., Bedi, G., Byma, G., Wang, X., Nagarajan, S., et al. (1996). Language comprehension in language-learning impaired children improved with acoustically modified speech. *Science, 271,* 81–84.

Templin, M. (1957). *Certain language skills in children.* University of Minnesota Institute of Child Welfare Monograph Series 26. Minneapolis: University of Minnesota Press.

Travis, L. E. (1931). *Speech pathology: A dynamic neurological treatment of normal speech and speech deviations.* New York: Appleton.

Vellutino, F., & Scanlon, D. (1987). Phonological coding: Phonological awareness, and reading ability: Evidence from a longitudinal and experimental study. *Merrill–Palmer Quarterly, 33,* 321–363.

CHAPTER 9

Number Sense
and Developmental Dyscalculia

Anna J. Wilson
Stanislas Dehaene

Claire is an 8-year-old girl in second grade who participated in a remediation study for dyscalculia that we recently conducted. Despite an average IQ and good motivation and attention, she struggles in school, especially in math. This does not seem to be due to her reading abilities; her reading speed is average, and although she has some trouble with comprehension, she already receives special education services for this difficulty, with no seeming improvement in her mathematical performance. Our tests confirm that her basic numerical skills are far behind those of her peers: She shows a developmental lag in counting, understanding of place value, and in addition and subtraction of one-digit numbers. The latter are only around 80 and 40% accurate, respectively, and both are carried out in a painstaking fashion using finger counting.

Claire is a fairly typical case of developmental dyscalculia, which is generally defined as a disorder in mathematical abilities presumed to be due to a specific impairment in brain function (Kosc, 1974; Shalev & Gross-Tsur, 1993, 2001). This definition is highly similar to that of "mathematics disorder" in the *Diagnostic and Statistical Manual of Mental Disorders—*

Fourth Edition (DSM-IV; American Psychiatric Association, 1994) and that of "mathematical learning disabilities" (Geary, 1993, 2004). Because of this similarity, and following Butterworth (2005a, 2005b), we take these constructs to be one and the same.[1]

Despite its professional and practical consequences (e.g., Rivera-Batiz, 1992) and a similar population prevalence of around 3–6% (Badian, 1983; Gross-Tsur, Manor, & Shalev, 1996; Kosc, 1974; Lewis, Hitch, & Walker, 1994), developmental dyscalculia is much less recognized, researched, and treated than its cousin developmental dyslexia. This neglect has partially been a consequence of the later development of our knowledge about the neural bases of numerical cognition, as opposed to reading. As research in the numerical cognition field has started to increase in volume, so has cognitive neuroscience research on dyscalculia, with several research teams conducting studies on its associated cognitive profile, brain bases, and genetics.

THE CORE DEFICIT HYPOTHESIS

An advantage provided by the 20-or-so-year lag between dyscalculia and dyslexia research is an opportunity to speed up research on the former by looking for analogies that may be made between the two disorders. One interesting and important analogy that has been made, for which we review evidence in this chapter, is that of a "core deficit." The core phonological deficit hypothesis is now accepted by many in the dyslexia field (Goswami, 2003; see also Goswami, Chapter 6, and Grigorenko, Chapter 5, this volume) and has resulted in many advances in prevention and remediation (Eden, 2002; Tallal et al., 1996; Temple et al., 2003). Importantly, the nature of the core deficit can be somewhat counterintuitive—who would have thought that training children in distinction of sounds would improve reading? However, this idea is now confirmed by our knowledge of the brain circuits involved in reading, especially the continuing role of phonological areas in reading in even practiced readers.

Could there be a similar core deficit in dyscalculia? Although our knowledge of its behavioral manifestations is incomplete, our knowledge of the adult circuits involved in numerical cognition is by now fairly advanced. It has been argued that the core aspect of numerical cognition is "number sense," which is a shorthand term for our ability to quickly understand, approximate, and manipulate numerical quantities (Dehaene, 1997, 2001). We now have a plausible candidate for a neural substrate of number sense: a specific region of the parietal cortex, the horizontal intraparietal sulcus (HIPS), which, based on neuroimaging results, is hypothesized to contain a nonverbal representation of numerical quantity analogous to a spatial map or "number line" (Dehaene, Piazza, Pinel, & Cohen, 2003).

Our knowledge of the intact adult system allows us, therefore, to make a prediction about the impaired system in the child. The behavioral hypothesis that a deficit in number sense is the cause of at least some types of dyscalculia has, in fact, been previously proposed by authors in the special education field (Gersten & Chard, 1999; Robinson, Menchetti, & Torgesen, 2002) and in the numerical cognition field (Butterworth, 1999). Here we propose a neural specification of this hypothesis: that at least some types of dyscalculia may be due to an impairment of functioning and/or structure in the HIPS and/or in its connections to other numerical cognition regions. In this chapter we examine how much evidence there is to support this hypothesis.

A COMPLEMENTARY HYPOTHESIS: MULTIPLE SUBTYPES OF DYSCALCULIA

As well as presenting and discussing the hypothesis of a core deficit, we present and discuss the possibility of multiple causes of dyscalculia. Although a majority of children might suffer from a core impairment in number sense, other sources of dyscalculia are likely to exist. Hypotheses about their nature may be generated from several sources, such as the adult neuroimaging literature, the developmental literature, and educational research on subtypes of dyscalculia. To take one example, in the adult neurological literature it is possible to find a "number sense" acalculia, in which the patient has lost all sense of the meaning of numbers, but it is also possible to find a "number fact retrieval" acalculia, in which the patient still understands the meaning of numbers but is unable to retrieve from memory basic multiplication or addition facts, and is thus forced to laboriously recalculate these facts each time by counting, or worse, retrieves the wrong result without noticing (Dehaene & Cohen, 1997). We also discuss whether there is evidence for a subtype of developmental dyscalculia similar to this latter type of patient.

OUTLINE OF THE CHAPTER

We begin by describing cases of adult-acquired dyscalculia and discussing what we know about the underlying numerical cognition systems in the adult. We then overview the developmental numerical cognition literature.

The combination of these two literatures allows us to elaborate some predictions about possible types and causes of developmental dyscalculia. Next we discuss in depth developmental dyscalculia: how it is identified, its characteristics and common comorbid disorders, and what we have learned from subtype research. We then discuss the extent to which this literature supports our hypotheses, in particular the behavioral and neural evidence for a deficit in number sense. Finally, we discuss future directions to be taken, the implications for education, and the construction of number sense remediation software in our laboratory.

ADULT NUMERICAL COGNITION

There are two important areas of adult numerical cognition research that can be used to shed light on the possible causes of developmental dyscalculia. The first is neuropsychological research on acquired dyscalculia (referred to here as *acalculia*), which may have similar causes and symptoms to developmental dyscalculia (referred to here as *dyscalculia*). The second is our knowledge of the functioning of the intact numerical cognition circuits in the adult brain, which gives us a clue as to what kind of deficits we might expect if developmental dyscalculia is caused by abnormalities in these circuits.

Acquired Dyscalculia or "Acalculia": Lesion Evidence

The adult neuropsychological literature supports a causative role of inferior parietal lesions in acalculia (see Cohen, Wilson, Izard, & Dehaene, in press, for a detailed review of this literature). Acalculia is often associated with Gerstmann syndrome, in which patients also present left–right disorientation, agraphia, and finger agnosia (Gerstmann, 1940). This syndrome is usually due to lesions around the region of the left angular gyrus (Jackson & Warrington, 1986; Rosselli & Ardila, 1989). However, the existence of a coherent syndrome has been questioned because it appears that the four deficits can be dissociated (Benton, 1992).

Dehaene and Cohen (1997) discuss two cases of acalculia (patients MAR and BOO) who together provide a double dissociation between a "number sense" type acalculia and a "verbal memory" type acalculia. Patient MAR, a left-hander with a right inferior parietal lesion and a pure Gerstmann syndrome, showed difficulties with tasks requiring quantity manipulation, such as choosing the larger of two digits, bisecting number lines, and subtraction. Patient BOO, a right-hander with a left subcortical lesion, showed a very different pattern with few difficulties in the former tasks but severe difficulties with more verbal or memory-related numerical tasks, such as multiplication. Other similar cases have also been reported more recently by Lemer, Dehaene, Spelke, and Cohen (2003), Cappeletti, Butterworth, and Kopelman (2001), and Delazer, Karner, Zamarian, Donnemiller, and Benke (2006).

To the extent that acquired and developmental dyscalculia are similar in their causes and manifestations, the acalculia literature suggests two important hypotheses for developmental dyscalculia: (1) that we should expect to find more than one type of dyscalculia, in particular, a number sense dyscalculia and a verbal memory dyscalculia; and (2) that we should expect to find a link between number sense dyscalculia and the inferior parietal lobes, particularly the angular gyrus. In the next section we show that the adult imaging literature supports these two suggestions and adds further precision to our hypothesis about anatomical location.

Imaging Evidence: Number Sense and the Horizontal Intraparietal Sulcus

Early PET imaging studies consistently showed activation in the parietal cortex during numerical tasks (Dehaene et al., 1996; Pesenti, Thioux, Seron, & De Volder, 2000; Zago et al., 2001), although only some of these early results (e.g., Dehaene et al., 1996) supported a dissociation between areas activated by quantity manipulation versus rote memory tasks, as would be expected from the neuropsychological literature.

Later fMRI studies provided much more precision, and in a recent meta-analysis of available data from this literature, Dehaene and colleagues (2003) put forward a more precise localization hypothesis, identifying three particular areas of the parietal lobe that appear to be differentially involved in representation and processing of numerical information (see Plate 9.1). The left angular gyrus—the classic Gerstmann lesion center—appears to be more active in more verbal numerical tasks such as multiplication and exact addition (Chochon, Cohen, van de Moortele, & Dehaene, 1999; Dehaene, Spelke, Pinel, Stanescu, & Tsivkin, 1999; Lee, 2000). The posterior superior parietal lobe (PSPL) appears to be activated in numerical tasks that may require the shifting of spatial attention, such as approximating, subtraction, and number comparison (Dehaene et al., 1999; Lee, 2000; Pinel, Dehaene, Riviere, & Le Bihan, 2001).

In contrast, the nearby HIPS appears to be more active in core quantity manipulation or number sense tasks, such as comparing the size of numbers, estimating, subtracting, and approximating (Chochon et al., 1999; Dehaene et al., 1999; Lee, 2000). This role of the HIPS in quantity representation has been further reinforced by subsequent imaging studies (Eger, Sterzer, Russ, Giraud, & Kleinschmidt, 2003; Pinel, Piazza, Le Bihan, & Dehaene, 2004), and by the recent finding by Piazza, Izard, Pinel, Le Bihan, and Dehaene (2004), using an fMRI habituation paradigm, that fMRI adaptation in this area shows tuning curves similar to those found in single neuron recordings from the analogous area of the monkey brain (Nieder & Miller, 2004).

Overall, the neuroimaging literature leads to the same hypotheses arrived at from the neuropsychological literature: We should expect to find a role of the inferior parietal lobes in dyscalculia, and we should be able to find different subtypes of dyscalculia. These subtypes should be a *number sense* dyscalculia linked to impairment (functional or structural) of the HIPS, a *verbal* dyscalculia linked to impairment of the angular gyrus, and a *spatial attention* dyscalculia linked to impairment of the PSPL.

However, one caveat is that these theoretical subtypes might be quite difficult to dissociate in developmental cases. Firstly, in a developmental context, any deficit in one of the numerical systems is likely to interfere with the normal development of the others, thus leading to an undifferentiated dyscalculic pattern, even if the underlying neurological damage is limited. Secondly, the physical proximity of the areas involved makes it likely that there is a high correlation between impairment in one area and impairment in another. As pointed out by Dehaene and colleagues (2003), this proximity explains why, in the neuropsychological literature, it is hard to find "pure" cases of verbal or number sense acalculia: areas that are close together are likely to be lesioned together. It is possible that this association of impairment could also occur in developmental dyscalculia; for instance, a gene-influenced growth factor could impact development in a whole subsection of the cortex, such as the inferior parietal lobule.

NORMAL INFANT AND CHILD NUMERICAL COGNITION

Of course, our ability to make predictions about developmental dyscalculia from the adult neuropsychology and imaging literature rests on the assumption that numerical cognition systems in the adult and the child are similar. However, it is not yet clear whether this is the case, and we have little knowledge of how the infant system develops into the child and then the adult system (Ansari & Karmiloff-Smith, 2002). In this section we briefly review some of our key knowledge about the infant and child systems.

Number Sense: Our Core Magnitude Representation

One obvious difference between the infant and adult numerical cognition system is that the infant is not born with an innate ability to process symbolic numerical codes, such as digits and number names. It was initially thought that all numerical knowledge had to be constructed through sensorimotor interaction with the environment (Piaget, 1952), but due to the many studies on infant numerical cognition in the past quarter of a century, we now know that infants are born with an ability to represent, discriminate, and operate on numerosities, although with only a limited degree of precision (for a recent review, see Feigenson, Dehaene, & Spelke, 2004). For instance, even with continuous visual cues such as luminance and occupied area controlled, 6-month-old infants can discriminate between groups of 8 and 16 or 16 and 32 dots, but not 16 and 24 dots (Xu & Spelke, 2000; Xu, Spelke, & Goddard, 2005). Recent work by McCrink and Wynn (2004) has shown that 9-month-olds can approximately add and subtract collections of objects (e.g., 5 + 5 or 10 − 5). These approximate representations of number in infants are constrained by the ratio of the two numbers and improve in precision during the first year of life (Lipton & Spelke, 2003).

Although no imaging evidence is available yet on the source of these representations in infants, due to the practical difficulties of conducting such studies, these characteristics are similar to the approximate representation present in animals (Gallistel & Gelman, 2000; Nieder, 2005) and in the HIPS of adult humans (see discussion above). Behavioral studies (and one ERP study) in preschool children also support this conclusion (Berch, Foley, Hill, & Ryan, 1999; Girelli, Lucangeli, & Butterworth, 2000; Huntley-Fenner, 2001; Rubinsten, Henik, Berger, & Shahar-Shalev, 2002; Siegler & Opfer, 2003; Temple & Posner, 1998; see Noël, Rousselle, & Mussolin, 2005, for a review). The fact that this number sense system matures in the first year of life and is a core aspect of adult numerical cognition makes it a likely candidate for a core deficit in dyscalculia.

A Second Nonsymbolic Core System: Object Files

For some time, opponents of the concept of an innate numerosity representation have argued that infants were able to represent number based on their visuospatial abilities (e.g., Simon, 1999). It has now become clear that to keep track of small quantities of objects, infants are also able to use a visuospatial "object file"–based system that allows them to keep references to up to three or four objects and also their continuous properties. Infants, in fact, may sometimes show a preference for using this system over the approximate magnitude system (Feigenson, 2005; Feigenson, Carey, & Hauser, 2002; Feigenson, Carey, & Spelke, 2002; Xu, 2003). It has been argued that adults may still use this system for subitizing (or rapidly identifying one to four objects; Trick & Pylyshyn, 1994), although this has not yet been proven to be the case (Feigenson et al., 2004). It is thus not certain whether, and to what extent, impairments in this second system could be responsible for developmental dyscalculia.

Development of Symbolic Capabilities

In addition to these two core systems children also develop (in the appropriate cultural context) the ability to represent numbers in a symbolic fashion, first using words and later using Arabic digits. This then allows them to extend their approximate abilities into the realm of exact arithmetic. Few developmental data are available on the neural foundations of developing symbolic representations, particularly on how these might be linked with the nonsymbolic core systems discussed above. However, it is clear that an impairment in symbolic representation or an impairment in the link between the nonsymbolic and the symbolic are both possible causes for dyscalculia.

The first key development that occurs between the ages of 2 and 4 years in normal children is the acquisition of counting. In order to make full use of the counting procedure, children need to learn the sequence of count words and to understand and execute their one-to-one mapping to a set of objects. Finally, they need to understand that this procedure gives the cardinality of the set. Some argue that it is only the language and procedural execution aspects of the task that need to be acquired and that the concept of one-to-one correspondence and the comprehension of cardinals are already present (Fuson, 1988; Wynn, 1990), whereas others claim that all of these need to be acquired (Cordes & Gelman, 2005; Gelman & Gallistel, 1978). Wynn (1990), in particular, demonstrates that between 2½ and 3½ years old, children exhibit a radical change in their understanding of counting and in their ability to use counting in simple quantity tasks.

Early work by Siegler and colleagues showed that prior to entering school, children spontaneously count on their fingers and thereby compute simple additions (Siegler & Jenkins, 1989; Siegler & Shrager, 1984). Preschool children also have usually mastered a strategy for exact addition, "counting all," in which, for example, to add 2 + 4 they would count out 2 on their fingers, count out 4 using other fingers, and finally count all the fingers to give 6. Eventually this strategy is replaced by a more advanced one, "counting on," in which children start at the first number and count up the second number of units, for instance, "2 . . . 3, 4, 5, 6." Finally, children learn the "min" strategy of starting at the largest number so that they have to count only the smallest distance, for example, "4 . . . 5, 6." As children get older, counting (with or without fingers) comes to play a decreasing role in addition as memory-based retrieval strategies take over. However, it has been shown that even adults still rely on backup strategies in the event of a retrieval failure, such as decomposition—for example, $8 + 6 \rightarrow (8 + 2) + 4 = 10 + 4 = 14$—or derivation from related facts—$8 + 6 \rightarrow (9 + 6) - 1 = 15 - 1 = 14$ (for a review, see LeFevre, Smith-Chant, Hiscock, Daley, & Morris, 2003).

Another possible candidate for dyscalculia is therefore an impairment in the symbolic system. Although, as mentioned earlier, there is little developmental evidence on the neural bases of this system, in the adult we know that at least part of it, especially that governing counting and retrieval of arithmetic facts, is verbal in nature (Spelke & Tsivkin, 2001). Neuroimaging evidence suggests that it is at least partially governed by perisylvian language areas (Stanescu-Cosson et al., 2000). In the case of strategy execution, there are currently no imaging data available even in the adult; however, we can tentatively say that this ability is likely to be linked to the frontal lobes. This then generates two hypotheses for dyscalculia: a subtype linked to verbal impairment and a subtype linked to executive dysfunction.

A further important hypothesis should be mentioned here. From the previous discussion it is evident that there are many bases for the representation of number, which can be divided into two broad categories: nonsymbolic and symbolic. These representations clearly come from different sources: Children are born with an approximate nonsymbolic representation of number that is similar to that present in animals, and then they later learn an exact symbolic representation. Another obvious hypothesis for dyscalculia is that of a disconnection syndrome: Children with dyscalculia could have an intact nonsymbolic representation of quantity but fail to make the link between this and their newly acquired symbolic representations.

SUMMARY OF HYPOTHESES
FOR DEVELOPMENTAL DYSCALCULIA

In summary of the previous sections, we now list the hypotheses put forward for developmental dyscalculia based on the neuropsychology, adult numerical cognition, and developmental numerical cognition literatures. There are two sets of questions to be addressed: first, whether or not there is a core deficit, and if so, what type of dyscalculia would be associated with it, and second, what other subtypes of dyscalculia might be found.

We propose that if there is a single core deficit that causes dyscalculia, it is likely to be due to one of the following:

1. *A deficit in number sense or nonsymbolic representation of number*. This deficit would be caused by structural or functional impairment to the HIPS. Its symptoms would include impaired understanding of the meaning of numbers, deficits in tasks that involve this area (nonsymbolic tasks such as comparison and approximate addition of dots, but also the symbolic tasks of numerical comparison, addition, and subtraction), and reduced automatic activation of quantity from number words and digits. Because these are such basic deficits, they would be likely to cause a developmental delay in all aspects of math, except the highly verbal processes of counting and fact retrieval.

2. *Impaired connections between symbolic and nonsymbolic representations*. In this case, we would expect to see the same pattern described above but with one important difference: little impairment on nonsymbolic tasks.

Based on our literature review, we might also expect several other subtypes of developmental dyscalculia:

1. *A deficit in verbal symbolic representation*, related to impairment in the angular gyrus, the left inferior frontal and/or temporal language areas, or the left basal ganglia. This impairment would result in difficulties learning and retrieving arithmetical facts (particularly for multiplication) and possibly also in learning the counting sequence.

2. *A deficit in executive dysfunction*, due to frontal dysfunction. This impairment would also be likely to result in difficulties in arithmetical fact retrieval, but would furthermore result in difficulties in strategy and procedure usage.

3. *A deficit in spatial attention*, due to posterior superior parietal dysfunction. This type of deficit could be linked to the object file tracking system and might therefore result in difficulties in subitizing (if this is the system underlying subitizing). It might also result in difficulties in perception of nonsymbolic quantity information and in quantity manipulation. However, due to the close intertwining of spatial and numerical representations, this subtype might be difficult to separate from a number sense subtype.

DEVELOPMENTAL DYSCALCULIA

Bearing in mind these hypotheses, we now turn to a review of the developmental dyscalculia literature and examine to what extent we find support for them. First we briefly discuss two important issues that should be borne in mind when thinking about this research and which can make it difficult to compare results across different studies.

Identification

In the introductory section we discussed the definition of developmental dyscalculia: a disorder in mathematical abilities presumed to be due to a specific impairment in brain function. In the educational field it has been traditional to identify learning disabilities by using standardized educational tests and defining dyscalculia as a significant lag in performance, taking into account age and IQ (e.g., Geary, Hamson, & Hoard, 2000; Jordan, Hanich, & Kaplan, 2003). Alternatively, some research laboratories studying dyscalculia have used their own tests based on neuropsychological batteries (e.g., Gross-Tsur et al., 1996). One important issue is the cutoff used to identify children as dyscalculic, which is essentially arbitrary, as in the case of dyslexia. This arbitrary cutoff point has led to important differences in the populations of children studied (see Butterworth, 2005b, for a detailed discussion), making it difficult to be certain of the true symptoms of dyscalculia.

Comorbid Disorders

Two important disorders that appear to be comorbid with dyscalculia are dyslexia and attention-deficit/hyperactivity disorder (ADHD; see Gatzke-Kopp & Beauchaine, Chapter 10; Grigorenko, Chapter 5; and Goswami, Chapter 6, this volume, for further discussion of these disorders). Estimations for the comorbidity rate of dyslexia vary wildly, possibly due to differences in criteria, methodology, and school year. For instance, a longitudinal prevalence study by Badian (1999) found that 60% of persistent low arithmetic achievers were also low reading achievers (using a cutoff of the 25th percentile on average achievement over a 7- to 8-year period). Lewis and colleagues (1994) found a comorbidity rate (64%) of a similar order in their prevalence study, in which they used a cutoff of the 16th percentile for reading and math difficulties. At the other extreme, Gross-Tsur and colleagues (1996) found a dyslexia–dyscalculia comorbidity of only 17% in their sample of children with dyscalculia. However, their cutoff for dyslexia was the 5th percentile on a standardized reading and spelling test, which was much more conservative than that of the previous authors. The comorbidity rate of dyscalculia and ADHD is no less certain, having been addressed in only one large prevalence study (Gross-Tsur et al., 1996). These authors found that 26% of their participants with dyscalculia showed symptoms of ADHD, as measured by Connor's questionnaire.

The presence of comorbid disorders in children with dyscalculia is important to keep in mind, because studies have not always controlled for, or reported, them and they may in fact be related to the symptoms observed.

Characteristics

Much work on the characteristics of dyscalculia has already been conducted in the educational field, although as we discuss later, this work can be difficult to compare to the numerical cognition field. Here we review key findings in the educational field briefly; for a more in-depth discussion, the reader is referred to excellent reviews by Geary (1993, 2004).

Several key characteristics of dyscalculia have been extensively studied and are generally agreed upon. First, Geary and colleagues (e.g., Geary, Bow-Thomas, & Yao, 1992; Geary et al., 2000; Geary, Hoard, & Hamson, 1999) have consistently found an early delay in understanding some aspects of counting (order irrelevance, detection of double counts) among first- and second-grade children with dyscalculia. It is unknown whether these deficits, or other deficits in counting, continue after this age. Second and probably related, many studies have reported a developmental delay in using counting strategies in simple addition; for instance, children with dyscalculia persist in using "counting all" strategies when their peers have learned to "count on" (e.g., Geary, 1990; Geary, Brown, & Samaranayake, 1991; Geary et al., 2000; Jordan & Montani, 1997). Finally, a delay and persistent deficit in acquiring and using verbal facts have been well documented: Children with dyscalculia tend to keep using time-absorbing finger-counting strategies for simple arithmetic facts that their peers have long since memorized (e.g., Ginsburg, 1997; Jordan & Montani, 1997; Kirby & Becker, 1988). A series of excellent longitudinal studies by Ostad (1997, 1999) suggests that this difference persists up until at least fifth grade for addition and seventh grade for subtraction.

A more controversial general deficit that has been proposed is a deficit in various components of working memory (Geary, 2004; Koontz & Berch, 1996; McLean & Hitch, 1999; Temple & Sherwood, 2002). Several studies have found impairment on central executive tasks (D'Amico & Guarnera, 2005; Gathercole & Pickering, 2000; McLean & Hitch, 1999; Passolunghi & Siegel, 2004), suggesting a possible frontal dysfunction, which fits with the procedural deficits discussed above. However, only some studies have found verbal working memory impairments (Wilson & Swanson, 2001), whereas others have not (McLean & Hitch, 1999; Passolunghi & Siegel, 2004). This discrepancy in findings may be due to different measures used for verbal working memory, particularly whether a digit-span task is used. A recent study by D'Amico and Guarnera (2005) examined children with a thorough battery of tests for all three types of working memory and found that children with dyscalculia showed a deficit in digit span, but not pseudo-word span, suggesting that the deficit is in the representation of numerical information, rather than the representation or rehearsal of verbal information in general. Most earlier studies did not examine spatial working memory; however, more recent studies have found deficits in this domain as well (D'Amico & Guarnera, 2005; Gathercole & Pickering, 2000; McLean & Hitch, 1999).

In our view, it is unlikely that working memory deficits in themselves are the core deficits in dyscalculia, but rather that both are co-occurring symptoms of other numerical, verbal, or spatial impairments.[2] For example, an impairment in the ability to store numerical information could result in dyscalculia, a reduced digit span, and possibly a lower central executive score (but solely for tasks involving numerical information). An impairment in the ability to shift spatial attention might result in dyscalculia, a reduced spatial span, and possibly a lower central executive score (for tasks involving spatial information). As we have seen, predictions such as these are starting to be examined, although it may be some time before the issue is clarified.

Dyscalculia Subtypes

It is important to note that not all children with dyscalculia show difficulties in all of the areas mentioned above, and that many authors have made the case for specific subtypes of developmental dyscalculia. Indeed the existence of known subtypes could lead to a clarification of symptoms: The current long list of characteristics might, in fact, be a mixture of many different subtypes. In this section we briefly review major subtype proposals that have been subject to, or are based on, several research studies.

Rourke and colleagues conducted much of the early subtyping research (see Rourke, 1993; Rourke & Conway, 1997 for reviews) and argued for two subtypes of mathematical disabilities: a verbal type, associated with left-hemispheric impairment, and a spatial type, associated with right-hemispheric impairment. They grouped children with dyscalculia based on whether they had concurrent reading and spelling deficits (RDSD) or isolated mathematical deficits (MD). Neuropsychological tests on these groups revealed a double dissociation: RDSD children performed better on visuospatial tests and worse on verbal tests, whereas MD children showed the opposite pattern (Rourke & Finlayson, 1978). Further studies found that MD children also showed deficits in psychomotor and perceptuotactile tasks, and on complex nonverbal abstract reasoning tasks (Rourke & Strang, 1978). However, not all independent studies have been able to find evidence for these two subtypes of dyscalculia; for example, Share, Moffitt, and Silva (1988) found this pattern only in boys, and Shalev, Manor, and Gross-Tsur (1997) failed to find it at all.

More recent studies by Jordan and colleagues (Jordan & Hanich, 2000; Jordan et al., 2003; Jordan & Montani, 1997) have also focused on grouping children into those with mathematical and reading disabilities (MDRD) and those with only MD. However, unlike in previous studies, these authors then measured performance on basic numerical and mathematical tasks. In general, the results reveal a single dissociation: MDRD children are consistently worse than MD children in exact calculation and solving story problems. However, there are no tasks at which MD children are worse than MDRD children, leaving open the possibility that the differences are simply due to the difficulty of the tasks. Furthermore, as of yet, other researchers, using core numerical cognition tasks, have failed to find a difference between the performance of children with MDRD and those with MD (e.g., Landerl, Bevan, & Butterworth, 2004).

A third influential proposal, based on a synthesis of the educational and neuropsychological literature, has been made by Geary (1993, 2004), who posits three key subtypes of mathematical disabilities. The first is a procedural subtype, in which children show a delay in acquiring simple arithmetic strategies, and which Geary proposes may be a result of verbal working memory deficits and perhaps also deficits in conceptual knowledge. The second is a semantic memory subtype, in which children show deficits in retrieval of facts, and which Geary proposes is due to a long-term memory deficit. As discussed earlier, there is much evidence for procedural and fact retrieval deficits in children with dyscalculia. The third subtype proposed by Geary is a visuospatial one, in which children show deficits in the spatial representation of number. However, there is little evidence for the existence of this subtype, although this absence may be due to the infrequency of testing for spatial abilities.

BEHAVIORAL AND NEURAL EVIDENCE FOR A NUMBER SENSE DEFICIT IN DYSCALCULIA

From this overview of the dyscalculia literature, we turn now to a more in-depth evaluation of the evidence for core cognitive deficits in dyscalculia, particularly that of number sense. However, first we note that it is difficult to use research in special education for this purpose because, as pointed out by other authors (e.g., Ansari & Karmiloff-Smith, 2002), many educational studies have not used basic measures of numerical cognition but rather higher-level tests. These tests are likely to involve many combinations of cognitive processes and thus may not reveal specific numerical deficits. When low-level tasks have been used, the authors have not always used reaction-time measures that may reveal abnormalities where accuracy does not (Butterworth, 2005b; Jordan & Montani, 1997). Thus below we discuss relevant research mostly from clinical neuropsychology.

An important exception to this rule is a recent study by Llanderl and colleagues (2004), whose results provide preliminary support for the number sense core deficit hypothesis. The authors tested a group of 8- and 9-year-old children with dyscalculia and compared their performance on core number processing tasks to that of controls. They found that the children with dyscalculia showed a deficit in speed of number comparison, although their performance on a nonnumerical comparison task was normal. They also found that children with dyscalculia showed a steeper increase in reaction time than controls when enumerating small quantities of dots, suggesting an impairment in subitizing, as had been suggested by earlier data (Koontz & Berch, 1996). In the counting range a similar steeper increase in reaction time was found.[3]

In the context of clinical neuropsychology, there are only a few published cases of developmental dyscalculia that support the core deficit hypothesis. For instance, Butterworth (1999) reports the case of "Charles," an adult with dyscalculia who, despite normal IQ and reasoning, showed a deficit in numerical comparison (even with a reverse distance effect) and in subitizing. Kaufmann (2002) reports a similar case of a 14-year-old boy who showed no distance effect (although he did show normal subitizing), even though he was perfectly able to complete multidigit calculation procedures. Both of these cases also showed a large amount of finger counting as opposed to using mental strategies and retrieval.

Other cases of developmental dyscalculia have been reported in the context of a developmental Gerstmann syndrome (Benson & Geschwind, 1970; Kinsbourne & Warrington, 1963), in which children show left–right disorientation, finger agnosia, agraphia, and dyscalculia, in the context of normal intelligence, although not always normal reading performance. Children with this syndrome show little difficulty with fact retrieval but clear difficulties in addition and (particularly) subtraction, which is consistent with a number sense deficit. However, as in the adult research, the existence of the syndrome as a coherent whole has been questioned (Miller & Hynd, 2004; Spellacy & Peter, 1978).

It should be noted that several case studies do support the possible existence of different subtypes of developmental dyscalculia. For instance, Kaufmann's (2002) case appears to have more than just a quantity representation deficit, because he also showed a large impairment in retrieval of arithmetical facts that seemed to be due to long-term memory interference, possibly caused by executive dysfunction. Three cases published by Temple (1989, 1991) support the existence of other subtypes of dyscalculia, seemingly independent of number sense: a procedural deficit related to frontal damage, a fact retrieval deficit in the presence of phonological dyslexia, and a transcoding deficit in the presence of impaired verbal working memory.

Finally, we turn to neural evidence of deficits in dyscalculia, which although in its infancy, is promising for the hypothesis of a number sense deficit. Several recent studies in specific subpopulations of subjects with dyscalculia have implicated abnormalities in the intraparietal sulcus (IPS), as would be predicted. Isaacs, Edmonds, Lucas, and Gadian (2001) selected two groups of 12 adolescents who had been born preterm (matched for IQ), one group showing impairment in arithmetic and the other, not. The authors compared the density of gray matter between the two groups of adolescents and found that only the left IPS showed reduced gray matter in the arithmetically impaired group, at the precise coordinates of the HIPS (see Plate 9.2, left panel).

Likewise, Molko and colleagues (Bruandet, Molko, Cohen, & Dehaene, 2004; Molko et al., 2003) studied women with Turner syndrome (X monosomy), for whom mathematical learning difficulties have been consistently reported (e.g., Mazzocco & McCloskey, 2005; Rovet, Szekely, & Hockenberry, 1994; Temple & Marriott, 1998). Bruandet and colleagues (2004) used a testing battery of symbolic and nonsymbolic tasks, and found that subjects with Turner syndrome showed deficits in number sense tasks, such as cognitive estimation, subitizing, addition, and subtraction. In a further imaging study, Molko and colleagues (2003) observed a disorganization of the right IPS, which was of abnormal depth. Furthermore, fMRI revealed reduced activation in the right IPS as a function of number size during exact calculation (see Plate 9.2, right panel).

A similar reduction in normal activation levels, extending to a broader parietoprefrontal network, has been observed in at least one other genetic condition associated with dyscalculia; fragile X syndrome (Rivera, Menon, White, Glaser, & Reiss, 2002). Other genetic conditions, such as velocardiofacial syndrome, may show similar impairments (Eliez et al., 2001; Simon et al., 2002, 2005).

SUMMARY

Although much research remains to be done, the preliminary evidence supporting the role of a number sense deficit in dyscalculia is promising. Behavioral evidence suggests that individuals with dyscalculia show impairments in numerical comparison and subitizing, which would be expected from an impairment in number sense. Neural evidence, although as of yet only from special populations, points to the role of the HIPS, which is believed to represent quantity. Furthermore, children with dyscalculia have been reported as showing persistent difficulties in learning simple addition and subtraction strategies—difficulties that would fit with a reduced understanding of the meaning of numbers or ability to manipulate them.

However, whether an impairment of number sense is a core deficit responsible for dyscalculia is not clear. Nor are we currently able to distinguish between a deficit in number sense itself or in its connections to symbolic representations of numerosity. The possibility of multiple types of dyscalculia remains an important one, with supporting information from special education research and clinical case studies. In particular, there is much evidence for fact retrieval deficits, which have been observed in isolation in case studies and which are consistently observed in populations with dyscalculia. Such deficits could be due to either a verbal memory deficit or a deficit in executive function. In the case of the former, the comorbidity between dyslexia and dyscalculia may be an important factor, whereas for the latter, that between ADHD and dyscalculia may be important. The possibility of a spatial attention-deficit subtype of dyscalculia remains an important one, which should be further investigated.

These possibilities should be borne in mind by researchers in the dyscalculia and mathematical disabilities fields. We suggest that future studies in these areas test children for dyslexia, ADHD, executive function, and spatial attention in order to allow for an analysis of results by possible subtypes.

IMPLICATIONS FOR EDUCATION AND INTERVENTION

In this final section we discuss recommendations for the field of education. We highlight the importance of the cognitive neuroscience and educational fields working more closely together in order to try and achieve three key aims: (1) the development of a "neurocognitive" description of dyscalculia; (2) the development, norming, and educational use of core tests based on numerical cognition research; and (3) the development and testing of new educational remediation methods.

Toward a "Neurocognitive" Description of Dyscalculia

By a *neurocognitive* description of dyscalculia, we mean a description that is based on, and ideally measured by, behavioral and neuroimaging paradigms previously studied in normal subjects, and with a theoretical basis in numerical cognition. Such a description would specify, at the neural level, the brain systems implicated in dyscalculia, and at the behavioral level, specific cognitive deficits that would be expected as a result of neural impairments. We argue that this focus would allow for better identification, better treatment, and the possibility of prevention. Better identification might one day mean being able to scan children for brain function and immediately identifying the subtype of dyscalculia present. Better treatment could mean designing a custom-built targeted remediation that would give each child the greatest chance of success. The possibility of prevention depends on early identification and on the plasticity of the brain circuits involved. Given that early identification may be possible for dyslexia (Lyytinen et al., 2005), this might also be the case for dyscalculia.

Core Ability Tests

To the extent that dyscalculia is caused by, or correlated with, deficits in core numerical cognition processes, it is important to test for it with batteries of basic numerical cognition tasks. These batteries should measure reaction time as well as accuracy and include symbolic and well as nonsymbolic tasks. The presence of personal computers in most Western classrooms now makes measures such as these feasible, and indeed, some countries are already starting to move to this system for testing for dyscalculia; for instance, in the United Kingdom, Brian Butterworth's "Dyscalculia Screener" (Butterworth, 2003) is now being used by some schools to identify children with dyscalculia on the basis of dot enumeration and number comparison. Which tests should be used in such instruments is still an issue that is under discussion and should be informed by ongoing research. Thus far, subitizing and number comparison are good candidates.

New Remediation Methods

Identifying neurocognitive deficits and subtypes of dyscalculia should allow for new remediation methods to be developed, as has already been the case in the field of dyslexia (as discussed in the introductory section). Based on what we know about dyscalculia, we hypothesize that remediation techniques based on number sense training should be effective. As of yet it is difficult to say whether techniques based on verbal memory training, visuospatial attention, or executive attention training would also be effective, but this is a possibility.

In our laboratory, we have developed and tested an adaptive computer game remediation, similar in concept to those used in dyslexia. This software, "The Number Race," is based on the number sense core deficit hypothesis and is designed to provide intensive training on the key number sense task of numerical comparison and to reinforce links between non-symbolic and symbolic representations of number (see Plate 9.3). The software adapts to children's performance by increasing the difficulty of the numerical comparison, by imposing a variable speed limit, and by increasing the ratio of symbolic to nonsymbolic stimuli according to performance. An early "open-trial" pilot study with this software shows promising results, with children showing significant improvements in subitizing, subtraction, and numerical comparison. Whether this tool will ultimately prove useful for all children with developmental dyscalculia is a matter for further research.

CONCLUSION

Developmental dyscalculia is a disorder in mathematical abilities presumed to be due to impaired brain function. It appears to have a similar prevalence to its equivalent in reading (dyslexia) but is vastly understudied in comparison. Its basic behavioral symptoms and neurological bases are only just starting to be investigated. In this chapter we proposed possible causes of dyscalculia from reviewing the literature on the neurological bases of adult numerical cognition and on development of numerical cognition in children. We identified two possible causes of a core deficit: (1) a deficit in number sense, or nonsymbolic representation of number, related to an impairment in the horizontal intraparietal sulcus area, and (2) a failure to build adequate connections between nonsymbolic and symbolic representations of number. We also identified three other possible causes of different subtypes of dyscalculia: deficits in verbal symbolic representation, executive dysfunction, or spatial attention.

We then reviewed what is currently known about dyscalculia to examine which of these hypotheses are supported by current data. Research conducted in the education field has identified several key deficits in dyscalculic children's acquisition of counting, counting-based strategies, and verbal facts. Some researchers in this field have argued that dyscalculia can be divided into verbal and nonverbal subtypes; however, research results have not always supported this proposal. One of the problems is that education research has typically used higher-level tasks composed of many component processes. We emphasize the need for future studies of dyscalculia symptoms to use a wide variety of tasks, including low-level numerical cognition tasks and nonsymbolic as well as symbolic tasks.

The evidence that is available from research using low-level numerical cognition tasks provides preliminary support for the number sense core deficit hypothesis. Children with dyscalculia show impairments in numerical comparison and subitizing, and research in special populations suggests that these impairments may be linked to an underfunctioning of the HIPS, which is known to represent quantity. However, this research is in its infancy, and much more investigation is needed for the issue to be resolved.

Finally, we discussed implications for education and intervention and emphasized three key aims. The first is the development of a neurocognitive description of dyscalculia, which would allow for better identification, treatment, and possibly prevention. The second is the development of core ability tests that would be based on the neurocognitive description developed. The third is the development of new remediation methods that target children's core deficits.

ACKNOWLEDGMENTS

We kindly acknowledge financial support from the Fyssen Foundation (to Anna J. Wilson), Institut National de la Santé et de la Recherche Médicale (INSERM), and a McDonnell Foundation centennial fellowship (to Stanislas Dehaene).

NOTES

1. See Geary and Hoard for a discussion of the similarities between the dyscalculia and mathematical learning disabilities literature.
2. Alternatively, an association could be purely circumstantial, due to the proximity of brain areas involved in working memory and numerical representation.
3. These results must be taken with caution, because the first was not significant, and the second only marginal, possibly due to a lack of statistical power.

REFERENCES

American Psychiatric Association. (1994). *Diagnostic and statistical manual of mental disorders* (4th ed.). Washington, DC: Author.

Ansari, D., & Karmiloff-Smith, A. (2002). Atypical trajectories of number development: A neuroconstructivist perspective. *Trends in Cognitive Sciences, 6*(12), 511–516.

Badian, N. A. (1983). Dyscalculia and nonverbal disorders of learning. In H. R. Myklebust (Ed.), *Progress in learning disabilities* (Vol. 5, pp. 235–264). New York: Stratton.

Badian, N. A. (1999). Persistent arithmetic, reading, or arithmetic and reading disability. *Annals of Dyslexia, 49,* 45–70.

Benson, D. F., & Geschwind, N. (1970). Developmental Gerstmann syndrome. *Neurology, 20*(3), 293–298.

Benton, A. L. (1992). Gerstmann's syndrome. *Archives of Neurology, 49*(5), 445–447.

Berch, D. B., Foley, E. J., Hill, R. J., & Ryan, P. M. (1999). Extracting parity and magnitude from Arabic numerals: Developmental changes in number processing and mental representation. *Journal of Experimental Child Psychology, 74*(4), 286.

Bruandet, M., Molko, N., Cohen, L., & Dehaene, S. (2004). A cognitive characterization of dyscalculia in Turner syndrome. *Neuropsychologia, 42*(3), 288–298.

Butterworth, B. (1999). *The mathematical brain.* London: Macmillan.

Butterworth, B. (2003). *Dyscalculia screener.* London: nferNelson.

Butterworth, B. (2005a). The development of arithmetical abilities. *Journal of Child Psychology and Psychiatry, 46*(1), 3–18.

Butterworth, B. (2005b). Developmental dyscalculia. In J. D. Campbell (Ed.), *Handbook of mathematical cognition* (pp. 455–467). New York: Psychology Press.

Cappelletti, M., Butterworth, B., & Kopelman, M. (2001). Spared numerical abilities in a case of semantic dementia. *Neuropsychologia, 39*(11), 1224.

Chochon, F., Cohen, L., van de Moortele, P. F., & Dehaene, S. (1999). Differential contributions of the left and right inferior parietal lobules to number processing. *Journal of Cognitive Neuroscience, 11*(6), 617–630.

Cohen, L., Wilson, A. J., Izard, V., & Dehaene, S. (in press). Acalculia and Gerstmann's syndrome. In O. Godefroy & J. Bogousslavsky (Eds.), *Cognitive and behavioral neurology of stroke.* Cambridge, UK: Cambridge University Press.

Cordes, S., & Gelman, R. (2005). The young numerical mind. In J. D. Campbell (Ed.), *Handbook of mathematical cognition* (pp. 127–142). New York: Psychology Press.

D'Amico, A., & Guarnera, M. (2005). Exploring working memory in children with low arithmetical achievement. *Learning and Individual Differences, 15*(3), 189–202.

Dehaene, S. (1997). *The number sense: How the mind creates mathematics.* Oxford, UK: Oxford University Press.

Dehaene, S. (2001). Précis of the number sense. *Mind and Language, 16*, 16–36.

Dehaene, S., & Cohen, L. (1997). Cerebral pathways for calculation: Double dissociation between rote verbal and quantitative knowledge of arithmetic. *Cortex, 33*(2), 219–250.

Dehaene, S., Molko, N., Cohen, L., & Wilson, A. J. (2004). Arithmetic and the brain. *Current Opinion in Neurobiology, 14*(2), 218–224.

Dehaene, S., Piazza, M., Pinel, P., & Cohen, L. (2003). Three parietal circuits for number processing. *Cognitive Neuropsychology, 20*, 487–506.

Dehaene, S., Spelke, E., Pinel, P., Stanescu, R., & Tsivkin, S. (1999). Sources of mathematical thinking: Behavioral and brain-imaging evidence. *Science, 284*, 970–974.

Dehaene, S., Tzourio, N., Frak, V., Raynaud, L., Cohen, L., Mehler, J., et al. (1996). Cerebral activations during number multiplication and comparison: A PET study. *Neuropsychologia, 34*(11), 1097–1106.

Delazer, M., Karner, E., Zamarian, L., Donnemiller, E., & Benke, T. (2006). Number processing in posterior cortical atrophy: A neuropsycholgical case study. *Neuropsychologia, 44*(1), 36–51.

Eden, G. F. (2002). The role of neuroscience in the remediation of students with dyslexia. *Nature Neuroscience, 5*(Suppl.), 1080–1084.

Eger, E., Sterzer, P., Russ, M. O., Giraud, A.-L., & Kleinschmidt, A. (2003). A supramodal number representation in human intraparietal cortex. *Neuron, 37*(4), 719.

Eliez, S., Blasey, C. M., Menon, V., White, C. D., Schmitt, J. E., & Reiss, A. L. (2001). Functional brain imaging study of mathematical reasoning abilities in velocardiofacial syndrome (del22q11.2). *Genetics in Medicine, 3*(1), 49–55.

Feigenson, L. (2005). A double-dissociation in infants' representations of object arrays. *Cognition, 95*(3), B37.

Feigenson, L., Carey, S., & Hauser, M. (2002). The representations underlying infants' choice of more: Object files versus analog magnitudes. *Psychological Science, 13*(2), 150–156.

Feigenson, L., Carey, S., & Spelke, E. (2002). Infants' discrimination of number vs. continuous extent. *Cognitive Psychology, 44*(1), 33–66.

Feigenson, L., Dehaene, S., & Spelke, E. (2004). Core systems of number. *Trends in Cognitive Sciences, 8*(7), 307–314.

Fuson, K. C. (1988). *Children's counting and concepts of number.* New York: Springer-Verlag.

Gallistel, C. R., & Gelman, R. (2000). Non-verbal numerical cognition: From reals to integers. *Trends in Cognitive Sciences, 4*(2), 59–65.

Gathercole, S. E., & Pickering, S. J. (2000). Working memory deficits in children with low achievements in the national curriculum at 7 years of age. *British Journal of Educational Psychology, 70*(2), 177–194.

Geary, D. C. (1990). A componential analysis of an early learning deficit in mathematics. *Journal of Experimental Child Psychology, 49*(3), 363–383.

Geary, D. C. (1993). Mathematical disabilities: Cognitive, neuropsychological and genetic components. *Psychological Bulletin, 114*(2), 345–362.

Geary, D. C. (2004). Mathematics and learning disabilities. *Journal of Learning Disabilities, 37*(1), 4–15.

Geary, D. C., Bow-Thomas, C. C., & Yao, Y. (1992). Counting knowledge and skill in cognitive addition: A comparison of normal and mathematically disabled children. *Journal of Experimental Child Psychology, 54*(3), 372–391.

Geary, D. C., Brown, S. C., & Samaranayake, V. A. (1991). Cognitive addition: A short longitudinal study of strategy choice and speed-of-processing differences in normal and mathematically disabled children. *Developmental Psychology, 27*(5), 787–797.

Geary, D. C., Hamson, C. O., & Hoard, M. K. (2000). Numerical and arithmetical cognition: A longitudinal study of process and concept deficits in children with learning disability. *Journal of Experimental Child Psychology, 77*(3), 236–263.

Geary, D. C., Hoard, M. K., & Hamson, C. O. (1999). Numerical and arithmetical cognition: Patterns of functions and deficits in children at risk for a mathematical disability. *Journal of Experimental Child Psychology, 74*(3), 213–239.

Gelman, R., & Gallistel, C. R. (1978). *The child's understanding of number.* Cambridge, MA: Harvard University Press.

Gersten, R., & Chard, D. (1999). Number sense: Rethinking arithmetic instruction for students with mathematical disabilities. *Journal of Special Education, 33*(1), 18–28.

Gerstmann, J. (1940). Syndrome of finger agnosia disorientation for right and left agraphia and acalculia. *Archives of Neurology and Psychiatry, 44,* 398–408.

Ginsburg, H. P. (1997). Mathematics learning disabilities: A view from developmental psychology. *Journal of Learning Disabilities, 30*(1), 20–33.

Girelli, L., Lucangeli, D., & Butterworth, B. (2000). The development of automaticity of accessing number magnitude. *Journal of Experimental Child Psychology, 76,* 104–122.

Goswami, U. (2003). Why theories about developmental dyslexia require developmental designs. *Trends in Cognitive Sciences, 7*(12), 534.

Gross-Tsur, V., Manor, O., & Shalev, R. S. (1996). Developmental dyscalculia: Prevalence and demographic features. *Developmental Medicine and Child Neurology, 38*(1), 25–33.

Huntley-Fenner, G. (2001). Children's understanding of number is similar to adults' and rats': Numerical estimation by 5–7-year-olds. *Cognition, 78*(3), B27–B40.

Isaacs, E. B., Edmonds, C. J., Lucas, A., & Gadian, D. G. (2001). Calculation difficulties in children of very low birthweight: A neural correlate. *Brain, 124*(9), 1701–1707.

Jackson, M., & Warrington, E. K. (1986). Arithmetic skills in patients with unilateral cerebral lesions. *Cortex, 22*(4), 611–620.

Jordan, N. C., & Hanich, L. B. (2000). Mathematical thinking in second-grade children with different forms of LD. *Journal of Learning Disabilities, 33*(6), 567–578.

Jordan, N. C., Hanich, L. B., & Kaplan, D. (2003). A longitudinal study of mathematical competencies in children with specific mathematics difficulties versus children with comorbid mathematics and reading difficulties. *Child Development, 74*(3), 834–850.

Jordan, N. C., & Montani, T. O. (1997). Cognitive arithmetic and problem solving: A comparison and children with specific and general mathematics difficulties. *Journal of Learning Disabilities, 30*(6), 624–634.

Kaufmann, L. (2002). More evidence for the role of the central executive in retrieving arithmetic facts: A case study of severe developmental dyscalculia. *Journal of Clinical and Experimental Neuropsychology, 24*(3), 302–310.

Kinsbourne, M., & Warrington, E. K. (1963). The developmental Gerstmann syndrome. *Archives of Neurology, 8,* 490–501.

Kirby, J. R., & Becker, L. D. (1988). Cognitive components of learning problems in arithmetic. *Remedial and Special Education, 9*(5), 7–16.

Koontz, K. L., & Berch, D. B. (1996). Identifying simple numerical stimuli: Processing inefficiencies exhibited by arithmetic learning disabled children. *Mathematical Cognition, 2*(1), 1–23.

Kosc, L. (1974). Developmental dyscalculia. *Journal of Learning Disabilities, 7*(3), 164–177.

Landerl, K., Bevan, A., & Butterworth, B. (2004). Developmental dyscalculia and basic numerical capacities: A study of 8–9-year-old students. *Cognition, 93*(2), 99–125.

Lee, K. M. (2000). Cortical areas differentially involved in multiplication and subtraction: A functional magnetic resonance imaging study and correlation with a case of selective acalculia. *Annals of Neurology, 48*(4), 657–661.

LeFevre, J.-A., Smith-Chant, B. L., Hiscock, K., Daley, K. E., & Morris, J. (2003). Young adults' strategic choices in simple arithmetic: Implications for the development of mathematical representations. In A. J. Baroody & A. Dowker (Eds.), *The development of arithmetic concepts and skills: Constructive adaptive expertise* (pp. 203–228). Mahwah, NJ: Erlbaum.

Lemer, C., Dehaene, S., Spelke, E., & Cohen, L. (2003). Approximate quantities and exact number words: Dissociable systems. *Neuropsychologia, 41*(14), 1942–1958.

Lewis, C., Hitch, G. J., & Walker, P. (1994). The prevalence of specific arithmetic difficulties and specific reading difficulties in 9- to 10-year old boys and girls. *Journal of Child Psychology and Psychiatry and Allied Disciplines, 35*(2), 283–292.

Lipton, J., & Spelke, E. (2003). Origins of number sense: Large-number discrimination in human infants. *Psychological Science, 14*(5), 396–401.

Lyytinen, H., Guttorm, T. K., Huttunen, T., Hamalainen, J., Leppanen, P. H. T., & Vesterinen, M. (2005). Psychophysiology of developmental dyslexia: A review of findings including studies of children at risk for dyslexia. *Journal of Neurolinguistics, 18*(2), 167–195.

Mazzocco, M. M. M., & McCloskey, M. (2005). Math performance in girls with Turner or fragile X syndrome. In J. D. Campbell (Ed.), *Handbook of mathematical cognition* (pp. 269–298). New York: Psychology Press.

McCrink, K., & Wynn, K. (2004). Large-number addition and subtraction by 9-month-old infants. *Psychological Science, 15*(11), 776–781.

McLean, J. F., & Hitch, G. J. (1999). Working memory impairments in children with specific arithmetic learning difficulties. *Journal of Experimental Child Psychology, 74*(3), 240–260.

Miller, C. J., & Hynd, G. W. (2004). What ever happened to developmental Gerstmann's syndrome? Links to other pediatric, genetic, and neurodevelopmental syndromes. *Journal of Child Neurology, 19*(4), 282–289.

Molko, N., Cachia, A., Riviere, D., Mangin, J. F., Bruandet, M., Le Bihan, D., et al. (2003). Functional and structural alterations of the intraparietal sulcus in a developmental dyscalculia of genetic origin. *Neuron, 40*(4), 847–858.

Nieder, A. (2005). Counting on neurons: The neurobiology of numerical competence. *Nature Reviews: Neuroscience, 6*(3), 177–190.

Nieder, A., & Miller, E. K. (2004). A parieto–frontal network for visual numerical information in the monkey. *Proceedings of the National Academy of Sciences USA, 101*(19), 7457–7462.

Noël, M.-P., Rousselle, L., & Mussolin, C. (2005). Magnitude representation in children: Its development and dysfunction. In J. D. Campbell (Ed.), *Handbook of mathematical cognition* (pp. 179–196).New York: Psychology Press.

Ostad, S. A. (1997). Developmental differences in addition strategies: A comparison of mathematically disabled and mathematically normal children. *British Journal of Educational Psychology, 67*, 345–357.

Ostad, S. A. (1999). Developmental progression of subtraction strategies: A comparison of mathematically normal and mathematically disabled children. *European Journal of Special Needs Education, 14*(1), 21–36.

Passolunghi, M. C., & Siegel, L. S. (2004). Working memory and access to numerical information in children with disability in mathematics. *Journal of Experimental Child Psychology, 88*(4), 348.

Pesenti, M., Thioux, M., Seron, X., & De Volder, A. (2000). Neuroanatomical substrates of Arabic number processing, numerical comparison, and simple addition: A PET study. *Journal of Cognitive Neuroscience, 12*(3), 461–479.

Piaget, J. (1952). *The child's conception of number.* New York: Norton.

Piazza, M., Izard, V., Pinel, P., Le Bihan, D., & Dehaene, S. (2004). Tuning curves for approximate numerosity in the human intraparietal sulcus. *Neuron, 44*, 547–555.

Pinel, P., Dehaene, S., Riviere, D., & Le Bihan, D. (2001). Modulation of parietal activation by semantic distance in a number comparison task. *NeuroImage, 14*(5), 1013.

Pinel, P., Piazza, M., Le Bihan, D., & Dehaene, S. (2004). Distributed and overlapping cerebral representations of number, size, and luminance during comparative judgments. *Neuron, 41*(6), 983.

Rivera, S. M., Menon, V., White, C. D., Glaser, B., & Reiss, A. L. (2002). Functional brain activation during arithmetic processing in females with fragile X syndrome is related to fmr1 protein expression. *Human Brain Mapping, 16*, 206–218.

Rivera-Batiz, F. L. (1992). Quantitative literacy and the likelihood of employment among young adults in the United States. *Journal of Human Resources, 27*(2), 313–328.

Robinson, C. S., Menchetti, B. M., & Torgesen, J. K. (2002). Toward a two-factor theory of one type of mathematics disabilities. *Learning Disabilities Research and Practice, 17*(2), 81–89.

Rosselli, M., & Ardila, A. (1989). Calculation deficits in patients with right and left hemisphere damage. *Neuropsychologia, 27*(5), 607–617.

Rourke, B. P. (1993). Arithmetic disabilities, specific and otherwise: A neuropsychological perspective. *Journal of Learning Disabilities, 26*(4), 214–226.

Rourke, B. P., & Conway, J. A. (1997). Disabilities of arithmetic and mathematical reasoning: Perspectives from neurology and neuropsychology. *Journal of Learning Disabilities, 30*(1), 34–46.

Rourke, B. P., & Finlayson, M. A. (1978). Neuropsychological significance of variations in patterns of academic performance: Verbal and visual–spatial abilities. *Journal of Abnormal Child Psychology, 6*(1), 121–133.

Rourke, B. P., & Strang, J. D. (1978). Neuropsychological significance of variations in patterns of academic performance: Motor, psychomotor, and tactile-perceptual abilities. *Journal of Pediatric Psychology, 3*, 62–66.

Rovet, J., Szekely, C., & Hockenberry, M.-N. (1994). Specific arithmetic calculation deficits in children with Turner syndrome. *Journal of Clinical and Experimental Neuropsychology, 16*(6), 820–839.

Rubinsten, O., Henik, A., Berger, A., & Shahar-Shalev, S. (2002). The development of internal representations of magnitude and their association with Arabic numerals. *Journal of Experimental Child Psychology, 81*(1), 74–92.

Shalev, R. S., & Gross-Tsur, V. (1993). Developmental dyscalculia and medical assessment. *Journal of Learning Disabilities, 26*(2), 134–137.

Shalev, R. S., & Gross-Tsur, V. (2001). Developmental dyscalculia. *Pediatric Neurology, 24*(5), 337–342.

Shalev, R. S., Manor, O., & Gross-Tsur, V. (1997). Neuropsychological aspects of developmental dyscalculia. *Mathematical Cognition, 3*(2), 105–120.

Share, D. L., Moffitt, T. E., & Silva, P. A. (1988). Factors associated with arithmetic-and-reading disability and specific arithmetic disability. *Journal of Learning Disabilities, 21*(5), 313–320.

Siegler, R. S., & Jenkins, E. A. (1989). *How children discover new strategies.* Hillsdale, NJ: Erlbaum.

Siegler, R. S., & Opfer, J. E. (2003). The development of numerical estimation: Evidence for multiple representations of numerical quantity. *Psychological Science, 14*(3), 237–243.

Siegler, R. S., & Shrager, J. (1984). Strategy choices in addition and subtraction: How do children know what to do? In C. Sophian (Ed.), *Origins of cognitive skill* (pp. 241–312). Hillsdale, NJ: Erlbaum.

Simon, T. J. (1999). The foundations of numerical thinking in a brain without numbers. *Trends in Cognitive Sciences, 3*(10), 363.

Simon, T. J., Bearden, C. E., Moss, E. M., McDonald-McGinn, D., Zackai, E., & Wang, P. P. (2002). Cognitive development in VCFS. *Progress in Pediatric Cardiology, 15*(2), 109.

Simon, T. J., Ding, L., Bish, J. P., McDonald-McGinn, D. M., Zackai, E. H., & Gee, J. (2005). Volumetric, connective, and morphologic changes in the brains of children with chromosome 22q11.2 deletion syndrome: An integrative study. *NeuroImage, 25*(1), 169.

Spelke, E. S., & Tsivkin, S. (2001). Language and number: A bilingual training study. *Cognition, 78*(1), 45–88.

Spellacy, F., & Peter, B. (1978). Dyscalculia and elements of the developmental Gerstmann syndrome in school children. *Cortex, 14*(2), 197–206.

Stanescu-Cosson, R., Pinel, P., van de Moortele, P.-F., Le Bihan, D., Cohen, L., & Dehaene, S. (2000). Understanding dissociations in dyscalculia: A brain imaging study of the impact of number size on the cerebral networks for exact and approximate calculation. *Brain, 123*(11), 2240–2255.

Tallal, P., Miller, S. L., Bedi, G., Byma, G., Wang, X., Nagarajan, S. S., et al. (1996). Language comprehension in language-learning impaired children improved with acoustically modified speech. *Science, 271*, 81–84.

Temple, C. M. (1989). Digit dyslexia: A category-specific disorder in development dyscalculia. *Cognitive Neuropsychology, 6*(1), 93–116.

Temple, C. M. (1991). Procedural dyscalculia and number fact dyscalculia: Double dissociation in developmental dyscalculia. *Cognitive Neuropsychology, 8*(2), 155–176.

Temple, C. M., & Marriott, A. J. (1998). Arithmetical ability and disability in Turner's syndrome: A cognitive neuropsychological analysis. *Developmental Neuropsychology, 14*(1), 47–67.

Temple, C. M., & Sherwood, S. (2002). Representation and retrieval of arithmetical facts: Developmental difficulties. *Quarterly Journal of Experimental Psychology A, 55A*(3), 733–752.

Temple, E., Deutsch, G. K., Poldrack, R. A., Miller, S. L., Tallal, P., Merzenich, M. M., et al. (2003). Neural deficits in children with dyslexia ameliorated by behavioral remediation: Evidence from functional MRI. *Proceedings of the National Academy of Sciences USA, 100*(5), 2860–2865.

Temple, E., & Posner, M. I. (1998). Brain mechanisms of quantity are similar in 5-year-old children and adults. *Proceedings of the National Academy of Sciences USA, 95*, 7836–7841.

Trick, L. M., & Pylyshyn, Z. W. (1994). Why are small and large numbers enumerated differently?: A limited-capacity preattentive stage in vision. *Psychological Review, 101*(1), 80–102.

Wilson, K. M., & Swanson, H. L. (2001). Are mathematics disabilities due to a domain-general or a domain-specific working memory deficit? *Journal of Learning Disabilities, 34*(3), 237–248.

Wynn, K. (1990). Children's understanding of counting. *Cognition, 36*, 155–193.

Xu, F. (2003). Numerosity discrimination in infants: Evidence for two systems of representations. *Cognition, 89*(1), B15–B25.

Xu, F., & Spelke, E. S. (2000). Large number discrimination in 6-month-old infants. *Cognition, 74*(1), B1–B11.

Xu, F., Spelke, E., & Goddard, S. (2005). Number sense in human infants. *Developmental Science, 8*(1), 88–101.

Zago, L., Pesenti, M., Mellet, E., Crivello, F., Mazoyer, B., & Tzourio-Mazoyer, N. (2001). Neural correlates of simple and complex mental calculation. *NeuroImage, 13*(2), 314–327.

CHAPTER 10

Central Nervous System Substrates of Impulsivity

IMPLICATIONS FOR THE DEVELOPMENT
OF ATTENTION-DEFICIT/HYPERACTIVITY DISORDER
AND CONDUCT DISORDER

Lisa M. Gatzke-Kopp
Theodore P. Beauchaine

Attention-deficit/hyperactivity disorder (ADHD) is among the most common childhood psychiatric conditions, affecting 3–7% of school-age children (American Psychiatric Association, 2000). Disruptions in behavior related to ADHD can lead to a host of difficulties, including academic underachievement, disturbed family relations, and peer rejection. Furthermore, disinhibition, the core behavioral trait underlying both the hyperactive/impulsive and combined subtypes of ADHD (see Barkley, 1997), confers risk for a host of adverse sequelae in adolescence and adulthood, such as occupational underachievement, substance abuses and dependencies, and disrupted interpersonal relationships (e.g., Johnston, 2002). Although medication is useful in alleviating hyperactive and impulsive symptoms for many of those afflicted with ADHD, a complete understanding of the neurobiological substrates of the disorder still eludes researchers.

Recently, several theories have been advanced toward delineating the specific neurological deficits underlying ADHD (e.g., Barkley, 1997;

Sagvolden, Johansen, Aase, & Russell, 2005), yet none of these theories is canonical. In part, disagreements regarding the neurobiological substrates of ADHD are likely the result of etiological heterogeneity among those afflicted with the behavioral syndrome. Different genetic polymorphisms and neurological deficits may result in similar behavioral profiles, and multiple combinations of risk may produce apparently similar diagnostic syndromes (Beauchaine & Marsh, 2006). Scientific advances in our understanding of complex disorders such as ADHD are therefore more likely to be realized by focusing on tightly defined traits and their central nervous system (CNS) correlates (endophenotypes) rather than exclusively on behavioral symptoms (phenotypes), which are imprecise by nature (Castellanos & Tannock, 2002; see also Grigorenko, Chapter 5, this volume). Following from this assumption, we provide an overview of brain structures that are likely implicated in the expression of impulsivity.

Before proceeding, it is important to note that the DSM-IV-TR (American Psychiatric Association, 2000) includes three subtypes of ADHD reflecting different combinations of hyperactivity/impulsivity and inattention. These subtypes are referred to as primarily inattentive, primarily hyperactive, and combined. Although debate exists regarding the degree to which these subtypes identify discrete behavioral syndromes, many ADHD researchers now believe that the primarily inattentive subtype is likely to be etiologically distinct from the hyperactive/impulsive and combined subtypes (see Milich, Balentine, & Lynam, 2001). Proponents of this view suggest that the inattention observed in combined cases is a behavioral manifestation of deficits that are not directly related to attentional allocation and processing. Rather, inattention in such cases is more likely a consequence of impulsivity (Barkley, 1997; Milich et al., 2001). Although space limitations preclude us from exploring these issues in detail, our assumption in writing this chapter is that the purely inattentive subtype is etiologically distinct. Given this assumption, our intent in the sections to follow is to discuss neurobiological models of the hyperactive/impulsive and combined subtypes of ADHD. Although models of the inattentive subtype could be discussed, this form of ADHD affects far fewer children and such models have been omitted due to space constraints.

In addition to subtype considerations, it should also be noted that children with ADHD experience high rates of comorbidity with other externalizing disorders, including oppositional defiant disorder (ODD) and conduct disorder (CD). This comorbidity presents additional challenges when attempting to identify unique etiological substrates of ADHD. Although ADHD clearly exists without ODD or CD behaviors, early-onset CD rarely, if ever, manifests without both prior and current ADHD symptoms. Furthermore, comorbidity of ADHD with ODD and CD has not been carefully controlled in most studies. Thus, if differences in CNS functioning exist among these conditions, such differences have not been isolated and may contribute to inconsistencies and complexities in findings reported for studies of ADHD that have not excluded participants with comorbid ODD and/or CD.

On the other hand, recent behavioral genetics studies have demonstrated that the spectrum of externalizing behaviors, including impulsivity, conduct problems, antisocial personality, and substance abuse, share a common genetic vulnerability conferred by a latent impulsivity trait, the behavioral expression of which is dictated by environmental opportunities (Krueger et al., 2002). To the extent that the theories discussed below relate to the neurobiological substrates of impulsivity, they are likely to extend to common genetic risks for disorders beyond ADHD. Such an interpretation is consistent with biosocial developmental models of CD, in which inherited impulsivity results in pure ADHD in protective familial environments but progresses to more serious conduct problems and delinquency in high-risk environments that include coercive and labile parenting practices, exposure to delinquent peers, and neighborhoods with high rates of violence and crime (see, e.g., Beauchaine, Gatzke-Kopp, & Mead, in press; Lynam et al., 2000; Patterson, DeGarmo, & Knutson, 2000). With these caveats in mind, our objective in writing this chapter is to discuss the neurobiological substrates of impulsivity and to advance a theory of dopaminergic deficiency that results in motivational deficits leading to the hyperactive/impulsive and combined forms of ADHD.

DOPAMINE NEUROBIOLOGY

Dopamine (DA) is widely considered to be directly involved in the pathophysiology of ADHD. One of the most compelling sources of evidence for this involvement is the effectiveness of methylphenidate (Ritalin) and other dopamine agonists in treating ADHD symptoms. Many animal models of ADHD also implicate central dopaminergic systems (Davids, Kehong, Tarazi, & Baldessarini, 2003; Sagvolden, 2001; Sullivan & Brake, 2003), and molecular genetics studies of ADHD have focused almost exclusively on genes involved in DA functioning (DiMaio, Frizenko, & Joober, 2003; Swanson & Castellanos, 2002). However, despite convergent evidence that DA is fundamentally involved in the expression of ADHD, the exact DA subsystem and the nature of the proposed dysfunction vary widely across competing theories.

Dopaminergic projections in the CNS are both extensive and complex and are usually grouped into three main subsystems: the mesocortical, mesolimbic, and nigrostriatal. These systems include neuroanatomical circuits that function in concert. Broadly speaking, the mesocortical system is associated with executive functioning, including maintenance of behavior in reference to specified goals or rule structures; the mesolimbic system is associated with motivated responding to reward; and the nigrostriatal system is associated with motoric responding (Kandel, 2000). Although these systems are often conceptualized as functionally distinct, interconnections among each are extensive, and functional integration of each is critical for appropriate execution of goal-directed behavior (Tisch, Silberstein, Limousin-Dowsey, & Jahanshahi, 2004). Moreover, each of these systems has been implicated in theories of ADHD. Nevertheless, it remains unclear whether or not there is widespread DA dysfunction across subsystems among ADHD probands, implicating all three systems, or if individual systems are compromised, with others remaining intact. A more detailed presentation of the neuroanatomical circuits comprising each system is presented below, along with evidence linking each to the pathophysiology of ADHD. This discussion is followed by a description of additional brain regions that have been implicated in the expression of ADHD, including the anterior cingulate cortex and the cerebellar vermis.

Nigrostriatal System

The nigrostriatal system consists of dopaminergic neurons originating in the substantia nigra pars compacta, which is located near the ventral tegmental area (VTA) in the midbrain (Saper, 2000). These neurons project to the dorsal striatum, consisting of the caudate nucleus and the putamen (Swartz, 1999), components of the basal ganglia. The nigrostriatal system has long been implicated in motor functions and is known to be dysfunctional in movement-related disorders such as Parkinson disease and Huntington's chorea (DeLong, 2000). However, the involvement of the basal ganglia in conjunction with motivational processes has also been suggested in research indicating that these structures may facilitate planned or goal-oriented movement by suppressing extraneous and unrelated activity (Marsden & Obeso, 1994). This possibility suggests a modulatory, but not primary, role in the execution of movement (Tisch et al., 2004), which may occur through integration of the multiple functions of the dopaminergic pathways. For instance, substantia nigra neurons appear to alter their firing patterns in response to predicted reward (Ljungberg, Apicella, & Schultz, 1992), a role typically governed by the nucleus accumbens. These neurons may not be responding to reward salience. Rather, they may provide input to the nigrostriatal system indicating that behavior needs to be modulated in reference to the cued reward. This conceptualization suggests that a DA deficiency in the nigrostriatal system could lead to an increase in indiscriminate movements that are unassociated with specific goals—behavior that is consistent with the observation that children with ADHD exhibit excess motor responses that interfere with goal achievement.

Neuroanatomical evidence also suggests the presence of dorsal striatal deficits in ADHD. Neuroimaging research has repeatedly demonstrated dysfunction in these regions, leaving little room for doubt regarding their involvement in ADHD symptoms. Specifically, structural neuroimaging studies have shown either volumetric abnormalities or abnormalities in asymmetry in the caudate nucleus in children with ADHD (Castellanos et al., 1996, 2003; Filipek et al., 1997; Hynd et al., 1993). Functional neuroimaging studies provide additional support for caudate dysfunction. Positron emission tomography (PET) studies completed at rest have demonstrated reductions in cerebral blood flow in dorsal striatal regions of participants with ADHD (Lou, Henriksen, Bruhn, Borner, & Nielsen, 1989). In addition, single photon emission computed tomography (SPECT) studies of ADHD indicate increased DA transporter density in the dorsal striatum (Krause, Dresel, Krause, la Fougere, & Ackenheil, 2003), which could result in increased DA uptake and a consequent reduction in receptor activation. This finding suggests that structural deficits may reflect reductions in DA function in this region. Functional magnetic resonance imaging (fMRI) studies are especially beneficial in that they are able to associate compromises in function directly with behavioral performance on selected tasks. Most fMRI studies have included tasks of motor inhibition, such as the stop-signal task or the go/no-go task, wherein participants are expected to inhibit a dominant motor response. Such tasks are designed to recruit dorsal striatal regions, and studies using these tasks routinely show functional deficiencies in nigrostriatal structures among ADHD samples (Rubia et al., 1999).

Although support for the involvement of the nigrostriatal system, primarily the dorsal striatum, in the pathology of ADHD has been fairly consistent, whether such deficiencies are primary to the expression of ADHD symptoms is uncertain. Rarely are the nigrostriatal system and its component structures implicated in isolation. Many theories of ADHD suggest that dysfunction within the nigrostriatal system may be a functional consequence of deficient feedback from other compromised DA systems and thus not necessarily the etiological source of the disorder. Most research supports an additional role for either the mesocortical or mesolimbic systems in ADHD pathology and their relationship to the dorsal striatum.

Mesocortical System

The mesocortical system is comprised of dopaminergic projections originating in the VTA and projecting to the dorsolateral prefrontal cortex, the temporal cortex, and the anterior cingulate cortex (Swartz, 1999). The dorsolateral prefrontal cortex is implicated in higher-level cognitive functions. Circuits within this system include connections with the head of the caudate nucleus, which is implicated in planning, organizing, and monitoring long-term goal-directed behaviors—actions that comprise "executive functioning" (Tisch et al., 2004). These higher-level tasks allow humans to maintain objectives and regulate behavior over long intervals, an ability that is often considered deficient in children with ADHD. This inability has led researchers to consider frontal dysfunction to be the primary deficit in the ontogenesis of ADHD (Barkley, 1997; Nigg, 2001). Barkley (1997) argues that the frontal lobe is responsible for governing behavior with respect to long-term goals and engaging self-imposed rules/structure in situations where immediate reinforcement is lacking and long-term objectives must be reached. Dysfunction in this system is offered as an explanation for the observation that ADHD children do not perform well when rewards are inconsistent and/or delayed. However, the absence of behavior provides only weak support for the neural structures involved; studies of neurological function are needed before firm conclusions can be drawn.

Neuroanatomically, this is a plausible theory. Frontal impairment could return control over goal-directed behavior to phylogenetically older motivational structures in the mesolimbic DA system, described below. In theory, this shift would result in a focus on immediate reinforcement, with no ability to modulate behavior over longer intervals. Sullivan and Brake (2003) describe a rodent model of ADHD that supports this supposition. This model proposes that the frontal cortex is the primary source of dysfunction leading to ADHD. A deficit in dopaminergic transmission in this area, the authors argue, results in hyperdopaminergic function in the ventral striatum, consisting of the nucleus accumbens, the primary structure responsible for reward-seeking behavior (see below). According to this model, tonic control over the ventral striatum, normally provided by the frontal cortex, is absent in ADHD, allowing the nucleus accumbens to fire in response to an exceedingly large variety of stimuli. Uncontrolled phasic firing of DA neurons in the accumbens is theorized to lead to increased behavioral responding and an overactive association of reward contingencies to irrelevant stimuli (Grace, 2001).

Evidence for frontal involvement in ADHD is also found in the neuroimaging literature. Structural neuroimaging studies have uncovered reduced prefrontal volume in children with ADHD (Castellanos et al., 1996; Filipek et al., 1997; Kates et al., 2002; Mostofsky, Cooper, Kates, Denckla, & Kaufmann, 2002). However, many of these studies focused exclusively on frontal and striatal systems and did not examine other cerebral areas (Durston, 2003). Recently, Castellanos and colleagues (2002) reported cortical volumetric reductions in ADHD participants in all four cerebral lobes, suggesting that, from a structural standpoint, the deficiencies are widespread. It is not entirely clear what the functional implications of such structural deficits are. Functional studies conducted at rest have demonstrated reduced activity in the prefrontal cortex among children with ADHD (Kim, Lee, Shin, Cho, & Lee, 2002). However, although structural studies continually demonstrate reduced prefrontal volumes, functional studies frequently show an increase in prefrontal activity during inhibition-related tasks (Schulz, Newcorn, Fan, Tangy, & Halperin, 2005; Schweitzer et al., 2004). The relative increase could suggest inefficiency or compensation, but a clear mechanistic explanation for this phenomenon is lacking.

According to mesocortical models of ADHD, DA agonists such as methylphenidate could function in one of two ways. Because methylphenidate increases synaptic DA levels by inhibiting reuptake (Patrick & Markowitz, 1997), we might assume that the site of action is in the region that is DA deficient—in this model, the frontal cortex. However, SPECT and PET studies demonstrate clearly that the primary site of methylphenidate action is on DA activity in the striatum (Vles et al., 2003; Volkow, Fowler, Wang, Ding, & Gatley, 2002). This finding argues against the frontal cortex as the site of therapeutic action. Moreover, given the assumption of this model that DA activity in the ventral striatum is excessive, the application of DA agonists should make symptoms worse, not better.

In order to render the therapeutic effect of methylphenidate consistent with mesocortical models of ADHD, it is necessary to describe DA functioning within the striatum in greater detail. According to Grace (2001), striatal DA has both tonic and phasic properties. *Tonic activity* refers to the regulatory control that frontal structures exert on the ventral striatum, which inhibits striatal cells from firing. When a rewarding stimulus is strong enough, the striatum fires *phasically*, activating dopaminergic postsynaptic receptors. This phasic activity is in direct response to a specific stimulus. Thus, tonic control is inhibitory, modulating excitatory phasic firing. These two functions are differentiated by alternative DA receptor subtypes. There are five dopamine receptors that have been identified to date, which are generally grouped as D1-like (excitatory) or D2-like (inhibitory) in nature (Laakso & Caron, 2004). The D1 subtypes are postsynaptic receptors that are activated by DA that is released from the presynaptic neuron into the synaptic cleft. Once activated, they potentiate neural activity. This is a phasic response. In contrast, D2 receptors are presynaptic, activated by extracellular DA that escapes the synapse. This action serves as an inhibitory feedback mechanism as DA concentrations reach levels exceeding reuptake capacity. Thus, when DA escapes the synaptic cleft, presynaptic receptors signal that DA release should cease. Under normal conditions, the striatum is thought to be suffused with extracelluar DA, which tonically inhibits the release of more DA unless a powerful action potential overrides this input (Grace, 2001). At low doses, DA agonists may inhibit phasic DA release by increasing inhibitory tonic control (Cooper, Bloom, & Roth, 2003).

Although this frontal dysfunction hypothesis has appeal, neuroimaging research has provided only modest support for it. Moreover, an interesting functional imaging experiment with children who had ADHD, which included conditions both on and off methylphenidate, calls into question the primary role of the frontal cortex. In this fMRI study, children with ADHD exhibited higher frontal activation and lower striatal activation when off medication, in direct contrast with the mesocortical deficiency theory (Vaidya et al., 1998). Methylphenidate administration resulted in increased frontal perfusion for both children with ADHD and normal controls, but only ADHD participants showed improved striatal perfusion. This finding questions whether deficits observed in the frontal lobe in neuroimaging studies indicate a core dysfunction in the frontal cortex, or whether input from other DA systems is deficient. Some measure of frontal dysfunction is implicated in nearly every psychological disorder, which is likely a reflection of the role that the frontal lobes play in monitoring and regulating most lower brain structures. It is possible that etiological deficits specific to ADHD reside in still another location.

Mesolimbic System

As with the mesocortical pathway, the mesolimbic pathway originates in the VTA. These DA neurons project to the ventral striatum (nucleus accumbens), the amygdala, the septum, and the hippocampus (Swartz, 1999). These structures are critical in motivated behavior. The nucleus accumbens is considered to be a primary structure involved in responding to cues for reward and incorporating reward contingencies into the behavioral profile of animals. Gray (1987) hypothesized that dopaminergic projections from the VTA to the nucleus accumbens (mesolimbic) are responsible for motivating an organism to respond to incentives, whereas dopaminergic projections from the substantia nigra to the dorsal striatum (nigrostriatal) are involved in executing the motivated response. Individual differences in the mesolimbic system have been implicated in the personality trait of novelty seeking (e.g., Cloninger, 1986) and in the predisposition to abuse drugs (Bardo, Donohew, & Harrington, 1996). Not surprisingly, a role for this system has been suggested in a variety of externalizing disorders, including ADHD. However, the exact nature of the role this system plays remains the topic of much debate.

Following from Gray's theory, behavioral researchers have proposed that overactivation of the mesolimbic DA system leads to increases in reward-seeking behavior, a hallmark of externalizing disorders (Matthys, van Goozen, de Vries, Cohen-Kettenis, & van Engeland, 1998; Quay, 1993). Anatomical support for this supposition derives from the rodent model of Sullivan and Brake (2003), who propose excess mesolimbic activation in response to mesocortical deficits. Despite the face validity of such a theory (an overactive ventral striatum leads to overactive behavior), several researchers have developed theories of DA hypoactivation in the nucleus accumbens as a direct etiological factor in ADHD (Beauchaine, 2002; Sagvolden, 2001; Sagvolden & Sergeant, 1998). The first of these theories was developed originally in a rodent model and focuses on the role of DA in learning (Sagvolden, 2001). Sagvolden and colleagues (2005) speculate that the tonic and phasic coupling of the mesocortical and mesolimbic systems becomes uncoupled in ADHD, and that both the frontal and the striatal dopaminergic systems are deficient. The result of this proposed deficit is a shortened reinforcement delay gradient, outlined in greater detail below.

Studies in which DA activity has been monitored in primates in response to incentives demonstrate that dopaminergic activity is critically involved in the learning of behavior/reward contingencies (Tremblay, Hollerman, & Schultz, 1998). When an animal encounters a reward, DA cells in the nucleus accumbens fire during the period in which the associative learning takes place. This process enables the animal to bring the reward within its own behavioral control. Sagvolden and colleagues (2005) have argued that this process is deficient in children with ADHD, leading to difficulty associating behavioral contingencies and reward because of a dopaminergic deficit in this region. This deficit reduces the amount of time in which a child with ADHD can associate behavioral contingencies with reward. Thus, if a child with ADHD is not rewarded for a behavior immediately, he or she will fail to learn the association between the behavior and the eventual reward, whereas normal children can make this association over longer intervals. As a result, the child with ADHD is unwilling to delay gratification and will work only for immediate rewards—a common behavioral pattern among these children (Sagvolden, Aase, Steiner, & Berger, 1998). The function of DA agonists such as methylphenidate in this model is to elevate DA in the nucleus accumbens directly, thereby lengthening the reinforcement gradient, allowing more time for associations between behavior and reward to develop. This point highlights the importance of behavioral treatment in addition to medication. According to this model, medication only serves to normalize reinforcement gradients that accommodate learning.

Mesolimbic DA dysfunction is also supported by a long history of motivational research suggesting decreased arousal as an etiological factor in externalizing behaviors (Ellis, 1987). Optimal arousal theory postulates that reductions in arousal are experienced as aversive, and that children are motivated to up-regulate chronically low arousal by engaging in sensation-seeking behaviors. Haenlein and Caul (1987) also speculated that children with ADHD require larger rewards to achieve behavioral performance comparable to that of normal children. Thus, the unbridled reward-seeking behavior characteristic of ADHD and other externalizing disorders may be driven by a need to achieve increases in mesolimbic DA tone. Consistent with this theory, low central DA activity is a predictor of trait irritability (Laakso et al., 2003). Furthermore, increases in central DA activity have been linked with pleasurable affective states and positive emotionality (Ashby et al., 1999). Following from this model, DA agonists should produce a calming effect by increasing mesolimbic DA activity, obviating the need to achieve the same result behaviorally. This theory is neuroanatomically supported by Sagvolden's model, but generates a slightly different explanatory function.

Additional support for the low mesolimbic DA theory comes from psychophysiological studies examining sympathetic nervous-system-linked cardiac reactivity to reward. Both the sympathetic and parasympathetic nervous systems (SNS and PNS, respectively) contribute to chronotropic (rate-related) cardiac activity (Berntson, Cacioppo, Quigley, & Fabro, 1994), and a growing body of research indicates that it is important to isolate the effects of each branch when participants respond to incentives. Studies in which both SNS and PNS activity are measured indicate that SNS reactivity is specific to conditions of reward, whereas PNS reactivity is observed across a wide range of stimuli (Brenner, Beauchaine, & Sylvers, 2005). In such studies, SNS-linked cardiac reactivity is indexed by cardiac pre-ejection period (PEP), a systolic time interval influenced solely by the sympathetic branch of the autonomic nervous system (see Sherwood et al., 1990). As the SNS is mobilized, increasing cardiac output in preparation for approach behaviors, PEP—the time between left-ventricular depolarization and ejection of blood into the aorta—shortens. Thus, PEP may represent a psychophysiological marker of mesolimbic DA activity in response to incentives. Consistent with this view, infusions of DA agonists into mesolimbic structures result in sympathetically mediated increases in blood pressure and cardiac output (van den Buusse, 1998).

If PEP is indeed a valid indicator of mesolimbic activation, using it as a peripheral marker during incentive tasks may help to resolve the debate between "overactive" and "underactive" mesolimbic theories of externalizing disorders. We have used PEP in three studies of externalizing psychopathology in children spanning preschool to adolescence. In the first, adolescents with ADHD and those with comorbid CD both showed significant reductions in electrodermal activity (Beauchaine, Katkin, Strassberg, & Snarr, 2001). This finding is consistent with the low-trait anxiety often observed among impulsive male samples. However, only adolescents with ADHD *and* comorbid CD exhibited attenuated PEP responses to reward. This finding may suggest that deficits in mesolimbic reactivity to incentives are more specific to aggressive externalizing behavior than to pure ADHD. In a later study, preschool children ages 4–6, who were deemed to be at high risk for developing CD because of early evidence of ADHD and ODD, also exhibited attenuated PEP responses to reward (Crowell et al., 2006). In a third study, similar findings were observed in a middle school sample of children high on both ADHD and CD symptoms (see Beauchaine et al., in press). Thus, deficiencies in PEP responding can be identified at multiple developmental time points with similar diagnostic implications. Lengthened PEP, or decreased SNS-linked cardiac reactivity to reward, appears to suggest hypofunctioning of the mesolimbic DA system in these children. Although this mechanism supports the underactive mesolimbic hypothesis among externalizing probands, a specific association with ADHD in the absence of comorbid disorders has not been established. However, two additional studies examining heart rate reactivity to reward among children with ADHD found deficiencies compared with controls (Crone, Jennings, & van der Molen, 2003; Iaboni, Douglas, & Ditto, 1997). Although SNS and PNS influences were not separated in these studies, the findings are consistent with the decreased sympathetic influences found by Beauchaine and colleagues. Unfortunately, neither study screened out probands with comorbid CD, so the specificity of the findings to ADHD is unknown. If such findings do apply to pure ADHD, combining motivational and learning models of mesolimbic dysfunction would suggest that children with ADHD are especially motivated to seek rewards, but less capable of learning how to increase reward probability. These theories contrast sharply with theories of (1) excess mesolimbic DA activity inducing reward-seeking behaviors and (2) an overattribution of reward salience to irrelevant stimuli.

Anterior Cingulate

Another neurological structure that has been implicated in ADHD is the anterior cingulate cortex (ACC). This structure is being discussed separately because it does not fall clearly into a mesocortical (cognitive) or a mesolimbic (motivational) theory of ADHD. Rather, the ACC appears to have complex functions that place it at the junction of both systems. The

ACC is a component of Posner's attention network (Posner & Petersen, 1990), giving rise to speculation that it may contribute to attentional symptoms in ADHD. In support of this conjecture, several neuroimaging studies have demonstrated reduced activation of the anterior cingulate in ADHD participants compared with controls during go/no-go and Stroop tasks (Bush et al., 1999; Durston et al., 2003).

In Posner and Petersen's original conceptualization, the ACC was involved in target detection (Posner & Petersen, 1990). Subsequent research revealed that the ACC is important in the performance of tasks such as the go-no/go and Stroop, in which participants are required to choose between competing responses. This finding led researchers to conclude that the ACC is implicated specifically in conflict resolution during behavioral decision making (Miller & Cohen, 2001). Such conceptualizations place a strong emphasis on the cognitive functions of the ACC. Traditionally, however, the ACC has been associated with motivational functions served by the mesolimbic system and limbic cortex, as evidenced by the profound apathy characteristic of ACC damage (Chow & Cummings, 1999).

More recent conceptualizations of the ACC reconcile these different functions by defining it as the "interface between emotion and cognition" (Allman, Hakeem, Erwin, Nimchinsky, & Hof, 2001, p. 107). Accordingly, functional subdivisions within the ACC are now recognized, with the dorsal region associated with cognitive functions and the ventral region associated with affective processing. Moreover, research has identified important interconnectivity between the affective and cognitive subdivisions, yet these are poorly understood at this time (Bush, Luu, & Posner, 2000). The ACC may interface these two functions by using information from afferent projections from the limbic system regarding errors in reward prediction to manage behavioral responding (Holroyd & Coles, 2002). Brown and Braver (2005) have proposed that rather than monitoring actual error commission rates, the ACC uses dopaminergic limbic input as a "training signal" to identify situations in which error is more likely to occur, thereby recruiting cognitive control over behavior to improve performance. This theory suggests that a deficit in the mesolimbic system could result in a temporal deficit in learning reward associations, leading to a failure of input to the ACC and a resulting decreased recruitment of cognitive control over vigilance in performance of tasks. In rodent models, lesions of the nucleus accumbens lead to impulsive choices, but lesions of the anterior cingulate do not (Cardinal, Winstanley, Robbings, & Everitt, 2004). This finding suggests that damage to the ACC in the absence of nucleus accumbens dysfunction is not likely to lead directly to impulsivity. According to this model, deficits in the ACC and the recruitment of executive control are consequences of mesolimbic dysfunction. However, the exact role of the ACC in the network of structures implicated in ADHD remains to be elucidated.

Cerebellum

A final dopaminergic theory of ADHD implicates the cerebellum, which functions to modulate both the timing and coordination of motor behavior and may be involved in the efficient shifting of attention and synchronization of neural activity across regions of the cerebral cortex (Ivry, 2003). Until recently, innervation of the cerebellum was assumed to be noradrenergic and serotonergic. However, it is now clear that there are extensive dopaminergic projections into the cerebellar vermis (Melchitzky & Lewis, 2000), which has received considerable attention as a region of interest in the study of ADHD (e.g., Castellanos & Tannock, 2002; Swanson & Castellanos, 2002). Deficiencies among children with ADHD in both motor coordination and temporal processing are well documented, and several studies have revealed volume reductions in the cerebellar vermis in ADHD probands (e.g., Berquin et al., 1998, Castellanos et al., 1996; Durston et al., 2003). These findings, coupled with the coordinative functions served by the region, have led some authors to suggest that the cerebellum may modulate mesocortical frontostriatal circuitry (Giedd, Blumenthal, Molloy, & Castellanos, 2001). However, cerebellar theories of ADHD are quite recent, and the neural mechanisms through which such modulation might occur have not been articulated. In contrast, theories of nigrostriatal, mesocortical, and mesolimbic dysfunction in ADHD are well elaborated, as indicated in previous sections. Because cerebellar theories of ADHD are emergent, and because cerebellar hypoplasia is probably not the neural substrate of impulsivity, the primary focus of this chapter, we do not consider these theories further.

CONCLUSIONS AND FUTURE DIRECTIONS

Research has led to a number of alternative theories of ADHD, some primarily frontal and others primarily limbic. Support for both types of theory suggests the potential for etiological heterogeneity among children with ADHD. ADHD is comprised of a variety of symptoms, including hyperactivity, impulsivity, forgetfulness, carelessness, cognitive distractibility, physical restlessness, and an increased need for behavioral activity. Too much emphasis may have been placed on associating brain function with the diagnostic syndrome, when the compilation of these symptoms into a single syndrome may be somewhat arbitrary. A diagnosis of ADHD can be achieved by a variety of different symptom combinations, even when only the hyperactive and combined subtypes are considered. Research to date has not focused on distinguishing characteristics, if any, among children who exhibit prefrontal deficits, striatal deficits, or both. Rather, the implicit assumption has been that all children who meet criteria for ADHD represent an etiologically homogenous group. Comparisons are then conducted with normal controls, and opportunities for examining subgroup distinctions are lost. Addressing the following questions could alter our research agenda.

Is There Etiological Heterogeneity?

It is possible that no single unifying theory of ADHD can be achieved and that within the DSM construct lie two or more distinct etiological pathways leading to similar behavioral manifestations. Considerable evidence suggests that frontal dysfunction does contribute to the impulsive behaviors associated with ADHD. However, functional deficiencies in lower brain structures that mediate motivational responding may lead to similar behaviors. If subgroups of children can be identified, through appropriate testing, who have primary deficits in specific regions of interest, researchers can then explore the behavioral profiles of these groups and examine whether or not they (1) exhibit distinct symptoms, (2) respond to different types of behavioral interventions, (3) respond to different types or different doses of pharmacological interventions, or (4) require different approaches to prevent the development of these symptoms.

Appropriate assessments of frontal lobe dysfunction may begin with neuropsychological test batteries, which have relatively low specificity but may nevertheless be useful as noninvasive markers to determine candidates for further assessment. Follow-up methods should include direct assessments of frontal lobe dysfunction using electroencephalography, or ideally, functional neuroimaging. Although structural imaging has been used repeatedly in ADHD, such studies are not as informative as functional neuroimaging research. Children with ADHD are at risk for multiple psychiatric disorders, particularly when placed in high-risk environments, and structural deficits may reflect underlying comorbidity rather than giving rise to information specific to ADHD pathology. Thus, functional imaging studies are crucial in highlighting specific structures that activate in concert and in response to specific, theoretically meaningful tasks that test hypotheses about dysfunctional systems. Motivational deficits appear to be readily indexed by psychophysiological functioning, when appropriately assessed in relevant reward contexts (Beauchaine et al., 2001; Crone et al., 2003; Fowles, 1980; Iaboni et al., 1997), but these findings await confirmation from neuroimaging assessments of CNS function.

Do Deficits in Certain Regions Explain Specific Symptoms of the ADHD Syndrome?

A second possibility is that the currently defined ADHD syndrome does identify a homogeneous group of impulsive children, but that each of the systems reviewed in this chapter contributes to different types of deficits. This possibility would suggest that isolated dysfunction in one region or another may result in subthreshold symptoms but that the combination of multiple deficiencies across systems would be required for functional impairment. In a recent study focusing specifically on caudate volume, asymmetry scores accounted for unique variance in parent-reported inattentive symptoms, but were much poorer at accounting for hyperactive/ impulsive symptoms (Schrimsher, Billingsley, Jackson, & Moore, 2002). This finding is consistent with those indicating that the caudate is intricately involved in executive functioning and cognition, and it suggests that mesocortical and nigrostriatal deficiencies may relate more to cognitive features of ADHD, whereas mesolimbic deficiencies may result in hyperactive and impulsive symptoms. Some researchers have speculated that hyperactive symptoms of ADHD in particular reflect sensation seeking (Antrop, Roeyers, Van Oost, & Buysse, 2000). Thus, hyperactivity symptoms should correlate with psychophysiological and neurological assessments of motivation, but specific comparison of symptoms with these measures has not been conducted.

A comment is also in order regarding neuroanatomical specificity in ADHD. Much has been written implicating the prefrontal cortex in explaining psychiatric disorders, which is unsurprising given the fundamental importance of this region in regulating lower brain structures. However, this extremely large region of the cortex consists of several subregions that are reliably differentiated in both structure and function (Chow & Cummings, 1999). The ventral and orbitofrontal regions have been implicated in reward processing in humans and provide inhibitory feedback to the ventral striatum (Chow & Cummings, 1999; Elliot, Friston, Dolan, 2000; Knutson, Fong, Adams, Varner, & Hommer, 2001; O'Doherty, Kringelbach, Rolls, Hornak, & Andrews, 2001; Tremblay & Schultz, 1999). Specifying exact locations of deficits will be critical in identifying etiologically homogeneous subgroups, because frontal deficiencies may include both executive and motivational components. Furthermore, assessment of orbitofrontal regions may require the use of brain imaging techniques, as less invasive strategies are not able to localize function in these regions.

Do Deficits in These Systems Reliably Differentiate Types of Externalizing Disorders?

Nigg (2003) has suggested that cortical deficits predispose to ADHD, whereas motivational deficits are more likely in CD. It is possible that isolated deficits produce impulsive, ADHD-like symptoms, whereas deficits across multiple systems increase the likelihood of developing additional externalizing disorders. Unfortunately, this possibility has not yet been examined in developmental paradigms. Psychophysiological research has suggested that motivational deficits may be specific to ADHD comorbid with CD (Beauchaine et al., 2001). Unfortunately, other studies relating motivational deficits to ADHD have not reported the incidence of CD in their samples (Crone et al., 2003; Iaboni et al., 1997). Evidence from the Multimodal Treatment Study of Children with ADHD trial already indicates that children with ADHD, with and without comorbid internalizing disorders, respond differently to pharmacological and behavioral interventions (Newcorn et al., 2001). Further understanding how comorbidity with externalizing disorders affects treatment remains to be achieved. Furthermore, no studies have systematically separated and compared ADHD and CD and examined them at the CNS level for potential functional differences, particularly in motivational processing. We are currently conducting an fMRI study that will address the CNS correlates of autonomic observations collected during reward responding in groups with ADHD and CD.

What Sort of Developmental Issues Should Be Considered?

Theories of ADHD rarely consider the importance of development in symptom expression. However, developmental context is important for several reasons. First, the developmental time point of neurological events can substantially alter behavioral outcomes. Rodent models of dopaminergic lesions demonstrate that the same DA-depleting lesion that produces severe motor impairment in mature rats can result in motor hyperactivity when induced in juvenile rats (Davids et al., 2003). Interestingly, adults with ADHD frequently show different deficits, both behaviorally and biologically, than younger probands (Ernst, Zametkin, Matochik, Jons, & Cohen,

1998), highlighting the importance of taking great care when extrapolating research findings to different developmental periods.

Second, neural activity reflects dynamic processes that may undergo substantial developmental changes. Plasticity in the CNS often allows compensation for nonoptimal functioning. For instance, a chronic abundance of DA may induce a reduction in receptor sites, increased reuptake, or increased inhibitory presynaptic feedback mechanisms, each of which may result in functional corrections for the DA increase. Thus, the state of dysfunction may not be static, and a better understanding of these dynamic developmental mechanisms is needed. This is especially true given our poor understanding of the long-term structural and functional changes incurred in response to prolonged treatment with DA agonists—a confound in many current studies of brain function in children with ADHD.

Finally, ADHD pathology itself is rarely static, and the relationship between neurological changes over development and related behavioral changes is poorly understood. Many cases of childhood ADHD are outgrown by late adolescence (American Psychiatric Association, 2000). This phenomenon is potentially informative regarding the role of CNS development in ADHD, yet it is rarely assessed directly. One study comparing adolescents diagnosed in childhood with ADHD but currently in partial remission, with those whose ADHD continued from childhood into adolescence, found that remitters showed significantly less widespread activation of ventrolateral prefrontal cortex than did those whose ADHD persisted. This improvement in ventrolateral prefrontal efficiency paralleled behavioral performance on a go/no-go task and was intermediate to full diagnostic ADHD and normal controls (Schulz et al., 2005).

The observed improvement in frontal lobe function is critical to understand, particularly given that the frontal lobe undergoes maturational processes through adolescence (Sowell, Thompson, Tessner, & Toga, 2001). It is possible that children who experience slower than average frontal lobe maturation will evidence impulsive behaviors and cognitive deficits compared with age-matched peers, but that they will catch up over time, thereby outgrowing the disorder. Moreover, children who have mesolimbic motivational deficits leading to hyperactivity, but who also have strong executive functioning, may be buffered from much of the risk associated with their impulsivity. Given that motivational deficits are thought to lead to sensation-seeking behaviors, research examining the degree to which the sensation-seeking behavior is outgrown versus channeled into more appropriate manifestations in children who fall below diagnostic threshold over time would be quite informative.

RELEVANCE FOR EDUCATION

ADHD represents a major challenge for teachers and school officials and can severely impair the academic success of afflicted children. As such, efforts to improve the accuracy of assessment and treatment are critical to dealing with the disorder. This chapter highlights the fact that multiple and complex brain systems may be involved in ADHD pathology. It is also possible that dysfunction in slightly different systems (prefrontal vs. limbic) results in behaviorally similar but neurologically unrelated subtypes of ADHD. As noted in the literature outlined above, the mechanism of action for psychostimulant efficacy in the treatment of ADHD has not been fully identified. However, according to the theory put forth by Sagvolden and colleagues (2005), medication may serve to normalize the reinforcement gradient of stimulus–response acquisition, allowing children with ADHD to learn behavioral contingencies over longer reinforcement intervals. This mechanism implies that medication alone should be insufficient to improve behavior in environments in which clear contingencies for appropriate behaviors are not established. Thus, effective parenting training and teacher training in implementing structured educational environments are necessary components in the treatment of ADHD, an assertion supported by evidence from both large-scale treatment–outcome studies and medication trials demonstrating that the most effective approaches to long-term success include behavioral contingency management (Beauchaine, Webster-Stratton, & Reid, 2005; Conners et al., 2001; Hinshaw, Klein, & Abikoff, 2002). Previous researchers studying classroom-based behavioral management have found success using frequent reinforcers in the form of tokens or points earned toward obtaining valued rewards (Kotkin, 1998). Optimal behavioral management of impulsivity among children with ADHD is likely to require both active awareness of positive behavior and response costs for negative behavior (e.g., Reid, O'Leary, & Wolff, 1994). This approach may represent a departure from traditional teaching techniques but may be especially effective in shaping the behavior of children with ADHD, who are high in reward-seeking behavior. Accordingly, effective management of ADHD will likely require schools to move beyond their traditional role in assessment and referral to include much more active participation, working in conjunction with parents to provide consistent reinforcement for desired behaviors. Children with ADHD should not be expected to be "cured" by the administration of stimulant therapy. By working with parents to modify inappropriate behaviors that may have become entrenched in children's response repertoires, school personnel are more likely to contribute to the social and academic success of children with ADHD.

REFERENCES

Allman, J. M., Hakeem, A., Erwin, J. M., Nimchinsky, E., & Hof, P. (2001). The anterior cingulate cortex: The evolution of an interface between emotion and cognition. *Annals of the New York Academy of Sciences, 935,* 107–117.

American Psychiatric Association. (2000). *Diagnostic and statistical manual of mental disorders* (4th ed., text rev.). Washington DC: Author.

Antrop, I., Roeyers, H., Van Oost, P., & Buysse, A. (2000). Stimulation seeking and hyperactivity in children with ADHD. *Journal of Child Psychology and Psychiatry, 41,* 225–231.

Ashby, F. G., Isen, A. M., & Turken, A. U. (1999). A neuropsychological theory of positive affect and its influence on cognition. *Psychological Review, 106,* 529–550.

Bardo, M. T., Donohew, R. L., & Harrington, N. G. (1996). Psychobiology of novelty seeking and drug seeking behavior. *Behavioural Brain Research, 77,* 23–43.

Barkley, R. A. (1997). Behavioral inhibition, sustained attention, and executive functions: constructing a unifying theory of ADHD. *Psychological Bulletin, 121,* 65–94.

Beauchaine, T. P. (2002). Autonomic substrates of heart rate reactivity in adolescent males with conduct disorder and/or attention-deficit/hyperactivity disorder. In S. P. Shohov (Ed.), *Advances in psychology research* (Vol. 18, pp. 83–95). New York: Nova Science.

Beauchaine, T. P., Gatzke-Kopp, L., & Mead, H. (in press). Polyvagal theory and developmental psychopathology: Emotion dysregulation and conduct problems from preschool to adolescence. *Biological Psychology.*

Beauchaine, T. P., Katkin, E. S., Strassberg, Z., & Snarr, J. (2001). Disinhibitory psychopathology in male adolescents: Discriminating conduct disorder from attention-deficit/hyperactivity disorder through concurrent assessment of multiple autonomic states. *Journal of Abnormal Psychology, 110,* 610–624.

Beauchaine, T. P., Webster-Stratton, C., & Reid, M. J. (2005). Mediators, moderators, and predictors of one-year outcomes among children treated for early-onset conduct problems: A latent growth curve analysis. *Journal of Consulting and Clinical Psychology, 73,* 371–388.

Berntson, G. G., Cacioppo, J. T., Quigley, K. S., & Fabro, V. T. (1994). Autonomic space and psychophysiological response. *Psychophysiology, 31,* 44–61.

Berquin, P. C., Giedd, J. N., Jacobsen, L .K., Hamburger, S. D., Krain, A. L., Rapoport, J. L., et al. (1998). Cerebellum in attention-deficit hyperactivity disorder: A morphometric MRI study. *Neurology, 50,* 1087–1093.

Brenner, S. L., Beauchaine, T. P., & Sylvers, P. D. (2005). A comparison of psychophysiological and self-report measures of BAS and BIS activation. *Psychophysiology, 42,* 108–115.

Brown, J. W., & Braver, T. S. (2005). Learned predictions of error likelihood in anterior cingulate cortex. *Science, 307,* 1118–1121.

Bush, G., Frazier, J. A., Rauch, S. L., Seidman, L. J., Whalen, P. J., Jenike, M. A., et al. (1999). Anterior cingulated cortex dysfunction in attention-deficit/hyperactivity disorder revealed by fMRI and the Counting Stroop. *Biological Psychiatry, 45,* 1542–1552.

Bush, G., Luu, P., & Posner, M. I. (2000). Cognitive and emotional influences in anterior cingulate cortex. *Trends in Cognitive Sciences, 4,* 215–222.

Cardinal, R. N., Winstanley, C. A., Robbins, T. W., & Everitt, B. J. (2004). Limbic corticostriatal systems and delayed reinforcement. *Annals of the New York Academy of Sciences, 1021,* 33–50.

Castellanos, F. X., Giedd, J. N., Marsh, W. L., Hamburger, S. D., Vaituzis, A. C., Dickstein, D. P., et al. (1996). Quantitative brain magnetic resonance imaging in attention-deficit hyperactivity disorder. *Archives of General Psychiatry, 53,* 607–616.

Castellanos, F. X., Lee, P. P., Sharp, W., Jeffries, N. O., Greenstein, D. K., Clasen, L. S., et al. (2002). Developmental trajectories of brain volume abnormalities in children and adolescents with attention-deficit/hyperactivity disorder. *Journal of the American Medical Association, 288,* 1740–1748.

Castellanos, F. X., Sharp, W. S., Gottesman, R. F., Greenstein, D. K., Giedd, J. N., & Rapoport, J. L. (2003). Anatomic brain abnormalities in monozygotic twins discordant for attention deficit hyperactivity disorder. *American Journal of Psychiatry, 160,* 1693–1696.

Castellanos, F. X., & Tannock, R. (2002). Neuroscience of attention-deficit/hyperactivity disorder: The search for endophenotypes. *Nature Neuroscience Reviews, 3,* 617–628.

Chow, T. W., & Cummings, J. L. (1999). Frontal–subcortical circuits. In B. L. Miller & J. L. Cummings (Eds.), *The human frontal lobes: Functions and disorders* (pp. 3–26). New York: Guilford Press.

Cloninger, C. R. (1986). A unified biosocial theory of personality and its role in the development of anxiety states. *Psychiatric Developments, 3,* 167–226.

Conners, C. K., Epstein, J. N., March, J. S., Angold, A., Wells, K. C., Klaric, J., et al. (2001). Multimodal treatment of ADHD in the MRA: An alternative outcome analysis. *Journal of the American Academy of Child and Adolescent Psychiatry, 40,* 159–167.

Cooper, J. R., Bloom, F. E., & Roth, R. H. (2003). Dopamine. In J. R. Cooper, F. E. Bloom, & R. H. Roth (Eds.), *The biochemical basis of neuropharmacology* (8th ed., pp. 225–270). New York: Oxford University Press.

Crone, E. A., Jennings, J. R., & van der Molen, M. W. (2003). Sensitivity to interference and response contingencies in attention-deficit/hyperactivity disorder. *Journal of Child Psychology and Psychiatry, 44,* 214–226.

Crowell, S., Beauchaine, T. P., Gatzke-Kopp, L., Sylvers, P., Mead, H., & Chipman-Chacon, J. (2006). Autonomic correlates of attention-deficit/hyperactivity disorder and oppositional defiant disorder in preschool children. *Journal of Abnormal Psychology, 115,* 174–178.

Davids, E., Kehong, Z., Tarazi, F. I., & Baldessarini, R. J. (2003). Animal models of attention-deficit hyperactivity disorder. *Brain Research Reviews, 42,* 1–21.

DeLong, M. R. (2000). The basal ganglia. In E. R Kandel, J. H. Schwartz, & T. M.

Jessell (Eds.), *Principles of neural science* (4th ed., pp. 853–867). New York: McGraw-Hill.

DiMaio, S., Frizenko, N., & Joober, R. (2003). Dopamine genes and attention-deficit hyperactivity disorder: A review. *Journal of Psychiatry and Neuroscience, 28,* 27–38.

Durston, S. (2003). A review of the biological bases of ADHD: What have we learned from imaging studies? *Mental Retardation and Developmental Disabilities Reviews, 9,* 184–195.

Durston, S., Tottenham, N. T., Thomas, K. M., Davidson, M. C., Eigsti, I.-M., Yang, Y., et al. (2003). Differential patterns of striatal activation in young children with and without ADHD. *Biological Psychiatry, 53,* 871–878.

Elliot, R., Friston, K. J., & Dolan, R. J. (2000). Dissociable neural response in human reward systems. *Journal of Neuroscience, 20,* 6159–6165.

Ellis, L. (1987). Relationships of criminality and psychopathy with eight other apparent behavioral manifestations of sub-optimal arousal. *Personality and Individual Differences, 8,* 905–925.

Ernst, M., Zametkin, A. J., Matochik, J. A., Jons, P. H., & Cohen, R. M. (1998). DOPA decarboxylase activity in attention deficit hyperactivity disorder adults. A [flourine-18]fluourdopa positron emission tomography study. *Journal of Neuroscience, 18,* 5901–5907.

Filipek, P. A., Semrud-Clikeman, M., Steingard, R. J., Renshaw, P. F., Kennedy, D. N., & Biederman, J. (1997). Volumetric MRI analysis comparing subjects having attention-deficit hyperactivity disorder with normal controls. *Neurology, 48,* 589–601.

Fowles, D. C. (1980). The three arousal model: Implications of Gray's two-factor learning theory for heart rate, electrodermal activity, and psychopathy. *Psychophysiology, 17,* 87–104.

Giedd, J. N., Blumenthal, J., Molloy, E., & Castellanos, F. X. (2001). Brain imaging of attention deficit/hyperactivity disorder. *Annals of the New York Academy of Sciences, 931,* 33–49.

Grace, A. A. (2001). Psychostimulant actions on dopamine and limbic system function: Relevance to the pathophysiology and treatment of ADHD. In M. V. Solanto, A. F. T. Arnsten, & F. X. Castellanos (Eds.), *Stimulant drugs and ADHD: Basic and clinical neuroscience* (pp. 134–157). New York: Oxford University Press.

Gray, J. A. (1987). The neuropsychology of emotion and personality. In S. M. Stahl, S. D. Iversen, & E. C. Goodman (Eds.), *Cognitive neurochemistry* (pp. 171–190). Oxford, UK: Oxford University Press.

Haenlein, M., & Caul, W. F. (1987). Attention deficit disorder with hyperactivity: A specific hypothesis of reward dysfunction. *Journal of the American Academy of Child and Adolescent Psychiatry, 26,* 356–362.

Hinshaw, S. P., Klein, R. G., & Abikoff, H. B. (2002). Childhood attention-deficit hyperactivity disorder: Non-pharmacological treatments and their combination with medication. In P. E. Nathan & J. M. Gorman (Eds.), *A guide to treatments that work* (2nd ed., pp. 3–23). New York: Oxford University Press.

Holroyd, C. B., & Coles, M. G. H. (2002). The neural basis of human error processing: Reinforcement learning, dopamine, and the error-related negativity. *Psychological Review, 109,* 679–709.

Hynd, G. W., Hern, K. L., Novey, E. S., Eliopulos, D., Marshall, R., Gonzalez, J. J., et al. (1993). Attention deficit-hyperactivity disorder and asymmetry of the caudate nucleus. *Journal of Child Neurology, 8,* 339–347.

Iaboni, F., Douglas, V. I., & Ditto, B. (1997). Psychophysiological response of ADHD children to reward and extinction. *Psychophysiology, 34,* 116–123.

Ivry, R. B. (2003). Cerebellar involvement in clumsiness and other developmental disorders. *Neural Plasticity, 10,* 143–155.

Johnston, C. (2002). The impact of attention deficit hyperactivity disorder on social and vocational functioning in adults. In P. S. Jenson & J. R. Cooper (Eds.), *Attention deficit hyperactivity disorder* (pp. 1–21). Kingston, NJ: Civic Research Institute.

Kandel, E. R. (2000). Disorders of thought and volition: Schizophrenia. In E. R Kandel, J. H. Schwartz, & T. M. Jessell (Eds.), *Principles of neural science* (4th ed., pp. 1188–1208). New York: McGraw-Hill.

Kates, W. R., Frederikse, M., Mostofsky, S. H., Folley, B. S., Cooper, K., Mazur-Hopkins, et al. (2002). MRI parcellation of the frontal lobe in boys with attention deficit hyperactivity disorder or Tourette syndrome. *Psychiatry Research: Neuroimaging, 116,* 63–81.

Kim, B.-N., Lee, J.-S., Shin, M.-S., Cho, S.-C., & Lee, D.-S. (2002). Regional cerebral perfusion abnormalities in attention deficit/hyperactivity disorder: Statistical parametric mapping analysis. *European Archives of Psychiatry and Clinical Neuroscience, 252,* 219–225.

Knutson, B., Fong, G. W., Adams, C. M., Varner, J. L., & Hommer, D. (2001). Dissociation of reward anticipation and outcome with event-related fMRI. *NeuroReport, 12,* 3683–3687.

Kotkin, R. (1998). The Irvine paraprofessional program: Promising practice for serving students with ADHD. *Journal of Learning Disabilities, 31,* 556–564.

Krause, K.-H., Dresel, S. H., Krause, J., la Fourgere, C., & Ackenheil, M. (2003). The dopamine transporter and neuroimaging in attention deficit hyperactivity disorder. *Neuroscience and Biobehavioral Reviews, 27,* 605–613.

Krueger, R. F., Hicks, B. M., Patrick, C. J., Carlson, S. R., Iacono, W. G., & McGue, M. (2002). Etiologic connections among substance dependence, antisocial behavior, and personality: Modeling the externalizing spectrum. *Journal of Abnormal Psychology, 111,* 411–424.

Laakso, A., & Caron, M. G. (2004). Dopamine receptors. In D. Robertson, I. Biaggioni, G. Burnstock, & P. A. Low (Eds.), *Primer on the autonomic nervous system* (2nd ed., pp. 39–43). New York: Elsevier.

Laakso, A., Wallius, E., Kajander, J., Bergman, J., Eskola, O. Solin, O., et al. (2003). Personality traits and striatal dopamine synthesis capacity in healthy subjects. *American Journal of Psychiatry, 160,* 904–910.

Ljungberg, T., Apicella, P., & Schultz, W. (1992). Responses of monkey dopamine neurons during learning of behavioral reactions. *Journal of Neurophysiology, 67,* 145–163.

Lou, H. C., Henriksen, L., Bruhn, P., Borner, H., & Nielsen, J. B. (1989). Striatal dysfunction in attention deficit and hyperkinetic disorder. *Archives of Neurology, 46,* 48–52.

Lynam, D. R., Caspi, A., Moffitt, T. E., Wikström, P. H., Loeber, R., & Novak, S. (2000). The interaction between impulsivity and neighborhood context on offending: The effects of impulsivity are stronger in poorer neighborhoods. *Journal of Abnormal Psychology, 109,* 563–574.

Marsden, C. D., & Obeso, J. A. (1994). The functions of the basal ganglia and the paradox of sterotaxic surgery in Parkinson's disease. *Brain, 117,* 877–897.

Matthys, W., van Goozen, S. H. M., de Vries, H., Cohen-Kettenis, P. T., & van Engeland, H. (1998). The dominance of behavioral activation over behavioral inhibition in conduct disordered boys with or without attention deficit hyperactivity disorder. *Journal of Child Psychology and Psychiatry, 39,* 643–651.

Melchitzky, D. S., & Lewis, D. A. (2000). Tyrosine hydroxylase- and dopamine transporter-immunoreactive axons in the primate cerebellum: Evidence for a lobular+ and laminar-specific dopamine innervation. *Neuropsychopharmacology, 22,* 466–472.

Milich, R., Balentine, A. C., & Lynam, D. R. (2001). ADHD combined type and ADHD predominantly inattentive type are distinct and unrelated disorders. *Clinical Psychology: Science and Practice, 8,* 463–488.

Miller, E. K., & Cohen, J. D. (2001). An integrative theory of prefrontal cortex function. *Annual Review of Neuroscience, 24,* 167–202.

Mostofsky, S. H., Cooper, K. L., Kates, W. R., Denckla, M. B., & Kaufmann, W. E. (2002). Smaller prefrontal and premotor volumes in boys with attention-deficit/hyperactivity disorder. *Biological Psychiatry, 52,* 785–794.

Newcorn, J. H., Halperin, J. M., Jensen, P. S., Abikoff, H. B., Arnold, L. E., Cantwell, D. P., et al. (2001). Symptom profiles in children with ADHD: Effects of comorbidity and gender. *Journal of the American Academy of Child and Adolescent Psychiatry, 40,* 137–146.

Nigg, J. T. (2001). Is ADHD a disinhibitory disorder? *Psychological Bulletin, 127,* 571–598.

Nigg, J. T. (2003). Response inhibition and disruptive behaviors: Toward a multiprocess conception of etiological heterogeneity for ADHD combined type and conduct disorder early-onset type. *Annals of the New York Academy Sciences, 1008,* 170–182.

O'Doherty, J., Kringelbach, M. L., Rolls, E. T., Hornak, J., & Andrews, C. (2001). Abstract reward and punishment representations in the human orbitofrontal cortex. *Nature Neuroscience, 4,* 95–102.

Patrick, K. S., & Markowitz, J. S. (1997). Pharmacology of methylphenidate, amphetamine enantiomers and pemoline in attention-deficit hyperactivity disorder. *Human Neuropharmacology, 12,* 527–546.

Patterson, G. R., DeGarmo, D. S., & Knutson, N. (2000). Hyperactive and antisocial behaviors: Comorbid or two points in the same process? *Development and Psychopathology, 12,* 91–106.

Posner, M. I., & Petersen, S. E. (1990). The attention system of the human brain. *Annual Review of Neuroscience, 13,* 25–42.

Quay, H. C. (1993). The psychobiology of undersocialized aggressive conduct disorder: A theoretical perspective. *Development and Psychopathology, 5,* 165–180.

Reid, M. J., O'Leary, S. G., & Wolff, L. S. (1994). Effects of maternal distraction and reprimands on toddlers' transgressions and negative affect. *Journal of Abnormal Child Psychology, 22,* 237–245.

Rubia, K., Overmeyer, S., Taylor, E., Brammer, M., Williams, S., Simmons, A., et al. (1999). Hypofrontality in attention deficit hyperactivity disorder during higher-order motor control: A study with functional MRI. *American Journal of Psychiatry, 156,* 891–896.

Sagvolden, T. (2001). The spontaneously hypertensive rat as a model of ADHD. In M. V. Solanto, A. F. Arnsten, & F. X Castellanos (Eds.), *Stimulant drugs and ADHD: Basic and clinical neuroscience* (pp. 221–237). London: Oxford University Press.

Sagvolden, T., Aase, H., Steiner, P., & Berger, D. (1998). Altered reinforcement mechanisms in attention-deficit/hyperactivity disorder. *Behavioural Brain Research, 94,* 61–71.

Sagvolden, T., Johansen, E. B., Aase, H., & Russell, V. A. (2005). A dynamic developmental theory of attention-deficit/hyperactivity disorder (ADHD) predominantly hyperactive/impulsive and combined subtypes. *Behavioral and Brain Sciences, 28,* 397–468.

Sagvolden, T., & Sergeant, J. A. (1998). Attention deficit/hyperactivity disorder—from brain dysfunction to behavior. *Behavioural Brain Research, 94,* 1–10.

Saper, C. B. (2000). Brain stem modulation of sensation, movement, and consciousness. In E. R Kandel, J. H. Schwartz, & T. M. Jessell (Eds.), *Principles of neural science* (4th ed., pp. 889–909). New York: McGraw-Hill.

Schrimsher, G. W., Billingsley, R. L., Jackson, E. F., & Moore, B. D. (2002). Caudate nucleus volume asymmetry predicts attention-deficit hyperactivity disorder (ADHD) symptomotology in children. *Journal of Child Neurology, 17,* 877–884.

Schulz, K. P., Newcorn, J., Fan, J., Tang, C. Y., & Halperin, J. M. (2005). Brain activation gradients in ventrolateral prefrontal cortex related to persistence of ADHD in adolescent boys. *Journal of the American Academy of Child and Adolescent Psychiatry, 44,* 47–54.

Schweitzer, J. B., Lee, D. O., Hanford, R. B., Zink, C. F., Ely, T. D., Tagamets, M. A., et al. (2004). Effect of methylphenidate on executive functioning in adults with attention-deficit/hyperactivity disorder: Normalization of behavior but not related brain activity. *Biological Psychiatry, 56,* 597–606.

Sherwood, A., Allen, M. T., Fahrenberg, J., Kelsey, R. M., Lovallo, W. R., & van Doornen, L. J. P. (1990). Committee report: Methodological guidelines for impedance cardiography. *Psychophysiology, 27,* 1–23.

Sowell, E. R., Thompson, P. M., Tessner, K. D., & Toga, A. W. (2001). Mapping continued brain growth and gray matter density reduction in dorsal frontal cortex: Inverse relationships during postadolescent brain maturation. *Journal of Neuroscience, 21,* 8819–8829.

Sullivan, R. M., & Brake, W. G. (2003). What the rodent prefrontal cortex can teach us about attention-deficit/hyperactivity disorder: The critical role of early developmental events on prefrontal function. *Behavioural Brain Research, 146,* 43–55.

Swanson, J. M., & Castellanos, F. X. (2002). Biological bases of ADHD— neuroanatomy, genetics, and pathophysiology. In P. S. Jenson & J. R. Cooper (Eds.), *Attention deficit hyperactivity disorder* (pp. 1–20). Kingston, NJ: Civic Research Institute.

Swartz, J. R. (1999). Dopamine projections and frontal systems function. In B. L. Miller & J. L. Cummings (Eds.), *The human frontal lobes: Functions and disorders* (pp. 159–173). New York: Guilford Press.

Tisch, S., Silberstein, P., Limousin-Dowsey, P., & Jahanshahi, M. (2004). The basal ganglia: Anatomy, physiology, and pharmacology. *Psychiatric Clinics of North America, 27,* 757–799.

Tremblay, L., Hollerman, J. R., & Schultz, W. (1998). Modifications of reward expectation-related neuronal activity during learning in primate striatum. *Journal of Neurophysiology, 80,* 964–977.

Tremblay, L., & Schultz, W. (1999). Relative reward preference in primate orbitofrontal cortex. *Nature, 398,* 704–708.

Vaidya, C. J., Austin, G., Kirkorian, G., Ridelhuber, H. W., Desmond, J. E., Glover, G. H., et al. (1998). Selective effects of methylphenidate in attention deficit hyperactivity disorder: A functional magnetic resonance study. *Proceedings of the National Academy of Sciences USA, 95,* 14494–14499.

van den Buuse, M. (1998). Role of the mesolymbic dopamine system in cardiovascular homeostasis: Stimulation of the ventral tegmental area modulates the effect of vasopressin in conscious rats. *Clinical Experimental Pharmacology and Physiology, 25,* 661–668.

Vles, J. S., Feron, F. J., Hendriksen, J. G., Jolles, J., van Kroonenburgh, M. J., & Weber, W. E. (2003). Methylphenidate down-regulates the dopamine receptor and transporter system in children with attention deficit hyperkinetic disorder. *Neuropediatrics, 34,* 77–80.

Volkow, N. D., Fowler, J. S., Wang, G., Ding, Y., & Gatley, S. J. (2002). Mechanism of action of methylphenidate: Insights from PET imaging studies. *Journal of Attention Disorders, 6,* S31–S43.

CHAPTER 11

Social Regulation of the Adrenocortical Response to Stress in Infants, Children, and Adolescents

IMPLICATIONS FOR PSYCHOPATHOLOGY AND EDUCATION

Emma K. Adam
Bonnie Klimes-Dougan
Megan R. Gunnar

In attempting to understand how social experiences impact both typical and atypical aspects of human social and emotional development, researchers have looked to the psychobiological stress response as a potential mediating and moderating mechanism (Chrousos & Gold, 1992). The neurological and physiological systems involved in the stress response are acutely sensitive to social events (Dickerson & Kemeny, 2004; Flinn & England, 1995). Individual differences in stress physiology have been related to social and emotional functioning within the normal range (e.g., temperamental variations; Gunnar, Sebanc, Tout, Donzella, & van Dulman, 2003) and have also been associated with abnormal functioning (psychopathology) in children (Kaufman, Martin, King, & Charney, 2001), adolescents (Klimes-Dougan, Hastings, Granger, Usher, & Zahn-Waxler, 2001), and adults (Chrousos & Gold, 1992).

Inclusion in social groups and successful negotiation of intimate personal relationships are vital features of successful child, adolescent, and adult functioning. It is therefore not surprising that social and interpersonal threats are among the most highly aversive of human experiences, serving to activate both negative emotion and stress-responsive physiological systems, including the sympathetic adrenal medullary (SAM) system and the hypothalamic–pituitary–adrenal (HPA) axis (Dickerson & Kemeny, 2004; Flinn & England, 1995). That social experiences may also have *long-term* effects on the organization and functioning of these physiological stress systems is perhaps less obvious. A growing body of evidence suggests that social experience may have important short- and long-term influences on the HPA axis, in particular, especially in the developing organism (Gunnar & Vazquez, 2006; Vazquez, 1998).

After a brief description of the historical foundations of HPA-axis research, we review current evidence regarding the role of social experiences in the regulation of HPA-axis physiology. We describe research on how social variables influence HPA-axis functioning in normal samples of infants, children, and adolescents, and we also describe variations in HPA-axis functioning observed in children exposed to atypical social experiences such as institutional rearing, maternal depression, and abuse and neglect. Data on the associations between exposure to social stress, HPA-axis functioning, and the development of psychopathology are then reviewed. We end by briefly describing data on the associations between HPA-axis activity and cognitive and memory performance and consider the potential implications of social regulation of the HPA axis for understanding educational performance.

SOCIAL INFLUENCES ON STRESS PHYSIOLOGY: HISTORICAL FOUNDATIONS

Stress research traces its history to Hans Selye's 1936 publication in the British journal *Nature*, in which he proposed that the body passes through three stages as it confronts and attempts to adapt to what he then termed *noxious agents* but later called *stressors*. Although many details of Seyle's theory have been challenged and revised, the idea that a wide variety of stressors can produce illness as a result of the body's *physiological stress response* forged a new field focused on biological stress and its effects. A young psychologist working in the newly minted field of neuroendocrinology forged the first links between stress biology and *development* and directed attention to the modulation of HPA-axis functioning and organization by social factors. In 1957, Seymour Levine demonstrated in *Science* that simply removing rat pups from their mother for a few moments daily (termed *handling)* permanently modified activity of what, then, was understood to be the core neuroendocrine system of the stress response, the HPA system. In the decades that followed, it became apparent that the brain was the primary site for the long-term alterations in HPA-axis functioning as a result of social experience; this discovery was due, in part, to McEwen's landmark work demonstrating that glucocorticoids (GCs; cortisol in humans and nonhuman primates, corticosterone in rats), the hormonal products of the HPA system, sustain normal brain function *and* paradoxically endanger nerve cells (McEwen, Weiss, & Schwartz, 1968). More recently, the link between early experience, brain development, and both normal and disordered functioning has become increasingly evident and better understood, due largely to evidence that early experience (especially deprivation experiences) reduces neural plasticity to stress experienced later in life (e.g., Mirescu, Peters, & Gould, 2004) and even permanently silences genes critical to the regulation of the stress response (e.g., Weaver et al., 2004). Truly, there is no way that this remarkable field and its implications for our understanding of healthy and disturbed neurodevelopment can be reviewed in a short chapter. Therefore, we focus our review primarily on the human data regarding social influences on the regulation of the HPA axis during development; this human literature primarily relies on measurement of CORT (cortisol in humans, corticosterone in many rodents) rather than the central nervous system (CNS) elements of HPA-axis regulation. We refer to rodent and nonhuman primate literatures when necessary to help interpret the human literature, particularly with regard to causation.

OVERVIEW OF HPA-AXIS PHYSIOLOGY

The two effector arms of the mammalian stress system are composed of the SAM system and the HPA axis (Gunnar & Vazquez, 2006). Generally speaking, the SAM system supports rapid mobilization and response, often described as "fight/flight" reactions. In contrast, the HPA system, through modulation of its basal activity, supports the efficacy of the SAM system and related CNS fight/flight responses. In addition, through elevation in response to stressors, the HPA axis counteracts or suppresses acute stress effects, including its own activation (Sapolsky, Romero, & Munck, 2000). The hormone produced by the HPA system, CORT, serves as a gene transcription factor that permits sculpting of the neural systems involved in learning, memory, and emotion (De Kloet, 2003). One function of CORT in stress is to alter the way the organism responds to a stressor the next time it is encountered (Sapolsky et al., 2000).

The HPA system is depicted in Figure 11.1. Briefly, the cascade of events resulting in elevations in CORT begins with the release of

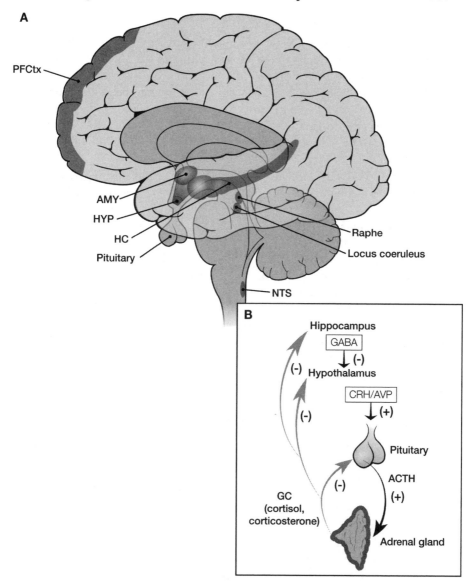

FIGURE 11.1. The limbic–hypothalamic–adrenal–pituitary axis. PFCtx, prefrontal cortex; AMY, amygdala; HYP, hypothalamus; HC, hippocampus; NTS, nucleus tractus solitarius; AVP, arginine vasopressin. Reprinted with permission of John Wiley & Sons, Inc. from Gunnar, M. R., & Vazquez, M., Stress neurobiology and developmental psychopathology. In D. Cicchetti & D. Cohen (Eds.), *Developmental psychopathology: Volume 2. Developmental neuroscience* (2nd ed., pp. 533–577). New York: Wiley. Copyright © 2006.

corticotropin-releasing hormone (CRH) and vasopressin (VP) from the paraventricular nuclei (PVN) in the hypothalamus. CRH and VP travel through small blood vesicles to the anterior pituitary (AP), where they stimulate the production and release of adrenocorticotropic hormone (ACTH). Of the two releasing hormones, CRH is the more potent, but VP appears to enhance the capacity of CRH to affect increases in ACTH production and release. Released into general circulation, ACTH interacts with receptors on the cortex of the adrenal glands to stimulate the production and release of CORT.

Multiple pathways are involved in the activation and inhibition of the HPA axis through regulating gamma-aminobutyric acid (GABA)-inhibition of CRH- and VP-producing cells in the PVN (for review, see Herman & Cullinan, 1997). With regard to activation, physical stressors that pose immediate threats to health and viability (e.g., cold stress, heat stress, blood loss) activate the HPA axis largely through norepinephrine (NE) neurons ascending from the brainstem. Psychological stressors (sometimes called processive stressors) activate the HPA axis through corticolimbic pathways, including pathways from the central nucleus of the amygdala (CEA). The HPA axis is under negative feedback control, meaning that increases in CORT result in inhibition of PVN, CRH, and VP production. This inhibition is effected by CORT-responsive cells in the hypothalamus, hippocampus, and, it now appears, medial regions of the prefrontal cortex (Herman & Cullinan, 1997; Sullivan & Gratton, 1999). None of these pathways is direct (i.e., they are multi-synaptic); thus, HPA regulation is multifactorial.

CORT acts by interacting with two classes of receptors: mineralocorticoid and glucocorticoid receptors (MRs and GRs, respectively; note that both receptors are responsive to CORT in the brain; de Kloet, Vreugdenhil, Oitzl, & Joels, 1998). MRs are high- and GRs are low-affinity CORT receptors. This means that when CORT is at low levels, MRs are activated, whereas GRs are only activated when CORT levels are high, as at the peak of the circadian cycle or during stress. MRs tend to mediate what have been termed "permissive" effects of CORT, which include maintaining the responsiveness of neurons to their neurotransmitters, maintaining the HPA circadian rhythm, and maintaining blood pressure. GRs mediate most of the effects of stress elevations in CORT. Presumably related to MR and GR activation, both chronically low and chronically high levels of CORT are associated with nonoptimal functioning. In contrast, moderate basal levels, a clear circadian rhythm in CORT, and rapid increases and then rapid reestablishment of basal levels in response to stressors tend to be associated with optimal physical and behavioral health.

MEASUREMENT, ANALYSIS, AND INTERPRETATION OF CORT ACTIVITY IN HUMAN POPULATIONS

Assessment of the HPA axis in humans has been accomplished in many ways, but it is important to distinguish between measures obtained under non-stimulated or basal conditions and measures obtained in response to specific stressors. In most human HPA-axis research, CORT levels are assessed noninvasively in small samples of saliva (Kirschbaum & Hellhammer, 1989).

Basal Activity

Researchers examining basal CORT activity are interested in identifying the typical, unstimulated level of CORT for individuals at a particular time of day or their typical pattern of CORT across the whole day. Although it has been common to use pretest measures of CORT in the laboratory as a basal or baseline measure (e.g., Vanyukov et al., 1993), recent evidence suggests that pretest measures are often significantly different from measures obtained in familiar (e.g., home) settings (Larson, Gunnar, & Hertsgaard, 1991; van Eck, Nicolson, Berkhof, & Sulon, 1996; Walker, Walder, & Reynolds, 2001). Increasing numbers of researchers are now taking advantage of the ease of having subjects collect home samples to examine basal CORT activity. Individual differences in CORT levels at particular times of the day, the pattern of CORT production across the waking day or across a 24-hour period (e.g., amplitude or slope of the diurnal rhythm), and the amount of within-person variability noted across multiple days are typical methods of assessing natural variation in basal cortisol activity. In some protocols, CORT is assessed at the same clock time across all subjects in an effort to control for the strong diurnal variability inherent in this neuroendocrine system. In other protocols, CORT is assessed at fixed periods following awakening in an effort to track activity of the HPA system in relation to the subject's own day–night behavior. Cortisol levels in humans are typically high in the morning upon waking, increase 50–60% in the first 30–45 minutes post-waking (known as the cortisol awakening response), drop rapidly over the first few hours after waking, and then more slowly across the day to reach a low point around midnight (Kirschbaum & Hellhammer, 1989; Pruessner et al., 1997). In infants and young children, this pattern is not quite as clear due to continued maturation of sleep-wake processes and the influence of daytime naps (Gunnar & Donzella, 2002). There is some evidence that CORT levels obtained early in the morning or in response to awakening reflect relatively stable traits of the HPA axis with high heritability quotients (e.g., Bartels, de Geus, Kirschbaum, Sluyter, & Boomsma, 2003), although the awakening response is also influenced by recent stressful experiences, includ-ing experiences occurring the prior day (Adam, Hawkley, Cacioppo, & Kudielka, 2006). Conversely, there is some evidence that levels assessed in the afternoon and evening are more influenced by state contributions to the system as it reacts to the cumulative challenges of the day. Nevertheless, the demarcation between state and trait contributions to CORT levels across the day is not distinct (e.g., Shirtcliff, Zahn-Waxler, & Klimes-Dougan, 2005). Other factors such as sleep, food, exercise, medication use, and menstrual timing also influence CORT levels and need to be measured and controlled in analyses (Kirschbaum & Hellhammer, 1989). Recent statisti-cal approaches (reviewed below) allow the isolation of variance associated with assay error, control factors, diurnal rhythms, and trait and state con-tributions to CORT activity. In general, researchers now recognize that sin-gle samples of CORT do not provide sufficient information to interpret CORT activity; multiple samples across the day and across multiple days provide the best characterization of basal activity, and measurement of CORT responses to stressors in addition to basal CORT provides a more complete picture of CORT functioning.

Cortisol Reactivity to Stressors

Assessment of the HPA axis may also involve examining reactivity to phar-macological probes and/or environmental stressors; however, pharmaco-logical probes are rarely used in studies of children. Developmental researchers tend to rely on laboratory stressor tasks or naturally occurring stressors such as the first day of school. Regardless, the optimal sampling protocol involves some home basal assessments, measures prior to the stressor, and multiple measures (often at 20- to 30-minute intervals) after the onset of the stressor to examine both reactivity and recovery. The clas-sic CORT stress response profile consists of moderate CORT levels at pre-test, high CORT levels in response to a stressor, and a subsequent return to near-pretest levels within 40–60 minutes after stressor termination. Because elevations in CORT may represent normative stress responses, the chal-lenges of defining disruptions in the stress reactivity cycle are consider-able. Typically, researchers consider individual differences in elevations of CORT in anticipation of a stressor (*anticipatory stress reaction*), the degree of elevation in response to a stressor (*reactivity*), and the degree of delay in returning to pretest levels following a stressor (*recovery*). Exaggerated lev-els of anticipatory stress or stress reactivity, a longer delay in returning to baseline, and a failure to show an HPA reaction in response to known stressors have all been considered disruptions of the expected HPA-axis response to stress. Recently, researchers have begun to note a potentially dysregulated pattern termed *declivity* in which rather than elevating, CORT decreases below not only pretest levels (which might be elevated in anticipation of testing) but also below home basal levels at the same time of day (Shirtcliff, Zahn-Waxler, & Klimes-Dougan, 2005; Van Goozen et al., 1998). At this point there is too little study of declivity to know whether it is associated with disordered functioning or is a normative pattern of response to laboratory stressors of a particular type.

Advanced Statistical Models

Advanced statistical approaches have recently been developed to help isolate and model separate aspects of HPA-axis activity, including trait variation in basal CORT levels and diurnal CORT patterning and day-to-day and moment-to-moment state variations in CORT in large samples. These approaches include latent state–trait modeling, which uses a latent variable approach to isolate and predict variance in CORT that is stable within individuals across time and is thus presumed to represent "trait" variance in CORT (Kirschbaum et al., 1990; Shirtcliff, Granger, Booth, & Johnson, 2005). Another approach, multilevel growth curve modeling, allows researchers to derive a latent estimate of each individual's basal pattern of CORT production across the day (presumably, trait cortisol variation), and to predict individual differences in these basal CORT patterns from trait variables of interest (Hruschka, Kohrt, & Worthman, 2005). It also allows researchers to model the effects of time-varying (state) factors such as mood and activity level on within-person changes in CORT (Adam, 2006; Adam & Gunnar, 2001; van Eck, Berkhof, Nicolson, & Sulon, 1996a), and conversely, to examine the effects of within-person changes in CORT on changes in subjective experience (Adam, Hawkley, et al., 2006). Using these approaches, associations between CORT and other parameters of interest, such as psychopathology, are much more robust than when trait and state variance in CORT are not isolated as effectively.

Now that the basic physiology, typical activity, and primary methods of examining HPA-axis activity have been described, research on the impact of social factors on HPA-axis functioning during development is reviewed.

SOCIAL REGULATION OF THE HPA AXIS IN INFANCY AND EARLY CHILDHOOD

Studies in rats and monkeys indicate that the HPA axis is under powerful social regulation early in development (for review, see Sanchez, Ladd, &

Plotsky, 2001). In rats, shortly after birth the axis enters a period described as the "stress hyporesponsive period" or SHRP. This period lasts until about postnatal day 14. During this time it is difficult to elevate CORT in response to many stressors, and it has been suggested that this period serves to protect the developing brain from adverse impacts of chronic CORT elevations. Removing the mother for 12–24 hours produces elevated CORT levels, but mimicking her stimulation of the pups (licking) by stroking them with a wet paintbrush and providing milk through a canula will keep CORT levels at baseline during maternal separation (Suchecki, Rosenfeld, & Levine, 1993). Thus it is social stimulation that maintains the axis in a nonstress state during development in the rat. Importantly, maternal licking also seems to regulate methlyation of the GR gene in the brain, such that pups who receive high levels of maternal licking have more GR receptors for CORT, as compared to those who receive low levels of licking and grooming (Weaver et al., 2004). More CORT receptors confer better negative feedback control of the HPA axis and less stress vulnerability.

Rats are less mature than primates at birth; therefore, it is not clear whether the mechanisms that mediate early experience effects in monkeys and humans are similar to those that operate in rats. What is clear, however, is that not long after birth in monkey infants, maternal availability and responsiveness serve as powerful CORT buffers. Capturing mother and infant from their social group produces behavioral expressions of distress from both parties, but if the infant can maintain contact with the mother, it exhibits only small increases in CORT (Levine & Wiener, 1988). Separation of mother and infant results in large increases in CORT and fear-related behaviors that may be regulated, at least in part, by CRH production in the amygdala and other extrahypothalamic areas (Kalin, Shelton, & Barksdale, 1989). Thus, in some ways similar to rats, nonhuman primate infants maintain basal CORT levels throughout most of early development through contact and proximity to attachment figures. The primate work, however, makes it clear that in some species alloparents can serve similar functions. That is, if the infant is separated from the mother but is then "mothered" by another female during separation, this intervention attenuates elevations in CORT and reduces behavioral distress (Levine & Wiener, 1988).

The human HPA axis also comes under strong social regulation or buffering during early development. In the earliest months of life, however, being held and soothed by the mother or other adults does little to reduce CORT responses to stressors such as being physically manipulated (e.g., during a doctor's exam) or experiencing a mildly painful stressor such as an inoculation, even though these caregiving actions do reduce crying (Gunnar, Marvinney, Isensee, & Fisch, 1988). As these studies demonstrate, although crying and CORT elevations are sometimes correlated in infancy, actions that reduce crying do not necessarily reduce the CORT response, and vice versa. Nonetheless, over the course of the first year it becomes increasingly difficult to elevate CORT to stressors such as brief separations (of a few minutes), wariness-eliciting stimuli, and inoculations (for review, see Gunnar & Donzella, 2002). The uncoupling of CORT responses and behavioral distress, which is often focused on eliciting contact with attachment figures, is particularly marked under acute threat conditions among toddlers who are in secure attachment relationships with the person who is available for immediate succor (Spangler & Schieche, 1998). Indeed, only in secure attachment relationships does the caregiver appear to be able to completely buffer CORT increases in distressed toddlers, as observed in laboratory (Nachmias, Gunnar, Mangelsdorf, Parritz, & Buss, 1996) and naturalistic contexts (Ahnert, Gunnar, Lamb, & Barthel, 2004). Insecurely attached toddlers show CORT responses to stressful events even with their attachment figure present, and toddlers who exhibit disorganized/disoriented attachment patterns may be particularly vulnerable to elevations in this hormone (Hertsgaard, Gunnar, Erickson, & Nachmias, 1995). Thus, over the course of the first year of life, the HPA axis comes under strong social regulation in human children, and the social buffer is more potent if the child is securely attached to his or her caregiver(s).

As in nonhuman primates, alloparents do appear to be capable of buffering CORT elevations in young children. This finding has been noted in studies of babysitters and child care providers (for review, see Gunnar & Donzella, 2002). Babysitters were instructed to provide sensitive, responsive care or more distant, neglectful care for brief (i.e., 30-minute) separations. Sensitive and responsive care by a babysitter, even if she were a stranger to the child, buffered or prevented elevations in CORT at least for brief periods. When young children are in group care settings, the quality of care provided by the alloparent appears to determine whether CORT levels rise or fall over the day. Typically, for young children, CORT levels average about the same in the midafternoon and midmorning, in contrast to the mature rhythm, which exhibits a decline over this period. The more mature adult rhythm emerges as children begin to outgrow their afternoon nap (Watamura, Donzella, Kertes, & Gunnar, 2004). Nonetheless, rising levels of CORT over the day suggest loss of adequate regulation of the HPA axis. Daytime increases in CORT have been observed frequently when children are in group or congregate care; however, CORT increases less in high-quality than low-quality settings (reviewed in Gunnar & Donzella, 2002). The pattern of CORT response in these settings, which is sometimes lower than home levels in the morning and then higher than home levels in the afternoon, suggests that these responses are not acute separation reactions (Gunnar & Donzella, 2002). Furthermore, CORT levels have been noted to decrease over nap periods at child care, even for children who simply lie on their cots and do not appear to fall asleep (Watamura, Sebanc, Donzella, & Gunnar, 2002). Such data suggest that whatever is happening while children are involved in activity at child care is responsible for stimulating the HPA axis. One reasonable possibility is *peer interactions*.

Over the toddler and preschool years, children become increasingly motivated to play with other children; meanwhile, their social skills are just emerging, making peer play challenging (Hartup, 1979). Social competence tends to be negatively correlated with the rise in CORT over the group care day, which is consistent with evidence that age correlates negatively with CORT when preschoolers are at child care but not when they are at home (reviewed in Gunnar & Donzella, 2002). The importance of peer relations is also demonstrated by evidence that as early as the preschool years, peer rejection is associated with chronic elevations in CORT when children are with their peers (Gunnar et al., 2003). This finding may explain why exuberant and undercontrolled as well as fearful and anxious children tend to be susceptible to producing higher CORT levels and rising CORT patterns over the child care day (Dettling, Gunnar, & Donzella, 1999; Gunnar et al., 2003; Watamura, Donzella, Alwin, & Gunnar, 2003). Thus, whereas temperament has been shown to correlate with CORT activity in infancy and early childhood, its associations may be both *mediated* by social relationships, as in exuberant, undercontrolled temperament influencing peer rejection that is more proximally related to elevated CORT, or *moderated* by social relationships, as when responsive caregiving prevents activation of the HPA axis in fearful children.

Although parents can clearly serve as buffers on the effects of social environments on young children's HPA-axis activity through positive, calming parenting behavior, they can also serve as a profound source of social strain if their behavior is threatening or fails to provide appropriate comfort. Conflict between two parents may be an especially powerful form of threat, because it combines exposure to anger and even violence with reduced access to parents who may be too preoccupied with their own problems to offer attention or comfort to the child. In a group of kindergarten-age children and their parents, Pendry and Adam (in press) found that young children living in homes characterized by higher levels of interparental conflict had significantly higher evening CORT levels and flatter diurnal cortisol slopes. Less effective parenting, defined by low levels of warmth and involvement, was independently associated with a flatter diurnal CORT rhythm.

SOCIAL REGULATION OF THE HPA AXIS
IN MIDDLE CHILDHOOD AND ADOLESCENCE

Although less evidence is available on the social regulation of CORT in the middle childhood and adolescent years, the evidence that does exist suggests that family and peer influences continue to play an important role. Beyond the results for young children mentioned above, several studies have found conflict in the family environment to be a powerful activator of CORT during middle childhood and adolescence, whereas a positive, stable, supportive home environment is associated with lower CORT levels (Flinn & England, 1995; Pendry & Adam, in press; see also Repetti, Taylor, & Seeman, 2002). In a sample of Caribbean children and adolescents, Flinn and England (1995, 1997) noted that high levels of family and peer conflict were among the most powerful activators of CORT. In terms of positive social influences, in the Caribbean study, the degree of support available to mothers in the home environment was also an important determinant of CORT levels in the children of this study. Children in single-mother homes without kin support and those living with distant relatives or in stepparent homes with nonrelated siblings had higher average CORT levels than those in biological parent homes and those living with biological mothers who had additional kin support.

Very few studies have examined social factors influencing HPA-axis activity specifically in adolescents—which is surprising, given the importance of changing peer and family relationships, combined with the many other changes in physical appearance, physiology, sexuality, and social roles of this age period. The convergence of all these changes in a short period of time is thought to contribute to the experience of high levels of stress in adolescence. Recent evidence also implicates ongoing brain development as a factor in the increased emotionality and risk taking that characterize the adolescent years (Dahl, 2004). A number of studies now suggest that a small increase in basal CORT levels occurs across mid to late adolescence, perhaps especially in adolescents girls (Elminger, Kuhnel, & Ranke, 2002; Jonetz-Mentzel & Wiedemann, 1993; Kenny, Gancayo, Heald, & Hung, 1966; Kenny, Preeyasombat, & Migeon, 1966; Kiess et al., 1995; Lupien, King, Meaney, & McEwen, 2001; Netherton, Goodyer, Tamplin, & Herbert, 2004 [in girls only]; Tornhage, 2002; Walker, Walder, & Reynolds, 2001). The origin and functional consequences of increasing basal CORT levels during adolescence are not yet known.

The combination of increased exposure to stressful circumstances and the ability of adolescents to report reliably on their own social experiences makes adolescence an attractive period during which to study the impact of social events on the HPA axis. Utilizing the experience sampling method (ESM), in which adolescents were signaled to complete diary reports as they went about their daily lives (see Larson, 1989), in conjunction with repeated sampling of salivary CORT, Adam (2006) found that adolescents' HPA axes were responsive to moment-to-moment changes in social and emotional experiences in their everyday environments. Controlling for the effects of time of day, momentary within-person increases in negative emotion were associated with significant within-person increases in CORT levels. In addition, being alone, rather than with other people, at the time of sampling was also associated with higher momentary CORT levels. Interestingly, being alone appeared to elevate CORT only for younger and not older adolescents.

In another sample of late adolescents, individuals who had recently experienced high levels of negative life events, those who were experiencing chronic strain in their interpersonal relationships (including family, peer, and romantic) were found to have flatter diurnal CORT curves (Adam, Doane, Mineka, Zinbarg, & Craske, 2006). Thus, as with infants and young children, important social relationships in the lives of children and adolescents, both within the immediate family environment and outside the home, are associated with individual differences in CORT activity.

HPA-AXIS ACTIVITY IN CHILDREN EXPOSED TO ABNORMAL SOCIAL ENVIRONMENTS

Situations in which extreme deviations from the expected social environment occur provide unfortunate illustrations of the importance of the environment for HPA-axis functioning. Studies of children reared in institutions or orphanages have provided important insights. Notably, infants and toddlers living in such institutions appear to lack the normal diurnal rhythm in CORT production (for review, see Gunnar, 2000). In particular, CORT levels are low early in the morning and fail to decline in the late evening. This atypical pattern has also been observed in rhesus infants raised on cloth surrogates (Boyce, Champoux, Gunnar, & Suomi, 1995). Lack of a consistent and supportive caregiver may be the factor that disrupts the normal diurnal CORT rhythm; indeed, similar disturbances have been noted in many young children placed in foster care (Fisher, personal communication). In contrast, permanently placing children in supportive adoptive families appears to allow the normal diurnal CORT rhythm to be reestablished (Gunnar, 2000). Several studies, however, suggest that not all children adopted from severely depriving conditions will reestablish completely normal patterns of HPA-axis regulation. Several studies now show elevated basal CORT levels in postinstitutionalized children many years after adoption (e.g., Gunnar, Morison, Chisholm, & Schuder, 2001). However, there is some evidence that long-term elevations in basal CORT levels may be restricted to children who experienced the most adverse early care, resulting in severe growth failure (Kertes, Gunnar, Madsen, & Long, in press).

In addition to children reared in institutions, researchers have also examined physically and sexually abused children who have experienced catastrophic failure of their caregiving system. There is some evidence of elevations in basal CORT among these children, particularly if they exhibit chronic posttraumatic stress disorder (PTSD) symptoms (Carrion et al., 2002; De Bellis et al., 1999). However, not all studies have reported altered HPA-axis activity, raising critical questions about the nature, duration, and severity of abuse necessary to produce long-term alterations (Cicchetti & Rogosch, 2001). Furthermore, the finding that PTSD pursuant to early abuse is associated with elevated basal CORT levels in childhood stands in contrast to the suppressed CORT levels reported for adults with PTSD. Some have suggested that the duration of PTSD symptoms may account for this discrepancy, with elevated CORT levels characterizing PTSD early in the disorder and suppressed levels emerging over time as the HPA system "down-regulates" or adjusts to chronic CORT elevations (Yehuda, Halligan, & Grossman, 2001). Taken together, the data on children exposed to severe deprivation early in life and those exposed to severe abuse suggest that such conditions increase the risk for long-term alterations in HPA-axis functioning. However, the pattern of effects observed also raises important questions about developmental changes in stress reactivity and regulation and individual difference factors that may determine whether and how long-term impacts are expressed.

Data presented thus far offer strong evidence for the influence of current social relationships on current HPA-axis activity and present the intriguing possibility that variations in social experience early in life may have organizational effects on HPA-axis activity in humans, supplementing the already convincing body of evidence on the long-term effects of early experience on the HPA axis in rodents and nonhuman primates. A critical question, however, is whether activity of the HPA axis mediates the impact of social environments on the development of psychopathology.

SOCIAL ENVIRONMENTS, HPA-AXIS FUNCTIONING, AND INTERNALIZING PSYCHOPATHOLOGY

Theoretical Models

Disruptions in the social environments of children are not only implicit to theories of HPA-axis functioning in abusive and neglectful family environments; they are also central to some of the core etiological theories of depression. Chronic exposure to stressful life events has long been considered an important risk factor for the development of depression (Tafet & Bernardini, 2003). Additionally, HPA-axis dysregulation among adults with major depressive disorder (MDD) is one of the most consistent findings in biological psychiatry (Chrousos & Gold, 1992; Pariante, 2003). Models pertaining to childhood depression have been based largely on a downward extension of research with clinically depressed samples of adults. A more developmental approach, and the approach taken in the current chapter, is to subsume anxiety and depressive symptomatology and disorders under the more inclusive class of internalizing problems (see Zahn-Waxler, Klimes-Dougan, & Slattery, 2000). This strategy is justified, in part, by (1) evidence that rates of comorbid anxiety and depression are high, (2) the fact that they have core negative affect features in common, and (3) the fact that anxiety disorders often precede the development of depression. It is even possible that in childhood, disruptions in the HPA axis are more closely linked to anxiety than depression (e.g., Feder et al., 2004; Granger, Weisz, & Kauneckis, 1996). Indeed, there are many parallels in the etiological models of anxiety and depression, and theories of stress and HPA-axis reactivity may be central to understanding the development of both.

Developmental models of depression and internalizing symptomatology focus on the effects of early experience on HPA-axis activity and the implications of normative variations in anxiety and fear reactions (Gunnar, 1992; Gunnar & Vazquez, 2006). The long history of early experience–stress studies in animals provides the basis for attempts to understand how variations in care early in life may impact individual differences in stress resilience and vulnerability, leading to psychiatric disorders (see Gunnar & Vazquez, 2006, for a recent review). Findings suggest that early experiences related to the quality of maternal care cause changes to extrahypothalamic, corticolimbic circuits that influence activity of the HPA axis. Briefly, this etiological model suggests that hippocampal alterations produced by prolonged stress and elevated CORT cause an impairment of the negative feedback loop and could account for alterations in basal CORT and stress reactivity in patients with MDD.

A second developmental approach focuses on individual differences. Pathological anxiety in animals and humans may reflect inhibited temperament, and an exaggeration of normal anticipatory HPA responses (Rosen & Schulkin, 1998) may be most characteristic of this group. In the presence of elevated GCs and CRH, a cascade of biomolecular events that includes increased expression of immediate-early genes (Makino, Gold, & Schulkin, 1994) increases the sensitivity of central fear circuits, heightens anxiety to distal danger cues, and supports the transition from normal to pathological anxiety. Thus, early social experiences, either on their own or in interaction with temperamental vulnerability, are thought to contribute to alterations in HPA-axis functioning associated with depression. What evidence exists for altered HPA-axis activity in children and adolescents with internalizing problems and for the contribution of social environments to the emergence of these differences?

Basal/Diurnal Functioning

In contrast with adults, children with internalizing problems are less likely to exhibit distortions in basal CORT or the HPA rhythm. Here the conclusions are based primarily on reviews by others (e.g., Brooks-Gunn, Auth, Petersen, & Compas, 2001; Dahl & Ryan, 1996; Goodyer, Park, & Herbert, 2001; Ryan, 1998), although more recent findings are duly noted. In clinical samples, children and adolescents with clinical levels of anxiety and depression do not consistently show alterations in their basal CORT. Disruptions are more likely to be noted for diurnal patterns, particularly with regard to sleep onset (Carrion et al., 2002; DeBellis et al., 1999; Feder et al., 2004; Klimes-Dougan et al., 2001; for recent exceptions, see Luby et al., 2003; Martel et al., 1999; Ronsaville et al., 2006). In addition, certain types of depression, including melancholic depression and depression with suicidal symptoms, are more likely to be linked to elevated basal cortisol levels (e.g., Dahl et al., 1991; Klimes-Dougan, Shirtcliff, & Zahn-Waxler, 2006; Luby et al., 2004).

Some researchers have considered within-person variability—a sign of erratic basal output—to be an important indicator of HPA-axis dysregulation and have examined this dysregulation in relation to the presence of MDD (Peeters, Nicholson, & Berkhof, 2004; Yehuda, Teicher, Trestman, & Siever, 1996). In one study that examined adolescents, more highly variable early-morning basal CORT levels (in particular, a spiking of these levels) across days predicted which adolescents would experience their first bout of clinical depression over the next months (Goodyer, Herbert, Tamplin, & Altham, 2000).

Several other studies suggest that premorbid differences in the axis precede and predict the development of depression in high-risk samples. Essex and colleagues (Essex, Klein, Cho, & Kalin, 2002; Smider et al., 2002) obtained salivary CORT samples in the afternoon when children were 4.5 years of age, and these measures predicted internalizing problems in them a year later, as kindergarteners, and both internalizing and externalizing problem behavior in first grade. Similar findings have been reported in studies of young adolescents (Granger, Weisz, & McCracken, 1996; Susman, Dorn, & Chrousos, 1991; Susman, Dorn, Inoff-Germain, Nottelman, & Chrousos, 1997). Higher CORT levels and higher CORT to dehydroepiandrosterone (DHEA; an adrenal androgen with effects that often counter those of CORT) ratios may also predict longer illness duration (Goodyer, Herbert, & Altham, 1998).

To what extent do early social experiences contribute to elevated cortisol levels and variability, and hence to risk of developing internalizing symptoms? In the Essex and colleagues (2002) study, the elevations in cortisol at age 4.5 that were found to predict internalizing and externalizing problems were, in turn, predicted by levels of maternal stress. Notably, however, concurrent maternal stress predicted high child CORT levels only if the currently stressed mother had also been highly stressed during the child's infancy. Furthermore, most of the association with maternal stress was carried by the effects of maternal depression symptoms. Maternal depression during the child's early years may seriously compromise the mother's capacity to provide sensitive, responsive, and supportive care to her child. However, in the Essex and colleagues study, it is not clear whether children with higher CORT levels had mothers who had been consistently depressed over the child's whole life. Work by Halligan, Herbert, Goodyer, and Murray (2004) suggests the importance of maternal depression in the child's early years, in particular. They found that adolescent children of mothers who were depressed postnatally had higher morning CORT levels and more variability in these levels, even after controlling for current life events and mothers' current levels of depression.

Stress Reactivity

Like the research on basal functioning, research on stress reactivity suggests that MDD in children and adolescents is less associated with endogenous dysregulation of the HPA axis than it is in adults. Nonsuppression of CORT to dexamethasone, a common finding in adults, is rare in children and adolescents with MDD, and ACTH and CORT responses to CRH are also typically normal, at least in children who have not also been physically abused (see Ryan, 1998). In contrast, children with clinical anxiety show elevations in CORT in response to some types of stressors, including a fear-potentiated startle paradigm in which a warning light is sometimes followed by an unpleasant blast of air (60 psi) to the throat (Ashman, Dawson, Panagiotides, Yamada, & Wilkinson, 2002).

Using experimental paradigms that involve some type of social stressor has also yielded mixed findings with regard to anticipation of, and reaction to, stress. Granger and his colleagues (e.g., Granger, Stansbury, & Henker, 1994; Granger, Weisz, & Kauneckis, 1994) used a conflict paradigm to assess stress reactivity with a clinic-referred sample of children and adolescents. They found that increased CORT reactivity was concurrently associated with higher levels of a number of internalizing symptoms, including social withdrawal, social anxiety, task inhibition, and low levels of perceived contingency. Using a similar conflict paradigm, Klimes-Dougan and colleagues (2001) found that moderate levels of CORT reactivity were associated with fewer internalizing and externalizing symptoms. A commonly used paradigm is the Trier Social Stress Test (TSST; Kirschbaum, Pirke, & Hellhammer, 1993) in which the participant gives a speech, then solves mathematics problems. Various adaptations of this procedure have also been used with children and adolescents. Although elevations in CORT are typically documented using this procedure, most studies have failed to find group differences in stress reactivity between children with internalizing disorders and comparison groups (e.g., Dorn et al., 2003; Klimes-Dougan et al., 2001; Martel et al., 1999). However, when parameters of stress reactivity and stress recovery were considered separately, the greatest increase in CORT reactivity for girls was associated with the highest levels of internalizing problems (Klimes-Dougan et al., 2001).

In addition to activation, understanding how children at risk for internalizing problems recover from a stressor is critical. In a few studies repeated CORT samples after a stressor have been considered (e.g., Klimes-Dougan et al., 2001). Another aspect of recovery—failure of CORT responses to habituate to familiar stressors—may be associated with internalizing symptomatology (Gunnar & Vazquez, 2006). Increasing CORT levels to novel stressors may not be unique to shy, inhibited, or anxious children and indeed may initially be associated with assertion and dominance, because more assertive children are often the first to approach challenging and uncertain circumstances. However, shy, inhibited, or anxious children may be less likely to habituate CORT responses as the situation becomes more familiar, and they may be less able to turn off the CORT response once they have left the novel situation. Several researchers have noted higher CORT levels among more anxious, introverted children, but only when the peer group setting was familiar (e.g., Bruce, Davis, & Gunnar, 2002; Davis, Donzella, Krueger, & Gunnar, 1999; Granger, Stansbury, & Henker, 1994; Legendre & Trudel, 1996). Failure to habituate, and the more frequent or prolonged elevations in CORT that go along with lack of habituation to stressors, may in turn increase risk for developing anxiety and depression (e.g., Pruessner et al., 1997; van Eck, Berkhof, et al, 1996a; van Eck, Nicolson, et al., 1996).

In addition to its cross-sectional association with symptoms of anxiety, CORT reactivity has been shown to predict subsequent internalizing symptoms. In one study, clinic-referred children participated in a conflict paradigm and were assessed for internalizing problems at the time of the conflict paradigm and 6 months later (Granger, Weisz, & McCracken, 1996). Those who exhibited high CORT reactivity at the time of the first assessment exhibited more internalizing symptoms at the second time point. Also, increases in internalizing problems were associated with higher CORT reactivity at the follow-up.

If disruptions in the HPA-axis system are related to internalizing symptomatology, attempts to normalize the HPA axis may provide us with critical information for diagnostic, preventive, and therapeutic purposes (Tafet & Bernardini, 2003). There is some preliminary evidence with adult samples to suggest that HPA-axis activity may be modified indirectly through psychotherapeutic processes, including cognitive-behavioral stress management (e.g., Gaab et al., 2003) and social support (e.g., Heinrichs, Baumgartner, Kirschbaum, & Ehlert, 2003; Kirschbaum, Klauer, Filipp, & Hellhammer, 1995). Given the importance of supportive peer affiliation, particularly in adolescence, more research is needed that examines the effects of support beyond the caregiving environment.

Thus, although evidence suggests that negative aspects of social circumstances may potentially place individuals at greater risk for the development of internalizing disorders through increased basal levels, variability, or CORT reactivity, positive social relationships may also offer the potential to protect against HPA dysregulation and the development of internalizing disorders.

HPA-AXIS FUNCTIONING AND EXTERNALIZING PSYCHOPATHOLOGY

Etiological models regarding HPA-axis functioning for externalizing problems center on core biological disruptions in the physiological response system. Raine (1996) suggests that systems implicated in HPA-axis functioning (e.g., central and autonomic nervous systems; CNS and ANS, respectively) are underaroused for some individuals (partially assumed to be genetically determined), and these response patterns may predispose some to criminality. Thus, the implication is that the HPA system is blunted or hyporesponsive in children with externalizing problems or disruptive behavior disorders (DBD). Consistent with this hypothesis, studies of response to serotonergic challenges in children with DBD have shown that these children exhibit blunted CORT reactions to fenfluramine (Soloff, Lynch, & Moss, 2000) and sumatriptan (Snoek et al., 2002), both of which typically elevate cortisol, suggesting that serotonergic regulation of the HPA axis is compromised.

There are various mechanisms that may account for low basal and reactivity CORT levels. Some possibilities include an unresponsive stress-reactivity system or a down-regulation of the axis following periods of elevated CORT. This latter hypothesis has been invoked by those who suggest that a chaotic and threatening family life may produce a down-regulated stress system in the children of antisocial parents, consistent with evidence of low basal cortisol in sons of substance-abusing fathers (Hardie, Moss, Vanyukov, Yao, & Kirillovac, 2002; Pajer, Gardner, Kirillova, & Vanyukov, 2001). Overregulation of the HPA axis may contribute to low basal CORT production. Alternatively, an increased threshold for stress reactivity may account for low levels of CORT reactivity. Finally, those exhibiting externalizing problems may be underreactive to threat stimuli, resulting in impaired avoidance learning and underarousal, which may encourage sensation seeking as a means of increasing arousal.

Basal, Pretest, and Diurnal HPA-Axis Functioning

Although low basal CORT has been observed in some samples of children with DBD (McBurnett, Lahey, Rathouz, & Loerber, 2000; van de Wiel, Van Goozen, Matthys, Snoek, & van Engeland, 2004; Van Goozen et al., 1998), this finding has not been consistent (Azar et al., 2004; Dabbs, Jurkovic, & Frady, 1991; Granger, Weisz, & Kauneckis, 1994; Scerbo & Kolko, 1994; Susman et al., 1999; Van Goozen, Matthys, Cohen-Kettenis, Buittelaar, & van Engeland, 2000). Unfortunately, these studies vary in the time of day when CORT levels were examined as well as in the conditions under which samples were obtained. Most do not involve a procedure for sampling CORT under highly familiar conditions (e.g., at home), but rather take samples when children come to the laboratory for testing, limiting our ability determine whether basal activity of the HPA axis is lower for children with disruptive behavior problems. Nevertheless, subgroup analyses within those studies to document basal—or, more accurately, baseline—differences in CORT for children with DBD in comparison to low-risk groups may be instructive. Thus, van de Wiel and colleagues (2004) noted lower baseline CORT levels only for those children with DBD who exhibited the most significant problem behavior. Similarly, McBurnett and colleagues (e.g., McBurnett, Pfiffner, Capasso, Lahey, & Loerber, 1997; McBurnett et al., 1991) found that boys with DBD who had the lowest CORT levels were described as the meanest by their peers, as the most aggressive by adults, and were more overtly rather than covertly aggressive. These results seem to suggest that only the children with the most severe DBD may exhibit abnormally low basal or baseline CORT.

Given this possibility, it is surprising to find that in both risk and community samples, low CORT has been found to correlate with scores of externalizing behavior (e.g., Pajer, Gardner, Kirillova, et al., 2001; Scerbo & Kolko, 1994; Vanyukov et al., 1993) and aggression (Flinn & England, 1995; Oosterlaan, Geurts, Knol, & Sergeant, 2005; Spangler, 1995; Tennes & Kreye, 1985; Tennes, Kreye, Avitable, & Wells, 1986). Many of these studies, however, assessed CORT in the early morning when levels are typically high, perhaps increasing the sensitivity to associations between externalizing problems and lower basal HPA activity. For example, using a very large community sample of children and adolescents, Shirtcliff, Granger, and colleagues (2005) applied latent state–trait modeling techniques to identify the trait component of early morning salivary CORT production. For boys, but not girls, they found a significant negative relation between trait CORT shortly after awakening and externalizing problems. In addition to these cross-sectional associations, several studies have demonstrated that low basal CORT levels predict heightened disruptive behavior several months or years later (e.g., Granger et al., 1996; McBurnett, Lahey, et al., 2000; Shoal, Giancola, & Kirrilova, 2003). Thus, in all, the data are suggestive, but not definitive, regarding low basal CORT activity and externalizing behaviors; more work is clearly needed to further investigate this relationship. This need is particularly salient because low basal CORT could contribute to low ANS and CNS reactivity, given that one function of basal cortisol is to maintain the responsiveness of neurons to their neurotransmitters (Sapolsky et al., 2000).

Stress Anticipation, Reactivity, and Recovery

Some researchers have suggested that disturbances in HPA activity in externalizing disorders may be most evident under stress as compared to baseline conditions (Snoek, Van Goozen, Matthys, Buitelaar, & Engeland, 2004). In examining this hypothesis, it is necessary to distinguish between failure to respond in anticipation of a threatening event, smaller elevations in CORT in response to such events, and/or more rapid return to baseline following termination of the event, because these distinctions could reflect different causes of low CORT reactivity. In this regard, there is growing evidence of blunted anticipatory responding. Specifically, in a number of studies, children with DBD or those at risk for DBD tend to exhibit low pretest CORT levels that do not change after exposure to a mild stressor, whereas nonrisk children tend to show higher pretest CORT levels that decrease over the period of stressor exposure (Hardie et al., 2002; King, 1998; Moss, Vanyukov, & Martin, 1995; Moss, Vanyukov, Yao, & Kirillova, 1999; Pajer, Gardner, Rubin, Perel, & Neal, 2001). The challenge in interpreting these findings is that, in most cases, the testing was conducted early in the morning; thus it is not clear whether children with DBD fail to exhibit an anticipatory response or simply have low early morning basal CORT levels. Clearly, these studies would have benefited from assessment of basal levels on nontest days (e.g., Klimes-Dougan et al., 2001).

There is also some evidence that children with DBD show less of a CORT increase in response to mild stressors (e.g., Jansen et al., 1999; Moss et al., 1995; Snoek et al., 2002; Targum, Clarkson, Magac-Harris, Marshall, & Skwerer, 1990). The implications for these findings are not clear, however, because in most of the studies the nonrisk group failed to elevate CORT to the stressor or actually showed decreasing CORT reactions over the stressor period (for an exception, see Snoek et al., 2002). To adequately examine whether children with DBD show a blunted CORT stress response, the paradigm should elevate CORT for the nonrisk comparison children. Van Goozen and colleagues (1998) employed such a paradigm; it involved a frustration/provocation task during which a peer (on audiotape) denigrated the target child's performance. They reported that children with oppositional defiant disorder (ODD) and those with comorbid attention-deficit disorder (ADD) showed decreased CORT in response to the provocation task, whereas nonrisk children tended to show an increase (see also Gatzke-Kopp & Beauchaine, Chapter 10, this volume). However, not all children with disruptive behavior problems exhibited blunted CORT reactivity; children with ODD comorbid for anxiety problems actually exhibited the highest CORT reactivity. This study suggests that blunted CORT reactivity may only be seen for children with DBD who are not comorbid for anxiety disorders, an interpretation also offered by McBurnett and colleagues (1991) and Snoek and colleagues (2004).

Finally, there is a paucity of research regarding CORT recovery following a stressor for children with externalizing problems. Van Goozen and colleagues (2000) found that children with DBD and nonrisk children tended to differ in CORT in the immediate poststress period, and children with DBD continued to show low CORT during a recovery period. Because the children with DBD did not show an elevation in CORT in response to the task, it is unlikely that this reflects a difference in negative feedback regulation of the HPA axis, as in PTSD (Yehuda et al., 2001).

The evidence of lower basal CORT and blunted CORT reactivity to frustration/provocation begs the question of whether these differences are meaningful. One way to address this question is to consider whether these reported effects have implications for responsivity to treatment. In a recent follow-up study, van de Wiel and colleagues (2004) examined effectiveness of treatment for children with DBD as a function of CORT baseline and reactivity, using a 9-month treatment window and multifaceted (medication, individual, and family therapy) intervention. Although pretest or baseline differences were not predictive and CORT reactivity was similar with regard to symptom severity at the pretest assessment, boys with more elevated CORT levels following the frustration/provocation paradigm were significantly more responsive to therapeutic intervention than were those with low CORT stress responsivity. A related question is whether CORT reactivity also can be altered by therapeutic interventions in children at risk for externalizing problems. A recent prevention study with low-income preschoolers who experienced the familial risk factors for conduct disorder addressed this question. Using a randomized prevention trial, Miller Brotman, Kiely Gouley, Pine, and Rafferty (2002) increased CORT reactions during a peer entry/interaction task among the children in the intervention group. Because this intervention focused on social-cognitive processes, the pattern of results suggests that low CORT reactivity among children at risk for DBD, at least, may not reflect dysregulation of the HPA axis as much as disturbances in psychological processes operating via corticolimbic circuits that activate the HPA axis. However, this conclusion is extremely tentative, given that it is based on only one study that was conducted on a risk group rather than children with DBD.

SUMMARY OF HPA ACTIVITY
IN CHILD CLINICAL DISORDERS

This brief review of research on HPA-axis activity in children with clinical disorders and subclinical behavior problems yields evidence of associations between internalizing and externalizing symptoms and basal CORT levels in children and adolescents. It also lends supportive evidence, but not universally so, for associations between internalizing disorders and CORT hyperactivity, and externalizing disorders and CORT hypoactivity in response to stressors. The control provided in animal studies and the growing literature on correlational studies with children and adolescents have enabled us to draw speculative conclusions that social–environmental factors play a role in regulating CORT levels and reactivity, and hence may play a role in the emergence and course of clinical symptoms and disorders associated with dysregulated HPA-axis activity.

SOCIAL AND NONSOCIAL CONTRIBUTIONS
TO HPA-AXIS FUNCTIONING: A MODEL

As illustrated by the above discussion of the literatures on externalizing and internalizing disorders, associations between psychopathology and HPA-axis activity are not straightforward, and inconsistencies abound. One explanation for these inconsistencies is that the design and measurement of most studies of psychopathology and CORT do not take into account the multiple influences on current HPA-axis functioning that exist, including influences of both a social and nonsocial nature. Figure 11.2 depicts some of the known influences on HPA-axis activity in humans, as measured by salivary CORT levels. Some of these influences are ongoing at the time of CORT assessment, whereas some are historical factors that have previously affected the organization of the HPA axis. We do not have space to review each component of the model in detail. The major point of Figure 11.2 is to illustrate the multiplicity of influences on current CORT levels and activity, and hence the complexity of the task of predicting individual differences in CORT.

Historical influences on CORT are critical (Figure 11.2, left-hand column). Recent research has suggested that prenatal stress exposure may play a role in the organization of the HPA axis and thus in CORT activity (Bertram & Hanson, 2002; Matthews, 2000; Wadhwa, Dunkel-Schetter, Chicz-DeMet, Porto, & Sandman, 1996). Early postnatal influences have also been shown to play a critical role, particularly in animal models, but also now in humans (Halligan et al., 2004). As noted in this review, an individual's prior history of stress exposure and of supportive relationships can modify current CORT activity (Essex et al., 2002; Pendry & Adam, in press); although less studied, health and lifestyle history also likely play a role in regulating current CORT activity.

Current influences on cortisol activity (Figure 11.2, right-hand column) include mood and cognitive biases present at the moment or on the days of testing (Adam, 2006), exposure to recent negative life events (Adam, Doane, et al., 2006), recent food, exercise, medication, nicotine or caffeine intake (Kirschbaum & Hellhammer, 1989, 1994), and, in the case of women, menstrual timing (Kirschbaum, Kudielka, Baab, Schommer, & Hellhammer, 1994). A variety of other physiological systems are in constant interaction with the HPA axis, including the activity of the sympathetic nervous system, immune and inflammatory systems, and adrenal, gonadal, and ovarian hormones (Heinrichs et al., 2003; Rosmond, 2005).

To complicate matters further, the effects of these multiple influences on HPA-axis functioning may change with ontogeny. In addition to age- and pubertal-stage-related changes in CORT levels (Netherton et al., 2004; Stroud, Papandonatos, Williamson, & Dahl, 2004), changes in other hormone systems (Cameron, 2004) and changes in the maturity and functioning of neural systems that interact with the HPA (Dahl, 2004; Spear, 2000; Stroud et al., 2004; Young & Altemus, 2004) have the potential to modify how experience and HPA-axis activity interrelate.

Basal CORT levels and reactivity to stressors have been found to be modified by gender (Kudielka & Kirschbaum, 2005; Stroud, Salovey, &

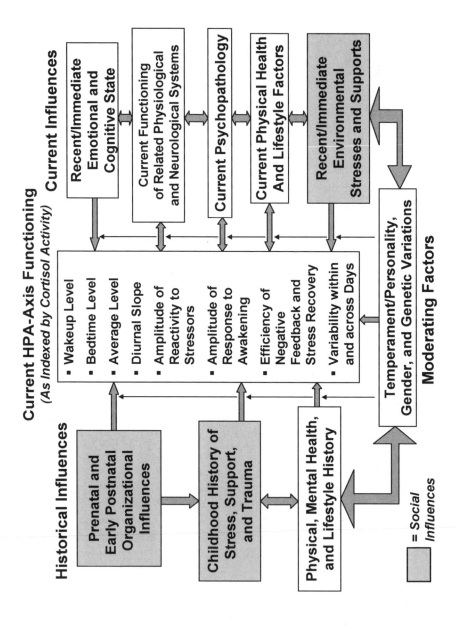

FIGURE 11.2. Historical and current influences on HPA-axis functioning, as indexed by salivary cortisol levels, highlighting the role of social factors.

288

Epel, 2002; Taylor et al., 2000) and by temperament or personality characteristics (Gunnar et al., 2003; Kirschbaum, Barussek, & Strasburger, 1992; Nachmias et al., 1996). Both behavioral genetic and molecular genetic studies have noted moderate to strong genetic contributions to aspects of basal CORT and also to CORT reactivity (Bartels, Van den Berg, Sluyter, Boomsma, & de Geus, 2003; Wüst, Federenko, Hellhammer, & Kirschbaum, 2000; Wüst, Federenko, et al., 2004a; Wüst, Van Rossum, et al., 2004b), providing evidence for a partial genetic basis for preexisting HPA-axis differences and differences in the reactivity and modifiability of the HPA with experience.

It is also important to note that the various influences identified in Figure 11.2 may have differential degrees of impact on the various parameters of CORT measurement, such as average levels, diurnal slopes, and the size of the CORT response to awakening or reactivity to laboratory stressors. For example, genetic predispositions may make a larger contribution to the size of the CORT response to awakening than to evening CORT levels (e.g., Wüst et al., 2000); social–environmental contributions may have a larger acute impact on evening CORT levels than they do on morning levels (e.g., Pendry & Adam, in press); and a history of trauma or childhood chronic stress may be more likely reflected in a current flattening of the diurnal rhythm than in an overall elevation of levels (Gunnar & Vazquez, 2006).

Rather than being discouraged by this complexity, our goal is to suggest that thorough measurement of each (or at least several) of these factors, in relation to multiple parameters of CORT functioning, should lead to better characterization and understanding of CORT activity, which should, in turn, reveal stronger and more consistent associations between CORT, behavior, and pathology. At the very least, it should make us more forgiving when only a small proportion of the variation in CORT levels is accounted for in any one study.

Also apparent in Figure 11.2 are many places in which *social variables* enter the model to influence both the developmental course and current activity of the HPA axis (see the darkly shaded boxes in the model). For example, social environments that influence the mother's emotional well-being and the hormonal environment of the pregnancy may alter the organization of the fetal HPA axis (Avishai-Eliner, Brunson, Sandman, & Baram, 2002; Wadhwa et al., 1996; Wellberg & Seckl, 2001). In a sophisticated set of rodent experiments (Weaver et al., 2004), early mother–pup interactions were shown to produce organizational effects on the structure and functioning of the offspring hippocampus, through permanent changes in the methylation of a portion of the DNA responsible for glucocorticoid receptor development. The long-term effects of early maternal depression (Halligan et al., 2004) and institutionalization (Gunnar et al., 2001), discussed previously, suggest the possibility of similar early social influences on the organization of HPA-axis functioning in humans.

Given the continuing plasticity and growth of the brain, however, it is likely that social experiences may continue to have organizational influences on the development of the HPA axis in early childhood and even into the adolescent years. Examining the cumulative effects of lifelong histories of social stress and support on HPA-axis activity, health, and development, using longitudinal data on social, behavioral, and physiological functioning, is a critical direction for future investigation. This need is beginning to be addressed by the incorporation of stress biomarkers in large-scale longitudinal studies in which social influences on CORT and other stress biomarkers will be studied from the prenatal period onward.

Another rich direction for future research involves the investigation of the impact of *macrosocial* or *macrosystemic* factors, such as poverty, lack of opportunity, and discrimination, on stress physiology, with racial and socioeconomic (SES) differences in stress exposure and stress system activation hypothesized to account partially for group disparities in adult functioning and health (Cohen et al., 2006; Flinn & England, 1997; Lupien et al., 2001; Sapolsky, 2004). Indeed, beyond its clear effects on social–emotional functioning, the known impacts of CORT on cognition, memory, immune system functioning, and physical health suggest possible pathways by which stress may jeopardize one important pathway to prosperity: educational performance.

IMPLICATIONS OF SOCIAL INFLUENCES ON HPA-AXIS ACTIVITY FOR EDUCATION

Research on the potential implications of individual differences in HPA-axis activity for educational functioning are only just beginning to be examined, but these differences represent a ripe area for future investigation. Existing research shows strong associations between experimental manipulations in CORT levels and cognition and memory processes in adults (Lupien, Gillin, & Hauger, 1999; Lupien & McEwen, 1997; Wolf, Schommer, Hellhammer, McEwen, & Kirschbaum, 2001). Associations between CORT levels and cognitive and memory functioning are thought to follow a reverse U-shaped curve, with too low and/or too high levels associated with impaired performance (note the similarity to CORT associations with emotional and physical health—in all cases, moderate and effectively regulated levels of this hormone are considered advantageous). More recently, some work on CORT and memory in children has suggested that negative effects of elevated CORT on memory are also present in preschool-age children (Heffelfinger & Newcomer, 2001; Lupien & McEwen, 1997).

In addition to direct effects on cognitive functioning, individual differences in HPA-axis functioning may have the potential to disrupt achievement through several indirect pathways. CORT levels may influence both the ability to fall asleep and the quality of sleep (Gillin, Jacobs, Fram, & Snyder, 1972). Decrements in number of hours of sleep have been shown to have strong effects on educational performance in middle school children (Sadeh, Gruber, & Raviv, 2003). In adults, high levels of CORT during sleep have been shown to impair declarative memory consolidation processes that typically occur during slow-wave sleep (Born & Wagner, 2004).

Another indirect pathway by which HPA-axis activity may influence educational performance is through its effects on physical and mental health. Increased absenteeism associated with the presence of physical health problems, and absenteeism and social problems associated with the presence of depression and anxiety could contribute to, and interact with, poor cognitive, attentional, and memory processing to cause additional impairments in educational functioning. Problems in classroom functioning and educational performance may then feed back to cause additional psychological strain and CORT elevations; failure experiences have been shown to be important activators of the HPA axis, particularly among individuals with low self-esteem (Pruessner, Hellhammer, & Kirschbaum, 1999).

Due to the relative lack of research in this area on children, much of our discussion on the potential educational implications of increased CORT has been based on extensions of experimental animal work and research with adult humans in laboratory settings. What do we know about how CORT levels relate to educational functioning in naturalistic academic settings? Initial findings by Adam and Snell (2006) show that CORT levels are typically lower when adolescents are productively engaged in academic activities than when they are engaged in nonacademic tasks (controlling for the effects of time of day and of being alone on CORT levels). Whether low CORT levels facilitate attention, focus, and achievement, or whether positive engagement in academic activities lowers CORT levels remains unclear from these correlational data; experimental research on CORT, attention, and performance in school-age children and adolescents is required to further explore these associations.

Another important implication for education emerges from Gunnar and Donzella's (2001) findings that individual differences in the quality of child care settings are important in determining the extent to which children will display increased HPA-axis activation in these environments. Whether CORT differences, in turn, relate to the degree of intellectual and social benefits children obtain from their day care settings remains to be examined, and whether the quality of elementary school, middle school, and high school classroom environments also influence CORT levels is another important direction for future research. Child attentional processes and readiness to learn upon entering the first grade are important determinants of later success in school (Alexander, Entwisle, & Dauber, 1993; Duncan et al., 2005; McClelland, Morrison, & Holmes, 2000). If elevated adrenocortical activity due to low-quality child care or learning environments does contribute to impairments in attention and social functioning in the classroom, this research would provide another important reason why the quality of these environments needs to be closely regulated, both in terms of the intellectual stimulation they offer and the quality of the social and emotional environment they provide.

In general, research on social influences on the HPA axis leads us to conclude what should already be obvious: that providing children with supportive social environments that promote positive emotion and feelings of safety and security is good for them and their development, and that adverse social environments can cause wounds that cut far beneath the skin, influencing children's mental and physical well-being and their cognitive potential.

ACKNOWLEDGMENTS

Writing of this review was facilitated by awards from the W. T. Grant Foundation and the Spencer Foundation to Emma Adam and by a K05 award (No. MH66208) to Megan Gunnar. We wish to thank Carol Worthman for her helpful comments on an earlier draft of the chapter.

REFERENCES

Adam, E. K. (2006). Transactions among trait and state emotion and adolescent diurnal and momentary cortisol activity in naturalistic settings. *Psychoneuroendocrinology, 31*(5), 664–679.

Adam, E. K., Doane, L. D., Mineka, S., Zinbarg, R., & Craske, M. (2006). *Cumulative affective strain and cortisol levels in adolescents at risk for mood and anxiety disorders.* Manuscript submitted for publication.

Adam, E. K., & Gunnar, M. R. (2001). Relationship functioning and home and work demands predict individual differences in diurnal cortisol patterns in women. *Psychoneuroendocrinology, 26*, 189–208.

Adam, E. K., Hawkley, L., Cacioppo, 1., & Kudielka, B. (2006). Day-to-day dynamics of experience-cortisol associations in a population-based sample of older adults. *Proceedings of the National Academy of Sciences, 103*, 17058–17063.

Adam, E. K., & Snell, E. (2006). *Schooling, parental involvement, adolescent emotion and cortisol.* Manuscript in preparation.

Ahnert, L., Gunnar, M., Lamb, M., & Barthel, M. (2004). Transition to child care: Associations with infant–mother attachment, infant negative emotion and cortisol elevations. *Child Development, 75,* 639–650.

Alexander, K. L., Entwisle, D. R., & Dauber, S. L. (1993). First grade classroom behavior: Its short- and long-term consequences for school performance. *Child Development, 64,* 801–514.

Ashman, S. B., Dawson, G., Panagiotides, H., Yamada, E., & Wilkinson, C. W. (2002). Stress hormone levels of children of depressed mothers. *Development and Psychopathology, 14,* 333–349.

Avishai-Eliner, S., Brunson, K. L., Sandman, C., & Baram, T. (2002). Stressed-out or in (utero)? *Trends in Neurosciences, 25,* 518–524.

Azar, R., Zoccolillo, M., Paquette, D., Quiros, E., Baltzer, F., & Tremblay, R. E. (2004). Cortisol levels and conduct disorder in adolescent mothers. *Journal of the American Academy of Child and Adolescent Psychiatry, 43*(4), 461–468.

Bartels, M., de Geus, E. J. C., Kirschbaum, C., Sluyter, F., & Boomsma, D. I. (2003). Heritability of daytime cortisol levels in children. *Behavior Genetics, 22,* 421–433.

Bartels, M., Van den Berg, M., Sluyter, F., Boomsma, D. I., & de Geus, E. J. C. (2003). Heritability of cortisol levels: review and simultaneous analysis oftwin studies. *Psychoneuroendocrinology, 28*(2), 121–137.

Bertram, C. E., & Hanson, M. A. (2002). Prenatal programming of postnatal endocrine responses by glucocorticoids. *Reproduction, 124,* 459–467.

Born, J., & Wagner, W. (2004). Memory consolidation during sleep: Role of cortisol feedback. *Annals of the New York Academy of Sciences, 1032,* 198–201.

Boyce, T., Champoux, M., Gunnar, M., & Suomi, S. (1995). Salivary cortisol in nursery-reared rhesus monkeys: Reactivity to peer interactions and altered circadian activity. *Developmental Psychobiology, 28,* 257–268.

Brooks-Gunn, J., Auth, J. J., Petersen, A. C., & Compas, B. E. (2001). Physiological processes and the development of childhood and adolescent depression. In I. Goodyer (Ed.), *The depressed child and adolescent* (2nd ed.). New York: Cambridge University Press.

Bruce, J., Davis, E. P., & Gunnar, M. (2002). Individual differences in children's cortisol response to the beginning of a new school year. *Psychoneuroendocrinology, 27*(6), 635–650.

Cameron, J. L. (2004). Interrelationships between hormones, behavior and affect during adolescence: Complex relationships exist between reproductive hormones, stress-related hormones, and the activity of neural systems that regulate behavioral affect. *Annals of the New York Academy of Sciences, 1021,* 134–142.

Carrion, V. G., Weems, C. F., Ray, R. D., Glaser, B., Hessl, D., & Reiss, A. L. (2002). Diurnal salivary cortisol in pediatric posttraumatic stress disorder. *Biological Psychiatry, 51,* 575–582.

Chrousos, G. P, & Gold, P. W. (1992). The concepts of stress and stress system disorders. Overview of physical and behavioral homeostasis. *Journal of the American Medical Association, 267,* 1244–1252.

Cicchetti, D., & Rogosch, F. A. (2001). Diverse patterns of neuroendocrine activity in maltreated children. *Development and Psychopathology, 13,* 677–693.

Cohen, S., Schwartz, J. E., Epel, E., Kirschbaum, C., Sidney, S., & Seeman, T. (2006). Socioeconomic status, race and diurnal cortisol decline in the coronary artery risk development in young adults (CARDIA) study. *Psychosomatic Medicine, 68,* 41–50.

Dabbs, J. M., Jurkovic, G. J., & Frady, R. L. (1991). Salivary testosterone and cortisol among late adolescent male offenders. *Journal of Abnormal Child Psychology, 19,* 469–478.

Dahl, R. E. (2004). Adolescent brain development: A period of vulnerabilities and opportunities. *Annals of the New York Academy of Sciences, 1021,* 1–22.

Dahl, R. E., & Ryan, N. D. (1996). The psychobiology of adolescent depression. In D. Cicchetti & S. L. Toth (Eds.), *Adolescence: Opportunities and challenges— Rochester symposium on developmental psychopathology* (Vol. 7, pp. 197– 232). Mahwah, NJ: Erlbaum.

Dahl, R., Ryan, N., Puig-Antich, J., Nguyen, N., Al-Shabbout, M., Meyer, V., et al. (1991). 24–hour cortisol measures in adolescents with major depression: A controlled study. *Biological Psychiatry, 30,* 25–36.

Davis, E. P., Donzella, B., Krueger, W. K., & Gunnar, M. R. (1999). The start of a new school year: Individual differences in salivary cortisol response in relation to child temperament. *Developmental Psychobiology, 35*(3), 188–196.

De Bellis, M. D., Baum, A. S., Birmaher, B., Keshavan, M. S., Eccard, C. H., Boring, A. M., et al. (1999). Developmental traumatology, Part 1: Biological stress systems. *Biological Psychiatry, 9,* 1259–1270.

de Kloet, E. R. (2003). Hormones, brain and stress. *Endocrine Regulations, 37,* 51– 68.

de Kloet, E. R., Vreugdenhil, E., Oitzl, M., & Joels, A. (1998). Brain corticosteroid receptor balance in health and disease. *Endocrine Reviews, 19,* 269–301.

Dettling, A. C., Gunnar, M. R., & Donzella, B. (1999). Cortisol levels of young children in full-day childcare centers: Relations with age and temperament. *Psychoneuroendocrinology, 24*(5), 505–518.

Dickerson, S. S., & Kemeny, M. E. (2004). Acute stressors and cortisol responses: A theoretical integration and synthesis of laboratory research. *Psychological Bulletin, 130,* 355–391.

Dorn, L. D., Campo, J. C., Thato, S., Dahl, R. E., Lewin, D., Chandra, R., et al. (2003). Psychological comorbidity and stress reactivity in children and adolescents with recurrent abdominal pain and anxiety disorders. *Journal of the American Academy of Child and Adolescent Psychiatry, 42,* 66–75.

Duncan, G. J., Dowsett, C. J., Brooks-Gunn, J., Claessens, A., Duckworth, K., Engel, M., et al., (2005). *School readiness and later achievement.* Manuscript submitted for publication.

Elmlinger, M. W., Kuhnel, W., & Ranke, M. B. (2002). Reference ranges for serum concentrations of flutropin (LH), follitropin (FSH), estradiol (E2), prolactin, progesterone, sex hormone-binding globulin (SHBG), dehydroepiandrosterone sulfate (DHEA), cortisol and ferritin in neonates, children and young adults. *Clinical Chemistry and Laboratory Medicine, 401*, 1151–1160.

Essex, M. J., Klein, M. H., Cho, E., & Kalin, N. H. (2002). Maternal stress beginning in infancy may sensitize children to later stress exposure: Effects on cortisol and behavior. *Biological Psychiatry, 52*(8), 776–784.

Feder, A., Coplan, J. D., Goetz, R. R., Mathew, S. J., Pine, D. S., Dahl, R. E., et al. (2004). Prepubertal children with anxiety or depressive disorders, *Biological Psychiatry, 56*, 198–204.

Flinn, M. V., & England, B. G. (1995). Childhood stress and family environment. *Current Anthropology, 36*, 854–866.

Flinn, M. V., & England, B. G. (1997). Social economics of childhood glucocorticoid response and health. *American Journal of Physical Anthropology, 102*, 33–53.

Gaab, J., Blattler, N., Menzi, T., Pabst, B., Stoyer, S., & Ehlert, U. (2003). Randomized controlled evaluation of the effects of cognitive-behavioral stress management on cortisol responses to acute stress in healthy subjects. *Psychoneuroendocrinology, 28*, 767–779.

Gillin, J. C., Jacobs, L. S., Fram, D. H., & Snyder, F. (1972). Acute effect of a glucocorticoid on normal human sleep. *Nature, 237*, 398–399.

Goodyer, I. M., Herbert, J., & Altham, P. M. (1998). Adrenal steroid secretion and major depression in 8- to 16-yr olds: III. Influence of cortisol/DHEA ratio at presentation on subsequent rates of disappointing life events and persistent major depression. *Psychological Medicine, 28*, 265–273.

Goodyer, I. M., Herbert, J., Tamplin, A., & Altham, P. M. (2000). First-episode major depression in adolescents: Affective, cognitive and endocrine characteristics of risk status and predictors of onset. *British Journal of Psychiatry, 176*, 142–149.

Goodyer, I. M., Park, R. J., & Herbert, J. (2001). Psychosocial and endocrine features of chronic first-episode major depression in 8–16 year olds. *Biological Psychiatry, 50*, 351–357.

Granger, D. A., Stansbury, K., & Henker, B. (1994). Preschoolers' behavioral and neuroendocrine responses to social challenge. *Merrill–Palmer Quarterly, 40*, 190–211.

Granger, D. A., Weisz, J. R., & Kauneckis, D. (1994). Neuroendocrine reactivity, internalizing behavior problems, and control-related cognitions in clinic-referred children and adolescents. *Journal of Abnormal Psychology, 103*, 267–276.

Granger, D. A., Weisz, J. R., & McCracken, J. T. (1996). Reciprocal influences among adrenocortical activation, psychosocial processes, and the behavioral adjustment of clinic-referred children. *Child Development, 67*(6), 3250–3262.

Gray, J. A. (1994). Three fundamental emotion systems. In P. Elkman & R. J. Davidson (Eds.), *The nature of emotion: Fundamental questions* (pp. 243–247). New York: Oxford University Press.

Gunnar, M. (1992). Reactivity of the hypothalamic–pituitary–adrenocortical system to stressors in normal infants and children. *Pediatrics, 80*(3), 491–497.

Gunnar, M. R. (2000). Early adversity and the development of stress reactivity and regulation. In C. A. Nelson (Ed.), *The effects of adversity on neurobehavioral development: Minnesota symposium on child psychology* (Vol. 31, pp. 163–200). Mahwah, NJ: Erlbaum.

Gunnar, M. R., & Donzella, B. (2002). Social regulation of the cortisol levels in early human development. *Psychoneuroendocrinology, 27,* 199–222.

Gunnar, M. R., Marvinney, D., Isensee, J., & Fisch, R. O. (Eds.). (1988). *Coping with uncertainty: New models of the relations between hormonal behavioral and cognitive processes.* Hillsdale, NJ: Erlbaum.

Gunnar, M. R., Morison, S. J., Chisholm, K., & Schuder, M. (2001). Long-term effects of institutional rearing on cortisol levels in adopted Romanian children. *Development and Psychopathology, 13*(3), 611–628.

Gunnar, M. R., Sebanc, A., Tout, K., Donzella, M. A., & van Dulman, M. (2003). Temperament, peer relationships, and cortisol activity in preschoolers. *Developmental Psychobiology, 43,* 346–368.

Gunnar, M. R., & Vazquez, D. M. (2006). Stress neurobiology and developmental psychopathology. In D. Cicchetti & D. Cohen (Eds.), *Developmental psychopathology: Vol. 2. Developmental neuroscience* (pp. 533–577). New York: Wiley.

Halligan, S., Herbert, J., Goodyer, I. M., & Murray, L. (2004). Exposure to postnatal depression predicts elevated cortisol in adolescent offspring. *Biological Psychiatry, 55,* 376–381.

Hardie, T. L., Moss, H. B., Vanyukov, M. M., Yao, J. K., & Kirillovac, G. P. (2002). Does adverse family environment or sex matter in the salivary cortisol responses to anticipatory stress? *Psychiatry Research, 111,* 121–131.

Hartup, W. W. (1979). Peer relations and the growth of social competence. In M. W. Kent & J. E. Rolf (Eds.), *Promoting social competence and coping in children* (Vol. 3, pp. 150–170). Hanover, NH: University Press of New England.

Heffelfinger, A. K., & Newcomer, J. W. (2001). Glucocorticoid effects on memory function over the human life span. *Development and Psychopathology, 13,* 491–513.

Heinrichs, M., Baumgartner, T., Kirschbaum, C., & Ehlert, U. (2003). Social support and oxytocin interact to suppress cortisol and subjective responses to psychosocial stress. *Biological Psychiatry, 54,* 1389–1398.

Herman, J. P., & Cullinan, W. E. (1997). Neurocircuitry of stress: Central control of the hypothalamo–pituitary–adrenocortical axis. *Trends in Neurosciences, 20,* 78–84.

Hertsgaard, L., Gunnar, M. R., Erickson, M., & Nachmias, M. (1995). Adrenocortical responses to the strange situation in infants with disorganized/disoriented attachment relationships. *Child Development, 66*(4), 1100–1106.

Hruschka, D. J., Kohrt, B. A., & Worthman, C. M. (2005). Estimating between- and within-individual variation in cortisol levels using multilevel models. *Psychoneuroendocrinology, 30,* 698–714.

Jansen, L. M. C., Gispen-deWied, C. C., Jasen, M. A., vander Gaag, R. J., Matthys, W., & van Engeland, H. (1999). Pituitary–adrenal reactivity in a child psychiatric population: Salivary cortisol response to stressors. *European Neuropsychopharmacology, 9,* 67–75.

Jonetz-Mentzel, L., & Wiedemann, G. (1993). Establishment of reference ranges for cortisol in neonates, infants, children and adolescents. *European Journal of Clinical Chemistry and Clinical Biochemistry, 31*, 525–529.

Kalin, N. H., Shelton, S. E., & Barksdale, C. M. (1989). Behavioral and physiologic effects of CRH administered to infant primates undergoing maternal separation. *Neuropsychopharmacology, 2*(2), 97–104.

Kaufman, J., Martin, A., King, R. A., & Charney, D. (2001). Are child-, adolescent-, and adult-onset depression one and the same disorder? *Biological Psychiatry, 49*, 980–1001.

Kenny, F. M., Gancayo, G., Heald, F. P., & Hung, W. (1966). Cortisol production rate in adolescent males at different stages of sexual maturation. *Journal of Clinical Endocrinology, 26*, 1232–1236.

Kenny, F. M., Preeyasambat, C., & Migeon, C. J. (1966). Cortisol production rate: II. Normal infants, children and adults. *Pediatrics, 37*, 34–42.

Kertes, D. A., Gunnar, M., Madsen, N. J., & Long, J. (in press). Early deprivation and home basal cortisol levels: A study of internationally-adopted children. *Development and Psychopathology.*

Kiess, W., Meidert, A., Dressendorfer, R. A., Schriever, K., Kessler, U., Konig, A., et al. (1995). Salivary cortisol levels throughout childhood and adolescence: Relation with age, pubertal stage, and weight. *Pediatric Research, 37*, 502–506.

King, J. A. (1998). Attention-deficit hyperactivity disorder and the stress response. *Biological Psychiatry, 44*, 72–74.

Kirschbaum, C., Barussek, D., & Strasburger, C. J. (1992). Cortisol responses to psychological stress and correlations with personality traits. *Personality and Individual Differences, 13*, 1353–1357.

Kirschbaum, C., & Hellhammer, D. H. (1989). Salivary cortisol in psychobiological research: An overview. *Neuropsychobiology, 22*, 150–169.

Kirschbaum, C., & Hellhammer, D. H. (1994). Salivary cortisol is psychoneuroendocrine research: Recent developments and applications. *Psychoneuroendocrinology, 19*(4), 313–333.

Kirschbaum, C., Klauer, T., Filipp, S. H., & Hellhammer, D.H. (1995). Sex-specific effects of social support on cortisol and subjective responses to acute psychological stress. *Psychosomatic Medicine, 57*, 23–31.

Kirschbaum, C., Kudielka, B. M., Gaab, J., Schommer, N., & Hellhammer, D. H. (1999). Impact of gender, menstrual cycle phase, and oral contraceptives on the activity of the hypothalamus–pituitary–adrenal axis. *Psychosomatic Medicine, 61*, 154–162.

Kirschbaum, C., Pirke, K., & Hellhammer, D. (1993). The "Trier Social Stress Test": A tool for investigating psychobiological stress responses in a laboratory setting. *Neuropsychobiology, 28*, 76–81.

Kirschbaum, C., Steyer, R., Eid, M., Patalla, U., Schwenkmezger, P., & Hellhammer, D. H. (1990). Cortisol and behavior: 2. Application of a latent state–trait model to salivary cortisol. *Psychoneuroendocrinology, 15*(4), 297–307.

Klimes-Dougan, B., Hastings, P. D., Granger, D. A., Usher, B. A., & Zahn-Waxler, C. (2001). Adrenocortical activity in at-risk and normally developing adolescents: Individual differences in salivary cortisol basal levels, diurnal variation, and responses to social challenges. *Development and Psychopathology, 13*, 695–719.

Klimes-Dougan, B., Shirtcliff, E., & Zahn-Waxler, C. (2006, August). *Diurnal and stress reactivity in the L-HPA axis for suicidal and nonsuicidal adolescents.* Paper presented at the annual meeting of the International Society of Psychoneuroendocrinology, Leiden, The Netherlands.

Kudielka, B. M., & Kirschbaum, C. (2005). Sex differences in HPA axis responses to stress: A review. *Biological Psychology, 69*, 113–132.

Larson, M., Gunnar, M., & Hertsgaard, L. (1991). The effects of morning naps, car trips, and maternal separation on adrenocortical activity of human infants. *Child Development, 62*(2), 362–372.

Larson, R. (1989). Beeping children and adolescents: A method for studying time use and daily experience. *Journal of Youth and Adolescence, 18*, 511–530.

Legendre, A., & Trudel, M. (1996). Cortisol and behavioral responses of young children coping with a group of unfamiliar peers. *Merrill–Palmer Quarterly, 42*(4), 554–577.

Levine, S. (1957). Infantile experience and resistance to physiological stress. *Science, 126*, 405–406.

Levine, S., & Wiener, S. G. (1988). Psychoendocrine aspects of mother-infant relationships in nonhuman primates. *Psychoneuroendocrinology, 13*(1–2), 143–154.

Luby, J. L., Heffelfinger, A., Mrakotsky, C., Brown, K., Hessler, M., & Spitznagel, E. (2003). Alterations in stress cortisol reactivity in depressed preschoolers relative to psychiatric and no-disorder comparison groups. *Archives of General Psychiatry, 60*, 1248–1255.

Lupien, S. J., Gillin, C. J., & Hauger, R. L. (1999). Working memory is more sensitive than declarative memory to the acute effects of corticosteroids: A dose–response study in humans. *Behavioral Neuroscience, 113*, 420–430.

Lupien, S. J., King, S., Meaney, M. J., & McEwen, B. S. (2001). Can poverty get under your skin? Basal cortisol levels and cognitive function in children from low and high socioeconomic status. *Development and Psychopathology, 13*, 653–676.

Lupien, S. J., & McEwen, B. S. (1997). The acute affects of corticosteroids on cognition: Integration of animal and human model studies. *Brain Research Review, 24*, 1–27.

Makino, S., Gold, P. W., & Schulkin, J. (1994). Effects of corticosterone on CRH mRNA and content in the bed nucleus of the stria terminals: Comparison with the effects in the central nucleus of the amygdala and the paraventricular nucleus of the hypothalamus. *Brain Research, 657*, 141–149.

Martel, F. L., Hayward, C., Lyons, D. M., Sanborn, K., Varady, S., & Schatzberg, A. F. (1999). Salivary cortisol levels in socially phobic adolescent girls. *Depression and Anxiety, 10*, 25–27.

Matthews, S. (2000). Antenatal glucocorticoids and the programming of the developing CNS. *Pediatric Research, 47*, 291–298.

McBurnett, K., Lahey, B. B., Frick, P. J., Risch, C., Loeber, R., Hart, E. L., et al.

(1991). Anxiety, inhibition, and conduct disorder in children: II. Relation to salivary cortisol. *Journal of the American Academy of Child and Adolescent Psychiatry, 30*(2), 192–196.

McBurnett, K., Lahey, B. B., Rathouz, P. J., & Loeber, R. (2000). Low salivary cortisol and persistent aggression in boys referred for disruptive behavior. *Archives of General Psychiatry, 57,* 38–43.

McBurnett, K., Pfiffner, L. J., Capasso, L., Lahey, B. B., & Loeber, R. (1997). Children's aggression and DSM-III-R symptoms predicted by parent psychopathology, parenting practices, cortisol, and SES. *NATO ASI Series: Series A: Life Sciences, 292,* 345–348.

McClelland, M., Morrison, F. J., & Holmes, D. L. (2000). Children at risk for early academic problems: The role of learning-related social skills. *Early Childhood Research Quarterly, 15,* 307–309.

McEwen, B. S., Weiss, J. M., & Schwartz, L. S. (1968). Selective retention of corticosterone by limbic structures in rat brain. *Nature, 220,* 911–912.

Miller Brotman, L., Kiely Gouley, K., Pine, D., & Rafferty, E. (2002, July). *Neuroendocrine functioning and behavior change among low-income, urban preschoolers at familiar risk for conduct problems: Preliminary results from a randomized prevention trial.* Paper presented at the Society for Research on Aggression, Montreal, Canada.

Mirescu, C., Peters, J. D., & Gould, E. (2004). Early life experience alters response of adult neurogenesis to stress. *Nature Neuroscience, 7*(8), 841–846.

Moss, H. B., Vanyukov, M. M., & Martin, C. S. (1995). Salivary cortisol responses and the risk for substance abuse in prepubertal boys. *Biological Psychiatry, 38,* 547–555.

Moss, H. B., Vanyukov, M. M., Yao, J. K., & Kirillova, G. P. (1999). Salivary cortisol responses in prepubertal boys: The effects of parental substance abuse and association with drug use behavior during adolescence. *Biological Psychiatry, 45,* 1293–1299.

Nachmias, M., Gunnar, M. R., Mangelsdorf, S., Parritz, R., & Buss, K. A. (1996). Behavioral inhibition and stress reactivity: Moderating role of attachment security. *Child Development, 67*(2), 508–522.

Netherton, C., Goodyer, I., Tamplin A., & Herbert J. (2004). Salivary cortisol and dehydroepiandrosterone in relation to puberty and gender. *Psychoneuroendocrinology, 29,* 125–140.

Oosterlaan, J., Geurts, H. M., Knol, D. L., & Sergeant, J. A. (2005). Low basal salivary cortisol associated with teacher-reported symptoms of conduct disorder. *Psychiatry Research, 134,* 1–10.

Pajer, K., Gardner, W., Kirillova, G. P., & Vanyukov, M. M. (2001). Sex differences in cortisol level and neurobehavioral disinhibition in children of substance abusers. *Journal of Child and Adolescent Substance Abuse, 10,* 65–76.

Pajer, K., Gardner, W., Rubin, R. T., Perel, J., & Neal, S. (2001). Decreased cortisol levels in adolescent girls with conduct disorder. *Archives of General Psychiatry, 58,* 297–302.

Pariante, C. M. (2003). Depression, stress and the adrenal axis. *Journal of Neuroendocrinology, 15,* 811–812.

Peeters, F., Nicholson, N.A., & Berkhof, J. (2004). Levels and variability of daily life cortisol secretion in major depression. *Psychiatry Research, 126,* 1–13.

Pendry, P., & Adam, E. K. (in press). Associations between interparental discord, parenting quality, parent emotion and cortisol levels in adolescent and kindergarten-aged children. *International Journal of Behavioral Development.*

Plihal, W., & Born, J. (1999). Memory consolidation in human sleep depends on inhibition of glucocorticoid release. *NeuroReport, 10*(13), 2741–2747.

Pruessner, J. C., Gaab, J., Hellhammer, D. H., Lintz, D., Schommer, N., & Kirschbaum, C. (1997). Increasing correlations between personality traits and cortisol stress responses obtained by data aggregation. *Psychoneuroendocrinology, 22,* 615–625.

Pruessner, J. C., Hellhammer, D. H., & Kirschbaum, C. (1999). Low self-esteem, induced failure, and the adrenocortical stress response. *Personality and Individual Differences, 27,* 477–489.

Pruessner, J. C., Wolf, O. T., Hellhammer, D. H., Buske-Kirschbaum, A., von Auer, K., Jobst, S., et al. (1997). Free cortisol levels after awakening: A reliable biological marker for the assessment of adrenocortical activity. *Life Sciences, 61,* 2539–2549.

Raine, A. (1996). *The psychopathology of crime: Criminal behavior as a clinical disorder.* San Diego, CA: Academic Press.

Repetti, R. L., Taylor, S. E., & Seeman, T. E. (2002). Risky families: Family social environments and the mental and physical health of offspring. *Psychological Bulletin, 128,* 330–366.

Ronsaville, D. S., Municchi, G., Laney, C., Cizza, G., Meyer, S. E., Haim, A., et al. (2006). Maternal and environmental factors influence the hypothalamic–pituitary–adrenal axis response to corticotropin-releasing hormone infusion in offspring of mothers with or without mood disorders. *Development and Psychopathology, 18*(1), 173–194.

Rosen, J. B., & Schulkin, J. (1998). From normal fear to pathological anxiety. *Psychological Review, 105,* 325–350.

Rosmond, R. (2005). Role of stress in the pathogenesis of the metabolic syndrome. *Psychoneuroendocrinology, 30,* 1–10.

Ryan, N. D. (1998). Psychoneuroendocrinology of children and adolescents. *Psychiatric Clinics of North America, 21,* 435–441.

Sadeh, A., Gruber, R., & Raviv, A. (2003). The effects of sleep restriction and extension on school-age children: What a difference an hour makes. *Child Development, 74,* 444–455.

Sanchez, M. M., Ladd, C. O., & Plotsky, P. M. (2001). Early adverse experience as a developmental risk factor for later psychopathology: Evidence from rodent and primate models. *Development and Psychopathology, 13,* 419–449.

Sapolsky, R. M. (2004). Social status and health in humans and other animals. *Annual Review of Anthropology, 33,* 393–418.

Sapolsky, R. M., Romero, L. M., & Munck, A. U. (2000). How do glucocorticoids influence stress responses? Integrating permissive, suppressive, stimulatory, and preparative actions. *Endocrine Reviews, 21,* 55–89.

Scerbo, A. S., & Kolko, D. J. (1994). Salivary testosterone and cortisol in disruptive children: Relationship to aggressive, hyperactive and internalizing behaviors. *Journal of the American Academy of Child and Adolescent Psychiatry, 33,* 1174–1184.

Schneider, M. L., & Moore, C. F. (2000). Effects of prenatal stress on development: A nonhuman primate model. In C. A. Nelson (Ed.), *The effects of early adversity on neurobehavioral development: The Minnesota Symposium on Child Psychology* (Vol. 31, pp. 201–244). Mahwah, NJ: Erlbaum.

Selye, H. (1936). A syndrome produced by diverse nocuous agents. *Nature, 38,* 32.

Shirtcliff, E. A., Granger, D., Booth, A., & Johnson, D. (2005). Low salivary cortisol level and externalizing behavior problems in youth. *Development and Psychopathology, 17,* 167–184.

Shirtcliff, E. A., Zahn-Waxler, C., & Klimes-Dougan, B. (2005, April). *Cortisol declivity during social challenge is related to stress and coping strategies in at risk adolescents.* Paper presented at the Society for Research in Child Development, Atlanta, GA.

Shoal, G., Giancola, P. R., & Kirrilova, G. (2003). Salivary cortisol, personality and aggressive behavior in adolescent boys: A 5-year longitudinal study. *Journal of the American Academy of Child and Adolescent Psychiatry, 42,* 1101–1107.

Smider, N. A., Essex, M. J., Kalin, N. H., Buss, K. A., Klein, M. H., Davidson, R. J., et al. (2002). Salivary cortisol as a predictor of socioemotional adjustment during kindergarten: A prospective study. *Child Development, 73,* 75–92.

Snoek, H., Van Goozen, S. H. M., Matthys, W., Buitelaar, J. K., & Van Engeland, H. (2004). Stress responsivity in children with externalizing behavior disorders. *Development and Psychopathology, 16,* 389–406.

Snoek, H., Van Goozen, S. H. M., Matthys, W., Sigling, H. O., Koppenschaar, H. P. F., Westenberg, H. G. M., et al. (2002). Serotonergic functioning in children with oppositional defiant disorder: A sumatriptan challenge study. *Biological Psychiatry, 51,* 319–325.

Soloff, P. H., Lynch, K. G., & Moss, H. B. (2000). Serotonin, impulsivity, and alcohol use disorders in the older adolescent: A psychobiological study. *Alcoholism, Clinical and Experimental Research, 24*(11), 1609–1619.

Spangler, G. (1995). School performance, type A behavior, and adrenocortical activity in primary school children. *Anxiety, Stress, and Coping, 8,* 299–310.

Spangler, G., & Schieche, M. (1998). Emotional and adrenocortical responses in infants to the Strange Situation: The differential function of emotion expression. *International Journal of Behavioral Development, 22,* 681–706.

Spear, L. P. (2000). The adolescent brain and age-related behavioral manifestations. *Neuroscience and Biobehavioral Reviews, 24,* 417–463.

Stroud, L. R., Papandonatos, G. D., Williamson, D. E., & Dahl, R. E. (2004). Sex differences in the effects of pubertal development on responses to a corticotropin-releasing hormone challenge: The Pittsburgh Psychobiologic Studies. *Annals of the New York Academy of Sciences, 1021,* 348–351.

Stroud, L. R., Salovey, P., & Epel, E. S. (2002). Sex differences in stress responses: Social rejection vs. achievement stress. *Biological Psychiatry, 52,* 318–327.

Suchecki, D., Rosenfeld, P., & Levine, S. (1993). Maternal regulation of the hypothalamic–pituitary–adrenal axis in the rat: The roles of feeding and stroking. *Developmental Brain Research, 75*(2), 185–192.

Sullivan, R. M., & Gratton, A. (1999). Lateralized effects of medial prefrontal cortex lesions on neuroendocrine and autonomic stress responses in rats. *Journal of Neuroscience, 19*, 2834–2840.

Susman, E. J., Dorn, E. D., Inoff-Germain, G., Nottelman, E. D., & Chrousos, G. P. (1997). Cortisol reactivity, distress behavior, and behavioral and psychological problems in young adolescents: A longitudinal perspective. *Journal of Research on Adolescence, 7*, 81–105.

Susman, E. J., Dorn, L. D., & Chrousos, P. (1991). Negative affect and hormone levels in young adolescents: Concurrent and predictive perspectives. *Journal of Youth and Adolescence, 20*(2), 167–190.

Susman, E. J., Schmeelk, K. H., Worrall, B. K., Granger, D. A., Ponirakis, A., & Chrousos, G. P. (1999). Corticotropin-releasing hormone and cortisol: Longitudinal associations with depression and antisocial behavior in pregnant adolescents. *Journal of the American Academy of Child and Adolescent Psychiatry, 38*, 460–467.

Tafet, G. E., & Bernardini, R. (2003). Psychoneuroendocrinological links between chronic stress and depression. *Progress in Neuro-Psychopharmacology and Biological Psychiatry, 27*, 893–903.

Targum, S. D., Clarkson, L. L., Magac-Harris, K., Marshall, L. E., & Skwerer, R. G. (1990). Measurement of cortisol and lymphocyte subpopulations in depressed and conduct-disordered adolescents. *Journal of Affective Disorders, 18*, 91–96.

Taylor, S. E., Klein, L. C., Lewis, B. P., Gruenewald, T. L., Gurung, R. A., & Updegraff, J. A. (2000). Biobehavioral responses to stress in females: Tend-and-befriend, not fight-or-flight. *Psychological Review, 107*, 411–429.

Tennes, K., & Kreye, M. (1985). Children's adrenocortical responses to classroom activities and tests in elementary school. *Psychosomatic Medicine, 47*(5), 451–460.

Tennes, K., Kreye, M., Avitable, N., & Wells, R. (1986). Behavioral correlates of excreted catecholamines and cortisol in second-grade children. *Journal of the American Academy of Child Psychiatry, 25*, 764–770.

Tornhage, C. J. (2002). Reference values for morning salivary cortisol concentrations in healthy school-aged children. *Journal of Pediatric Endocrinology and Metabolism, 15*, 197–204.

Van De Wiel, N. M., Van Goozen, S. H., Matthys, W., Snoek, H., & van Engeland, H. (2004). Cortisol and treatment effect in children with disruptive behavior disorders: A preliminary study. *Journal of the American Academy of Child and Adolescent Psychiatry, 43*, 1011–1018.

van Eck, M., Berkhof, H., Nicolson, N., & Sulon, J. (1996). The effects of perceived stress, traits, mood states, and stressful daily events on salivary cortisol. *Psychosomatic Medicine, 58*, 447–458.

van Eck, M., Nicolson, N. A., Berkhof, H., & Sulon, J. (1996). Individual differences in cortisol responses to a laboratory speech task and their relationship to responses to stressful daily events. *Biological Psychology, 43,* 69–84.

Van Goozen, S. H., Matthys, W., Cohen-Kettenis, P. T., Buittelaar, J. K., & van Engeland, H. (2000). Hypothalamic–pituitary–adrenal axis and autonomic nervous system activity in disruptive children and matched controls. *Journal of the American Academy of Child and Adolescent Psychiatry, 39,* 1438–1445.

Van Goozen, S. H., Matthys, W., Cohen-Kettenis, P. T., Gispen-de Wied, C., Wiegant, V. M., & van Engeland, H. (1998). Salivary cortisol and cardiovascular activity during stress in oppositional defiant disordered boys and normal controls. *Biological Psychiatry, 43,* 531–539.

Vanyukov, M. M., Moss, H. B., Plial, J. A., Blackson, T., Mezzich, A. C., & Tarter, R. E. (1993). Antisocial symptoms in preadolescent boys and in their parents: Associations with cortisol. *Psychiatry Research, 46*(1), 9–17.

Vazquez, D. M. (1998). Stress and the developing limbic–hypothalamic–pituitary–adrenal axis. *Psychoneuroendocrinology, 23,* 663–700.

Wadhwa, P. D., Dunkel-Schetter, C., Chicz-DeMet, A., Porto, M., & Sandman, C. A. (1996). Prenatal psychosocial factors and the neuroendocrine axis in human pregnancy. *Psychosomatic Medicine, 58,* 432–446.

Walker, E. F., Walder, D. J., & Reynolds, F. (2001). Developmental changes in cortisol secretion in normal and at-risk youth. *Development and Psychopathology, 13,* 721–732.

Watamura, S. E., Donzella, B., Alwin, J., & Gunnar, M. (2003). Morning to afternoon increases in cortisol concentrations for infants and toddlers at child care: Age differences and behavioral correlates. *Child Development, 74*(4), 1006–1020.

Watamura, S., Donzella, B., Kertes, D., & Gunnar, M. (2004). Developmental changes in baseline cortisol activity in early childhood: Relations with napping and effortful control. *Developmental Psychobiology, 45,* 125–133.

Watamura, S., Sebanc, A., Donzella, B., & Gunnar, M. (2002). Naptime at childcare: Effects on salivary cortisol levels. *Developmental Psychobiology, 40,* 33–42.

Weaver, I. C., Cervoni, N., Champagne, F. A., D'Alessio, A. C., Sharma, S., Seckl, J. R., et al. (2004). Epigenetic programming by maternal behavior. *Nature Neuroscience, 7*(8), 847–854.

Wellberg, L. A., & Seckl, J. R. (2001). Prenatal stress, glucocorticoids, and the programming of the brain. *Journal of Neuroendocrinology, 13,* 113–128.

Wolf, O. T., Schommer, N. C., Hellhammer, D. H., McEwen, B. S., & Kirschbaum, C. (2001). The relationship between stress induced cortisol levels and memory differs between men and women. *Psychoneuroendocrinology, 26,* 711–720.

Wüst, S., Federenko, I., Hellhammer, D. H., & Kirschbaum, C. (2000). Genetic factors, perceived chronic stress, and the free cortisol response to awakening. *Psychoneuroendocrinology, 25,* 707–20.

Wüst, S., Federenko, I., Van Rossum, E., Koper, J. W., Kumsta, R., Entringer, S., et al. (2004). A psychobiological perspective on genetic determinants of hypothalamic–pituitary–adrenal axis activity. *Annals of the New York Academy of Sciences, 1032,* 52–62.

Wüst, S., Van Rossum, E., Federenko, I., Koper, J. W., Kumsta, R., & Hellhammer, D. H. (2004). Common polymorphism in the glucocorticoid receptor gene are associated with adrenocortical responses to psychosocial stress. *Journal of Clinical Endocrinology and Metabolism, 89*(2), 565–573.

Yehuda, R., Halligan, S. L., & Grossman, R. (2001). Childhood trauma and risk for PTSD: Relationship to intergenerational effects of trauma, parental PTSD, and CORT excretion. *Development and Psychopathology, 13,* 733–753.

Yehuda, R., Teicher, R. L., Trestman, R., & Siever, L. J. (1996). Cortisol regulation in posttraumatic stress disorder and major depression: A chronobiological analysis. *Biological Psychiatry, 40,* 79–88.

Young, L. A., & Altemus, M. (2004). Puberty, ovarian steroids, and stress. *Annals of the New York Academy of Sciences, 1021,* 124–133.

Zahn-Waxler, C., Klimes-Dougan, B., & Slattery, M. (2000). Internalizing disorders of childhood and adolescence: Progress and prospects for advances in understanding anxiety and depression. *Development and Psychopathology, 12,* 443–466.

CHAPTER 12

Child Maltreatment and the Development of Alternate Pathways in Biology and Behavior

Catherine C. Ayoub
Gabrielle Rappolt-Schlichtmann

Approximately one million cases of child abuse are substantiated through child protective services in the United States each year, but experts indicate that this figure is actually an underestimate of child maltreatment (U.S. Department of Health and Human Services, 2005). The effects of child maltreatment are not only acute distress, but also lasting changes in psychological and physiological functioning throughout childhood and into adulthood (Briere, 1992a). Child maltreatment is a risk factor for psychiatric illness, including depression, suicide, borderline personality disorder, posttraumatic stress disorder (PTSD), dissociative disorders, and somatization disorders (Walker et al., 1999), violence and criminal behavior, substance abuse, learning and school problems, and poor physical health (Felitti et al., 1998).

Over the past decade researchers have begun to document an association between the experience of trauma related to maltreatment and neuroanatomical and neurophysiological differences (Cicchetti & Toth, 2005; DeBellis, 2001; Teicher, 2000). Such differences might be related to the stress associated with the experience of maltreatment; there is now good evidence that exposure to severe stress early in life leads to atypical neurodevelopment (e.g., see Adam, Klimes-Dougan, & Gunnar, Chapter 11, this volume). As a result of severely stressful experiences early in life, a stress-sensitive and atypical neurodevelopmental pathway may emerge that appears to be adaptive for the child in the context of a high-stress environment, but which is maladaptive in the context of more benign environments the individual may face later in life.

The study of alternative developmental pathways is based in the new field of *developmental traumatology,* a term coined by DeBellis (2001) to describe the interface of development and biology in the context of interpersonal violence. Developmental traumatology synthesizes knowledge from developmental psychology, developmental psychopathology, and trauma research to offer hypotheses about the brain–behavior connections, over time, that influence human functioning. The field focuses on children with complex developmental disorders that result from environmental influences; child maltreatment is one of the most pervasive and powerful of such influences (DeBellis, 2001).

In this chapter we describe a framework for understanding the psychobiological impact of maltreatment on children's development within the field of developmental traumatology. Our framework, called a *developmental pathways model,* emphasizes the highly complex and adaptive nature of maltreated children's behavior and biology. We extend earlier writing regarding the psychological and behavioral effects of maltreatment (Fischer et al., 1997) to include a discussion of the biological effects of such experiences. We outline hypotheses regarding the link between aspects of the atypical developmental pathway associated with maltreatment and specific brain functions.

ALTERNATE DEVELOPMENTAL PATHWAYS AND THE EMERGENCE OF ADAPTIVE SKILLS

Traditional views on psychopathology resulting from early maltreatment experiences have posited that such experiences lead to immaturity or developmental delay characterized by fixation or regression (Freud, 1966). In fact, evidence has not supported the notion that maltreated children are delayed, fixated, or regressed in their development. Instead, evidence suggests that maltreated children demonstrate complex skills, requisite to their particular, unique experience, which are on par with their nonmaltreated age-mates, even when psychopathology is evident (Ayoub et al., 2006; Fischer et al., 1997). Our research applies this alternate lens to trauma, focusing on how seemingly atypical behavior and biology among maltreated children can be both adaptive and complex.

Rather than viewing development as unidirectional and domain general, with one universal and normative developmental trajectory, the developmental pathways approach is one in which development is viewed as multidimensional and increasingly complex over time. Through this lens of ever-increasing complexity involving integrative and differentiating developmental functions over time, variation among individuals is dependent upon the interface of the timing and nature of individuals' experiences with their developmental processes. In turn, the nature and context of traumatic experiences have the potential to change physiological and psychological functioning in a manner that leads these children on an alternative developmental trajectory.

Consider, for example, the effects of maltreatment on the development of attachment. Research has shown that abusive or neglectful parental behavior often results in the formation of insecure attachment on the part of the child (Crittenden, 1985; Egeland & Sroufe, 1981; Schneider-Rosen, Braunwald, Carlson, & Cicchetti, 1985; Schneider-Rosen & Cicchetti, 1984). As a result, in the context of attachment situations, maltreated children's behavior toward their parents tends to be disorganized and erratic, shifting between approach and avoidance behaviors (Cicchetti, 1991; Crittenden, 1988). This pattern of interaction with parents may later generalize and become elaborated in the individuals' other relationships with adults and peers, such that individuals who have experienced abuse may appear unpredictable, volatile, and rigid (Darwish, Esquivel, Houtz, & Alfonso, 2001; Mueller & Silverman, 1989). The pattern of approach–avoidance exhibited by abused children, however, is likely adaptive in a high-risk context, serving a self-regulatory and self-protective function. In the context of an environment in which the primary caregiver might be alternatively nurturing and abusive, such behavior can be considered both complex and organized (Ayoub, Fischer, & O'Connor, 2003). Moreover, these adaptive attachment behaviors likely become even more sophisticated as the maltreated children hone their defenses over time. In this way, children who have experienced maltreatment remain on par with nonabused peers with respect to the relative complexity of skills but are nevertheless at significant risk for psychopathology (Briere, 1992b; Putnam, 1994). Thus, abused children's behavior is both adaptive and maladaptive, making survival in the home possible but survival in other contexts challenging.

As demonstrated in this example, the developmental pathways framework places emphasis on the unique experiences of maltreated children and the resulting organization of their behavior into adaptive and complex skill sets. The pathways view is based on the theoretical perspective of Fischer and Bidell (1998), which emphasizes the existence and nature of the many varied pathways traversed by individuals as they grow in diverse environments, developing complex and adaptive skills. Skills are constructed gradually over the course of development through practice in real activities during interaction with others and independently (Fischer & Granott, 1995); an individual may develop a skill to ride a bike, understand metaphor, make new friends, or interpret facial expressions. A developmental pathway forms a web of multiple growing skills, rather than a single ladder of stages that is the classical developmental assumption (Fischer, 1980; Fischer & Bidell, 1998). This web structure is the norm for children's full range of developing skills.

The web construct allows for more than linear associations of skills across domains. Each strand can be separate or connected at any given point in the child's development. This concept is illustrated in Figure 12.1. Here we see the development of two children, one following a normative integrative pattern and the other demonstrating a pattern resulting from dissociative coping strategies, a typical adaptive mechanism of some maltreated children (see also Ayoub & Fischer, 2006). Specifically, the trauma of child maltreatment can affect the coordination of skills across development. In the case of abuse or neglect, children often actively separate, rather than coordinate, events and anxieties as an adaptive strategy to avoid being overwhelmed by fear and anxiety. In essence, fragmentation of

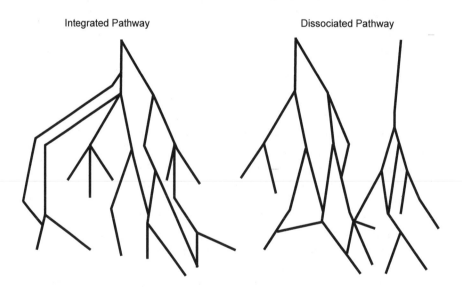

FIGURE 12.1. Two developmental webs illustrating relatively integrated (*left*) and dissociated (*right*) pathways. Courtesy of Kurt Fischer.

thoughts and feelings serves an adaptive function, allowing the child to limit the experience of severe anxiety and helplessness and to maintain functioning in order to survive. If maltreatment is recurrent, which it often is, these traumatogenic responses become habitual and generalized. The routine and generalized use of these different ways of thinking and feeling mark what we call a *traumatogenic alternative developmental pathway*.

Although the behavioral and psychological literature on child maltreatment has shifted to allow for the consideration of maltreated children's behavior as adaptive and complex, the research literature on the neurobiological sequelae of child maltreatment has not. In particular, researchers have characterized the excessive stress of child maltreatment as a toxic agent, interfering with normal brain development and resulting in altered and impaired brain function (e.g., Bremner et al., 1997; DeBellis et al., 1999; Schiffer, Teicher, & Papanicolaou, 1995). Although it is true that early stress can affect developmental processes at both the biological and behavioral levels, we argue that the result is not an impaired brain but rather a unique brain, actively adapted to survive in a malevolent social world. In the remaining sections of this chapter we elaborate the developmental pathways framework to include the neurobiological level of analysis, beginning with a review of the literature on the neurobiological consequences and corresponding behavioral correlates of child maltreatment.

THE NEUROBIOLOGY OF CHILD MALTREATMENT

To date, very few prospective, longitudinal, or even cross-sectional studies of the neurodevelopment of maltreated children have been conducted. Rather, most studies have been correlational in design, and as such, we caution against taking a causal view of the neurobiological findings reported here. As more prospective and cross-sectional studies are completed, the nature of the effects described here will become clearer. In the meantime understanding how the neurobiology of maltreated children, particularly those with negative behavioral and psychiatric outcomes, is different from that of their healthy agemates will provide a preliminary lens for interpreting the alternate developmental pathways maltreated children exhibit, informing both future research and our understanding of clinical outcomes. The evidence for brain correlates of maltreatment suggests several hypotheses about relations between alternate pathways, illustrated through behavioral studies and possible brain functions.

Neuroimaging studies comparing maltreated and nonmaltreated children have demonstrated variable structural and functional differences (see Teicher et al., 2003, for a review), providing evidence for one or more alternative neurodevelopmental pathways in maltreated children. Among the differences found in maltreated children are a smaller corpus callosum; attenuation of the development of the left neocortex, hippocampus, and amygdala; enhanced electrical activity in the limbic system; and reduced activity of the cerebellar vermis. For example, Carrion and colleagues (2001) assessed the frontal lobe asymmetry of 24 children with trauma histories and PTSD symptoms. They found that the maltreated children had attenuated frontal lobe asymmetry. In 2003, Teicher and his colleagues measured the regional corpus callosum from magnetic resonance imaging (MRI) scans in 52 children admitted for psychiatric evaluation, of whom 28 were identified as abuse or neglect victims. These children were compared to 115 healthy children. The researchers found that the corpus callosum of the maltreated children was 17% smaller than in the comparison children. The greatest difference was evident in the neglected children and was associated with a 15–18% reduction in regions 3, 4, 5, and 7 of the corpus callosum. These two studies are examples of recent advances in the field; such findings suggest ways in which a combination of new imaging techniques can support the associations between behavioral observations and brain activity to better understand the development of alternative pathways.

To generalize advances from a neurodevelopmental perspective, we have begun to identify brain regions that have a high density of glucocorticoid receptors and a long period of postnatal development as those that are particularly vulnerable to the stress of early maltreatment. Such findings help to explain the structural and functional differences observed across individuals based on their exposure to traumatic experiences.

The Hippocampus, Memory, and Behavioral Inhibition

The hippocampus plays a central role in the verbal recall aspect of explicit memory; stress experiences strongly shape such memory (Teicher et al., 2003). The stress of abuse trauma influences a number of functions related to the hippocampus, including changes in the creation of semantic memory, specifically memory deficits (e.g., amnesia), and alterations in memory (e.g., intrusive memories) and concentration (e.g., increased dissociation)—which are all common in PTSD (Joseph, 1999; Newport & Nemeroff, 2000). It comes as no surprise, then, that the hippocampus seems to have a particular vulnerability to severe stress experiences (Gould & Tanapat, 1999; Sapolsky, Uno, Rebert, & Finch, 1990). Specifically, the hippocampus has a long postnatal developmental period and a high density of glucocorticoid receptors, making it vulnerable to cortisol neurotoxicity and thus severe stress (Patel et al., 2000; Sapolsky, McEwen, & Rainbow, 1983). Studies investigating the effect of childhood abuse on the structure and function of the hippocampus have yielded mixed results in different age groups. A reduction in left hippocampal volume has been reported in adults with a childhood history of trauma and current PTSD (Bremner et al., 1997; Stein, 1977). Bilateral reduction in hippocampal volume has been reported in women with a history of child abuse and borderline personality disorder (Driessen et al., 2000). In contrast, studies of maltreated children and adolescents consistently report no reduction in hippocampal volume in comparison to healthy controls (Carrion et al., 2001; DeBellis et al., 1999; Teicher et al., 2003).

These discrepancies in the data may reflect a developmental trend in which the effects of early abuse on hippocampal structure emerge over the course of development (Sapolsky, Krey, & McEwen, 1985; Teicher et al., 2003), or it may be the case that preexisting small hippocampal volume is a risk factor among adult individuals for the development of PTSD and other psychiatric illnesses following child abuse (Teicher et al., 2003). It is also possible that the psychological and behavioral sequelae of early stress and abuse may play a direct role in the effects on hippocampal volume seen in adults. Specifically, the onset of psychiatric illness and risky coping behaviors such as alcohol and drug abuse in adolescence may precipitate the reduction in hippocampal volume that has been reported among adult survivors of child maltreatment (Dunn, Ryan, & Dunn, 1994; Ellason, Ross, Sainton, & Mayran, 1996; van der Kolk, & Fisler, 1994). More research is needed to decipher the nature of the relationship between early severe stress and later hippocampal structure. However, concern remains because damage to the hippocampus may affect an individual's ability to form new memories and access or organize previously formed memories (Newport & Nemeroff, 2000; Teicher et al., 2003).

The behavioral and psychological sequelae of alterations to hippocampal functioning among maltreated children may manifest primarily as disruptions to the encoding and retrieval of episodic memories, and secondarily as the inhibition of ongoing behavior that is inappropriate to the environment (Teicher et al., 2003). We have documented these behaviors among maltreated children in our laboratory. Specifically, we have examined maltreated toddlers' performance in a structured task for negative and positive storytelling (Ayoub et al., 2006). In this study, children were asked to retell and/or act out a series of stories involving interactions that were nice, mean, or a combination of nice and mean. The stories began simply with a nice interaction between the self doll and a friend doll—or a child doll and a parent doll—at the developmental level of single representations, defined in terms of dynamic skill theory (Fischer, 1980; Fischer, Shaver, &

Carnochan, 1990). Stories were told in order of increasing complexity, forming a developmental sequence based on skill complexity. Children's performance on each story was coded on two variables. First, each story was coded on whether the participant successfully retold it. To successfully pass a story task at a particular level of complexity the participant had to attend to the story and accurately represent the characters as nice or mean, including the various component parts of the story. The representations could be performed either verbally or nonverbally. Each child received a skill level score for correct completions. Second, the children's stories were coded for complexity of representation regardless of whether or not the story was retold correctly. For example, a child might fail to accurately retell the story by switching the mean and nice characters, or by making a nice story mean, but his or her story might be highly complex nonetheless. In this procedure, children were scored according to the complexity of the story with which they exhibited the highest skill level, regardless of whether they recounted the story correctly. These two forms of coding made it possible to separate the developmental level of performance that matched the modeled stories from the developmental level in general.

Hierarchical regression analyses were conducted in order to investigate whether having a history of maltreatment affected children's complexity of performance in the nice and mean storytelling tasks. Among both maltreated and nonmaltreated participants, older children correctly retold higher-level stories and told more complex stories regardless of passing. There was an effect of having a maltreatment history on children's complexity of storytelling performance, but only for the structured component of the assessment. That is, children with a maltreatment history tended to successfully complete fewer story tasks prior to three failures than did their nonmaltreated peers. This "gap" between the maltreated and nonmaltreated performances was larger among older children. Importantly, there were no differences in the complexity of stories told between maltreated and nonmaltreated participants when correctness was not taken into account. These effects are illustrated in Figure 12.2.

Maltreated children's alternate developmental pathway in this domain is clearly illustrated in this example. In Figure 12.2A we see that older children, whether maltreated or nonmaltreated, tend to exhibit higher skill levels in correctly representing nice/mean interactions during this structured storytelling task. However, in comparison, the maltreated and nonmaltreated groups exhibit different developmental trajectories. Specifically, young maltreated children tend to produce more complex stories when correct early on, but the rate at which they become more complex and correct over time is slower in comparison to their nonmaltreated peers. This devel-

(A) Only correct performances count

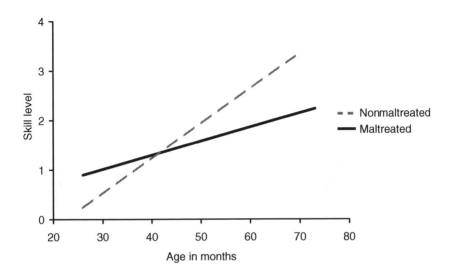

(B) Any performance counts

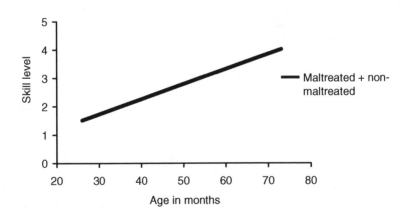

FIGURE 12.2. Maltreated and nonmaltreated children's cognitive performance under two conditions: performance, accuracy, and complexity on the structured storytelling task when (A) only correct performances count and when (B) any performance counts.

opmental trajectory results in a large "gap" in performance by 5 years of age, with the nonmaltreated children tending to retell more complex nice and mean stories correctly.

From these findings it would seem that the traditional characterization of maltreated children as "delayed" might be correct at least in part, but there is more to this story—as evidenced by the performance of children who have been maltreated on incorrect and negative stories. In Figure 12.2B we see that without the constraint of having to correctly retell the story, there are no differences in the maltreated and nonmaltreated children's performances throughout early childhood. The maltreated children tell mean and nice relationship stories just as complex as their peers, but only under particular conditions. On closer examination of the data we found that the maltreated children were more distractible, often refusing to do the task as presented, and tended to "switch" the content of nice stories to mean. They also tended to "fail" at telling the nice stories and to spend much more time and energy than their counterparts telling richly detailed negative stories. Overall, they had difficulty inhibiting their negative impulses in the stories.

Our behavioral data illustrate that it is not that the maltreated children are "delayed"; rather, they exhibit an alternate developmental path commensurate with their early experience, demonstrating more skill with, and selective attention to, negative situations and relationships (Fischer et al., 1997). Our work, like that of others, demonstrates that this developmental pathway seems to render attention and persistence on structured school-like tasks difficult (Porter, 2003), especially for tasks that do not capitalize on these children's honed skills around threat-related signals (Pollak & Tolley-Schell, 2003). These findings support those noted in older maltreated children. For example, Pollak and Sinha (2002) found that school-age, physically abused children detected angry emotions at lower steps in a visual sequence of increasingly angry facial expressions than their nonmaltreated counterparts, but showed no differences when responding to other facial displays. Similarly, Dodge and his colleagues (Dodge, Pettit, Bates, & Valente, 1995) found that school-age abused children attributed hostility to others in situations in which most people would not make such an attribution. All of these behavioral findings of memory-related differences in maltreated children, including both intrusive memories that distract the child from responding to the current surroundings and avoidance of painful memories that skew the child's responses to daily interactions, can be linked to changes in hippocampal functioning. Future studies of the interface will strengthen the brain–behavior argument and provide further support for a pathways model of alternative development.

The Amygdala, the Cerebellar Vermis, Negative Affect, and Complex Behavior in Alternate Pathways

The amygdala has also been identified as a structure affected by the trauma of childhood abuse, although findings pertaining to the association between maltreatment and abnormal amygdala volume are even less consistent than those reported for the hippocampus. The amygdala is a component of the limbic system and is believed to play a key role in emotions, particularly in fear and vigilance (Pollak, Cicchetti & Klorman, 1998). Although most studies of amygdala volume have revealed no differences between adults with a childhood history of abuse and age-matched controls (Bremner et al., 1997; DeBellis et al., 1999; Stein, 1997), Driessen and colleagues (2000) reported an 8% reduction in amygdala volume bilaterally in adult female survivors of child abuse who also were diagnosed with borderline personality disorder. Other studies have reported that adults with a history of combined physical and sexual abuse and children with concurrent psychiatric issues showed abnormal and hyperactive amygdala activity (Ito et al., 1993; Teicher, Glod, Surrey, & Swett, 1993).

The functioning of the cerebellar vermis may also be affected by the experience of child maltreatment. The cerebellar vermis is a narrow structure that links the two hemispheres of the cerebellum; it is one of the last brain structures to fully develop in the postnatal period and is vulnerable to glucocorticoid toxicity and thus severe stress (Giedd et al., 1999). It is thought to play an inhibitory role in limbic system activation (Anderson, Teicher, Polcari, & Renshaw, 2002). Abnormalities of the cerebellar vermis have been linked to a wide array of psychiatric disorders, including schizophrenia (Andreasen, Paradiso, & O'Leary, 1998), autism (Courchesne, 1991), attention-deficit/hyperactivity disorder (Mostofsky, Reiss, Lockhart, & Denckla, 1998), and depression (Lauterbach, 1996). Anderson and colleagues (2002) found the activity of the cerebellar vermis to be lower in adults with a history of child abuse and neglect as compared to healthy controls. They used steady-state functional magnetic resonance imaging (fMRI) to assess resting blood flow in the vermis of 24 young adults, a third of whom had a history of repeated child sexual abuse. Child sexual abuse survivors had higher T2 relaxation times when compared to the community controls. The vermal T2-RT also correlated strongly with Limbic System Checklist–33 (LSCL-33) ratings of temporal lobe epilepsy-like symptomatology. These findings, however promising, have not yet been replicated. Much more research on the effects of child maltreatment on the development of the cerebellar vermis is needed before implications can be drawn definitively.

Altered amygdala or cerebellar vermis functioning may have an impact on children's emotional functioning; specifically, alterations to amygdala or cerebellar vermis functioning among severely maltreated children and adolescents may result in frequent impulsive violence, increased fear and negativity, and may contribute to the development of PTSD and depression (Teicher et al., 2003). Abuse victims frequently show violence, depression, and PTSD, all of which are consistent with disturbances in the amygdalae and the cerebellar vermis (Newport & Nemeroff, 2000).

Findings from our behavioral and psychiatric studies of girls who have been abused might also be related to alterations in amygdalar and cerebellar functioning. In our laboratory, we have examined sexually and physically abused adolescent girls' perceptions of themselves and their relationships in an effort to identify behaviors that were associated with given abuse experiences. In addition, we reviewed each girl's psychiatric diagnoses and compared them to those of girls who were depressed but had not experienced abuse (Ayoub, Hong, Wright, Fischer, & Noam, 2004). To measure self-perception, we used the Self-in-Relationship Interview (Calverley, Fischer, & Ayoub, 1994). This interview supports adolescents and adults in characterizing themselves in relationships. It also is designed to detect the full range of a person's cognitive developmental levels and to assess the effects of variation in contextual support. Each girl was interviewed using a semistructured format that asked her to describe what she was like—her perception of self—in various important relationships: those with mother, father, best girlfriend, romantic friend, and "the real you no matter who you are with." For each relationship, the girls were asked to write down five self-descriptions on separate pieces of self-sticking paper, thus coming up with a total of 25 different descriptions of self in relationships. The girls then assigned each description a valence: either positive,[1] negative,[2] or mixed valence. Each label was placed on a "self-diagram" consisting of three concentric circles representing the core, middle, and outer self. Self-descriptions placed in the core circle were labeled most important, whereas those placed in the outer circle were labeled least important.

We coded all maltreated adolescents for the type, severity, frequency, duration, and timing of maltreatment and perpetrator's identity by episode on the basis of the Maltreatment Classification System developed by Barnett, Manly, and Cicchetti (1993). Psychiatric diagnoses were obtained from the clinician's discharge report and the Diagnostic Interview Schedule for Children (DISC-C).[3] The psychiatric diagnoses were based on DSM-III-R, which was in use at the time of data collection. Psychiatric background variables were obtained from each girl's medical records, including the admission and discharge reports, treatment team conference summaries, social worker's notes, clinician's individual and group therapy notes, and psychoeducational reports. These variables included the number of psychiatric hospitalizations, number of psychoactive medications taken while hospitalized, whether they had received outpatient psychotherapy prior to hospitalization, and psychiatric history of the family.

Girls were divided into groups that differentiated their specific and cumulative maltreatment status, including girls who experienced sexual abuse only and girls with co-occurring sexual and physical abuse/neglect. Two additional groups of depressed girls were identified, one group with no maltreatment history and a second group of girls with a history of physical abuse/neglect but no sexual abuse history.

First, we found that the frequency of negative perceptions of self was highest among sexually abused girls. Furthermore, sexually abused girls were much more likely to rank their negative perceptions of themselves and their relationships as most important to their "true" or core self, whereas girls who had been physically abused or experienced no abuse saw negative perceptions as much less important. Those sexually abused girls with co-occurring physical abuse were the most negative in their perceptions of self, followed by the group of girls with sexual abuse only, as illustrated in Figure 12.3. In spite of significant differences in the organization of their perceptions of themselves in relationships, the sexually abused girls and the remaining girls in the sample evidenced normal levels of cognitive complexity across their descriptions (Fischer et al., 1997).

This work led us to describe at least two distinctive characteristics of alternative developmental pathways of abuse: representations of self and others that center on negative evaluation rather than positive, and dissociative splitting that develops at complex and sophisticated levels (Calverley et al., 1994; Fischer & Ayoub, 1994). As we hypothesized, these behavioral findings are consistent with the biological changes noted in studies of the amygdala and the cerebellar vermis mentioned above. The behavioral characteristics of the two key components of our proposed traumatogenic developmental pathway found in the abused girls include symptoms of increased negativity, dissociation, and PTSD symptoms that may be attributed to the amygdala, because it plays a central role in consolidating the emotional significance of traumatic events, and to the cerebellar vermis because it modulates stress in maltreated children and adolescents.

In a second set of findings, the sexually abused girls—both those with sexual abuse as their sole form of maltreatment and those with sexual abuse as one of multiple forms of maltreatment—experienced a similar constellation of symptoms unique to their sexual abuse categorization. We have combined these self-destructive behaviors into an interaction style we call *self-focused aggression*. Such self-focused aggressive indicators include

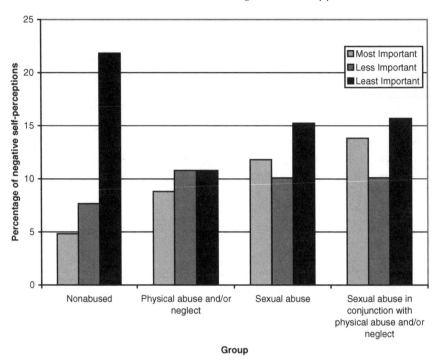

FIGURE 12.3. Average percentage of negative self-perceptions of adolescent girls assigned to each category of importance to the self, out of total number of negative self-perceptions by maltreatment classification.

histories of suicide attempts, self-mutilation, PTSD, and substance abuse. Thirty-nine percent of the sexually abused girls were diagnosed with borderline personality disorder, which is described by the American Psychiatric Association (2000) as a pervasive pattern of instability in interpersonal relationships, self-image, and affect, marked by impulsivity and a tendency to view relationships in the extreme. A core characteristic of this disorder is a tremendous fear of loss of relationships and anticipation of such loss in everyday encounters.

In summary, sexually abused girls, on average, are aggressive toward themselves more than toward others, putting them at serious risk for suicide, substance abuse, self-mutilation, and other self-destructive behavior. These serious self-destructive behaviors can be interpreted as attempts to escape from the intense pain and anxiety of posttraumatic hyperarousal or to assert the need to "feel real" in the context of chronic numbing and avoidance. These findings support the work of Shipman, Zeman, Penza, and Champion (2000) that demonstrates that sexually abused girls anticipate more conflict and less support in relationships. Recent work in trauma and psychopathology supports a connection between the repeated trauma of abuse and a pervasive array of changes in thinking and emotion that involve serious disturbance in perceptions of self (Cole & Putnam, 1992; Herman, 1992; Terr, 1991). Such approach–avoidance mechanisms are an example of what we have call *polarized affective skills* for splitting or dissociating across domains, in this case, from hypervigilance to numbing. The other girls, in spite of being depressed like their sexually abused counterparts, did not see themselves as negative in this way nor did they show dramatic switching in patterns of activity across contexts.

These behavioral and psychiatric findings are consistent with the patterns associated with reported alterations to the amygdala and cerebellar vermis among female sexual abuse survivors as reported in the neurobiological literature. The emergence of enhanced fight or flight reactions, aggression, hypervigilance, negative worldview, and even complex psychopathology in the form of PTSD and borderline personality disorder can be viewed from the pathways perspective as physiological and psychological self-protective and adaptive mechanisms present in the context of the abusive environment. Such an alternative pathway appears to persist so that once the child is in a more benign environment, these adaptations to the abusive context become detrimental or less functional than nontraumatic coping strategies. In some cases, as is evident with the sexually abused girls, long-term patterns of thinking and feeling become the primary patterns of interaction and are classified as trauma-related characterological disorders such as borderline personality disorder.

The Corpus Callosum, the Frontal Cortex, Cerebral Lateralization, and Maltreated Children's Negativity Bias and Affective Splitting and Merging

The corpus callosum, the frontal cortex, and cerebral lateralization also appear to be affected by the severe stress of child maltreatment. The corpus callosum connects the right and left cerebral hemispheres (Berrebi et al., 1988; Juraska & Kopcik, 1988; Lauder, 1983). Most communications between regions of the cortex in different hemispheres are carried across the corpus callosum. Several studies have found a volume reduction in sections of the corpus callosum in children with substantiated histories of abuse and concurrent psychiatric disorder (DeBellis et al., 1999; Teicher et al., 1997, 2000). These studies highlight gender differences: boys overall and more markedly boys with a history of neglect, as well as sexually abused girls, seem to be particularly susceptible to the effects of abuse on the corpus callosum. These findings are potentially serious because reduced size of the corpus callosum is associated with reduced communication between the hemispheres (Yazgan, Wexler, Kinsbourne, Peterson, & Leckman, 1995).

In addition, prefrontal maturation and cerebral lateralization appear to be affected by the early severe stress of child abuse and neglect. The cerebral cortex and especially the prefrontal cortex are late to develop, with myelination continuing through adolescence and midadulthood (Fuster, 1980), and are sensitive to glucocorticoid toxicity (Diorio, Viau, & Meaney, 1993). Several studies suggest that maltreated children's cortical development is attenuated and asymmetrical, especially for those with PTSD (DeBellis, Keshavan, Spencer, & Hall, 2000; Ito, Teicher, Glod, & Ackerman, 1988; Thatcher, 1992). Specifically, the frontal cortex, particularly in the left hemisphere, has been shown to lag behind in development for children with a history of abuse, in comparison to nonabused controls (Ito et al., 1988; Teicher et al., 1997). One convenient means of assessing lateralized hemispheric activity is through probe auditory evoked potentials. In Schiffer's study (Schiffer et al., 1995) adult participants with a history of trauma showed a marked suppression of the evoked potential response over the left hemisphere during recall of a neutral memory, while demonstrating a suppressed evoked potential response over the right hemisphere during recall of a difficult or disturbing memory. Nontraumatized comparison participants demonstrated equal probe-evoked amplitudes between hemispheres on both tasks.

These findings raise concerns for maltreated individuals because the prefrontal and frontal cortex regulate key aspects of the planning, coordination, and control of behavior as well as other executive function skills (for reviews, see DeBellis, 2001; Teicher et al., 2003). Alterations in these functions, coupled with possible asymmetrical development in response to trauma, may result in changes in the child's ability to integrate executive functions across context. For example, we have hypothesized that the tendency of abused children to split rather than to integrate when problem solving, especially when the topic or emotion cues memories of past trauma, is one way that this dysynchrony between hemispheres may present behaviorally. These differences may be observed through the development of polarized problem-solving schemas that are applied in specific contexts but are contradictory when examined in the context of integrated planning and problem-solving skills. This hallmark of the alternative developmental pathway model we have described may be explained, in part, through changes in the development and functioning of the frontal cortex along with the tendency of maltreated children to demonstrate asymmetrical use of the right and left hemispheres.

Functionally, alterations to the corpus callosum following child maltreatment would affect the integration of information across the two hemispheres. The two cerebral hemispheres are specialized in their information-processing abilities. For example, in most people the right hemisphere has a specialized role in the expression and perception of emotion, especially negative emotion. In the case of child maltreatment the reduced size of the corpus callosum as well as the increased dominance of the right hemisphere may manifest as a negativity bias in emotion expression and perception (DeBellis, 2001).

Such a negativity bias is well documented in research among maltreated children and adolescents, and it contrasts markedly with the normal, strong positivity bias that pervades behavior among most people (Fischer & Ayoub, 1994; Fischer et al., 1990; Greenwald et al., 2002). Using both the biological and the behavioral frameworks as models, we examined narratives of young maltreated children. In their earliest narratives about interactions with peers and caregivers, maltreated toddlers demonstrate a negativity bias, commonly initiating or choosing negative interactions, demonstrating a richer understanding of negative interactions, and characterizing themselves in predominantly negative terms (Ayoub & Raya, 1993). Specifically, they tend to spontaneously enact negative social interchanges even when offered a positive model for interaction and when scaffolded with social support for producing such a story. For example, 2.5-year-old Donald, a child in our lab, when asked to model a nice interaction of the self doll with the other friend doll, said forcefully, "Guy, you wanna fight? I'll knock you down. He fight him. They fight. You wanna fight? I'm gonna fight you. Fuck my butt, fuck it." When he is supported by the examiner who reminds him that the task is to tell a nice story, Donald tries again to replicate the nice story he has heard. With this social support, Donald is able to say, "Have some Playdough, guy, don't leave me, please don't leave me." To review, Donald at first is unable to repeat a nice story; instead, he describes an elaborate mean interaction. Support from a caring examiner helps Donald to replicate a positive response, but this nice story is followed by an abandonment theme ("don't leave me, please don't leave me"). Even at this young age, children such as Donald, who have experienced repeated maltreatment trauma, have come to expect aggression and loss rather than kindness and sustained care.

The maltreated toddlers in our lab describe their interpersonal worlds in terms of three primary schemas: (1) positive relationships are conventionalized and relatively bland; (2) positive relationships are reconstructed or converted into negative relationships (as with Donald); and (3) negative relationships are richly textured, dynamic, and often aggressive or violent (Ayoub & Raya, 1993).

In a pathways model the tendency to choose negative stories, to convert neutral and positive situations to negative ones, to worry about the loss of positive caring, and the need to be the powerful one in the interaction constitute an adaptive but vigilant approach to recurrent overwhelming negative maltreatment experiences (Crittenden, 1985; Fischer et al., 1997; Westen, 1994). Our work confirms the findings of Shields, Ryan, and Cicchetti (1991), who found that increased negative representations of preschoolers affected their relationships with peers, and those of Macfie, Cicchetti, and Toth (2001), who demonstrated that maltreated children exhibited higher levels of dissociative or splitting experiences than their nonabused counterparts. Such cumulative works reinforce both a behavioral and biological framework for understanding hypervigilance, a characteristic prominent in the alternative pathways in maltreated children. That is, if the world is threatening and dangerous, it is only reasonable to become hypervigilant to guard against such threats. The experience of trauma leads the young maltreated child to anticipate threat and danger. This altered worldview, when applied to daily living, results in a child with a dramatically divergent perspective on the world at large.

These adaptive patterns are markedly different from those of non-maltreated toddlers, who routinely produce a kind of positivity bias in which they represent themselves as nice or good and someone else as mean or bad, whether or not the circumstances warrant that evaluation (Ayoub & Fischer, 1994; Fischer, Shaver, & Carnochan, 1990). Findings of differences in critical structures (such as the corpus callosum) that support coordination across hemispheres may help to explain the negative perspectives and hypervigilant presentations of the maltreated children we evaluated. If, as in adults (Schiffer et al., 1995), there is differential use of each hemisphere, depending on the threatening nature of the events perceived, as well as increased negativity expressed by the abused participants, then use of the left hemisphere in more prominent ways would support a case for increased negativity in maltreated children. Clearly, this is a beginning hypothesis that needs further study, but may have promise for understanding the relationship between brain and behavior within the developmental pathways model.

CONCLUSION: CHILD MALTREATMENT AND THE FORMATION OF ALTERNATE DEVELOPMENTAL PATHWAYS: BRAIN–BEHAVIOR CONNECTIONS

A prevailing view drawn from the current literature on the neurobiology of child maltreatment is that the excessive stress of child maltreatment acts as a toxic agent, interfering with normal development and resulting in an altered and impaired brain. Implicit in this view is the assumption that there is one "right," "normal," "universal" developmental course, which has been altered by this extreme social condition. We have argued that development does not occur in a domain-general and unidirectional way, without regard for context (Fischer & Bidell, 1998). To accurately describe and begin to understand maltreated children's development, a framework that emphasizes the enormous variation in human development and the role of the environment in that variation is necessary. Variation is not noise or error in the data but an essential and important component of development to be studied. That premise is the starting point for the developmental pathways approach.

Through the pathways lens, maltreated children's neurodevelopmental profile looks very different. The brain is not impaired by maltreatment, but it adapts to a malevolent environment. When a child is born into a stress-filled world, he or she forms an alternate developmental pathway that includes both behavioral and brain changes as adaptations to exposure to high levels of stress hormones and other aspects of stress, moving brain and behavior to organize early in life along a stress-sensitive pathway (Seckl, 1998; Seckl, Cleasby, & Nyirenda, 2000; Welberg & Seckl, 2001). This stress-sensitive pathway allows maltreated children to protect themselves by demonstrating an acutely sensitive fight-or-flight response system in the face of environmental challenge. Unfortunately this adaptation comes at a high price. The same developmental pathway that allows for survival in a malevolent world leaves the individual at increased risk of serious health problems and psychopathology. Furthermore, these stress-sensitive adaptations become detrimental and maladaptive when the affected individuals find themselves in a more benign environment.

Shifting to the pathways approach is not simply a matter of semantics. It potentially can change the way therapists treat children and their families. In addition, it offers a different theoretical perspective for scientists studying the process of change and development in childhood, influencing the research questions asked, the methods used, and the conclusions drawn. The pathways approach encourages both researchers and therapists to understand the multiple domains and transactional nature of development and to explore the tremendous variation inherent in developmental processes and the adaptations of maltreated children. For example, there is now mounting evidence that the stable and predictable non-normative biological and behavioral patterns exhibited by maltreated children undergo a rapid reorganization toward a more normative biobehavioral response pattern after transition into sensitive and responsive care (Bruce, Kroupina, Parker, & Gunnar, 2000; Gunnar & Cheatham, 2003). Dismissing variation as error or viewing maltreated children as disordered may result in overlooking the role of plasticity and change in understanding children's ever-changing behavioral, psychological, and biological adaptations and outcomes. A maltreated child may exhibit predictable, relatively stable, non-normative biobehavioral patterns, but at the same time he or she shows much variation around this state both biologically and behaviorally (Gunnar & Donzella, 2002). These variations within the system provide the potential for new adaptation over time in response to changes in the environment.

Although the study of the neurodevelopment of maltreated children is in its infancy, with current findings needing further study and replication, early results suggest that there are likely neurobiological consequences to the experience of early maltreatment trauma. Studying child maltreatment from the biological point of view holds great promise to inform both the overall knowledge base and approaches to treatment and intervention. Research to date suggests several hypotheses about relations between biology and behavior in developmental pathways arising from maltreatment:

1. Effects on memory and behavioral inhibition may relate to changes in the hippocampus, which develops gradually over time.
2. The negative bias in behavior and the development of especially complex negative constructions of self and relationships may correspond to alterations in the amygdala and the cerebellar vermis.
3. Maltreated children's merging of positive and negative affect, combined with their strong negativity bias, may relate to changes in components of the brain that facilitate coordination, especially the corpus callosum, the frontal cortex, and hemispheric lateralization.

Of course, these three hypotheses about brain–behavior correlations are only a rough start in understanding the complex relations between brain and behavior in maltreatment. However, it is important to note that each one does support the hypothesis of an alternative developmental pathway that results from brain–behavior–environment interactions in the context of childhood maltreatment.

Effective understanding of maltreated children, involving both treatment and research, requires moving beyond misunderstanding them as delayed and dysregulated as a result of their maltreatment. Effective understanding of both the behavior and biology of children who have been maltreated requires recognizing that they develop along alternate pathways in adaptation to their maltreating, stressful world. A clear and complex picture of maltreated children becomes possible only when their development is understood as combining complex strengths and weaknesses that vary by context and are based in the worlds that they experience with their family, community, body, and brain (Fischer et al., 1997).

ACKNOWLEDGMENTS

We thank Kurt Fischer, Erin O'Connor, Pamela Raya, Elizabeth Nelson, Kyung-wha Hong, Travis Wright, and Gil Noam for their contributions to the work on which this chapter is based. The research described in this chapter was made possible in part by the Roche Relief Fund, the Milton Fund, the National Institutes of Health, and the Harvard Graduate School of Education.

NOTES

1. "Something I like about myself." A positive self-description of a girl's relationship with someone does not necessarily indicate that her relationship with that person is positive. For example, one of the girls who identified all her self-descriptions as positive had "I'm cranky," "I'm mad," "I scream," "I cry," "I want to die" for her relationship with her father. She indicated that she likes the fact that she is like this with her father and that that is why she identified these self-descriptions as positive.
2. "Something I do not like about myself."
3. DISC-C is a standardized instrument that elicits information directly from the child about the presence or absence of symptoms, behaviors, and emotions that correspond to the DSM-III diagnostic criteria for Axis 1 disorders of childhood and adolescence (Calverley, 1995, p. 70).

REFERENCES

American Psychiatric Association. (2000). *Diagnostic and statistical manual of mental disorders* (4th ed., text rev.). Washington, DC: Author.

Anderson, C., Teicher, M., Polcari, A., & Renshaw, P. (2002). Abnormal T2 relaxation time in the cerebellar vermis of adults sexually abused in childhood: Potential role of the vermis in stress-enhanced risk for drug abuse. *Psychoneuroendocrinology, 27*(1–2), 231–244.

Andreasen, N., Paradiso, S., & O'Leary, D. (1998). Cognitive dysmetria as an integrative theory of schizophrenia: A dysfunction in cortical–subcortical–cerebellar circuitry? *Schizophrenia Bulletin, 24*(2), 203–218.

Ayoub, C., & Fischer, K. (2006). Intersections among domains of development. In K. McCartney & D. Phillips (Eds.), *The Blackwell handbook of early child development* (pp. 62–82). Oxford, UK: Blackwell.

Ayoub, C., Fischer, K., & O'Connor, E. (2003). Analyzing development of working models for disrupted attachments: The case of family violence. *Attachment and Human Development, 5*(2), 97–120.

Ayoub, C., Hong, K., Wright, T., Fischer, K., & Noam, G. (2004, April). *Developmental impact of sexual abuse on adolescent girls: Negative self and self-destructive aggression.* Paper presented at the annual conference of the Society for Research in Adolescence, Baltimore, MD.

Ayoub, C., O'Connor, E., Rappolt-Schlichtmann, G., Fischer, K., Rogosh, F., Toth, S., et al. (2006). Cognitive and emotional differences in young maltreated children: Application of dynamic skill theory. *Development and Psychopathology, 18*(3), 679–706.

Ayoub, C., & Raya, P. (1993, April). *Social interactions in young maltreated toddlers: The development of self in relationships.* Paper presented at the meetings of the Society for Research in Child Development, New Orleans.

Barnett, D., Manly, J. T., & Cicchetti, D. (1993). Defining child maltreatment: The interface between policy and research. In D. Cicchetti & S. L. Toth (Eds.), *Child abuse, child development, and social policy* (pp. 7–74). Norwood, NJ: Ablex.

Berrebi, A., Fitch, R., Ralphe, D., Denenberg, J., Friedrich, V., & Denenberg, V. (1988). Corpus callosum: Region-specific effects of sex, early experience and age. *Brain Research, 438*(1–2), 216–224.

Bremner, J., Randall, P., Vermetten, E., Staib, L., Bronen, R., Mazure, C., et al. (1997). Magnetic resonance imaging-based measurement of hippocampal volume: Posttraumatic stress disorder related to childhood physical and sexual abuse—a preliminary report. *Biological Psychiatry, 41*(1), 23–32.

Briere, J. (1992a). *Child abuse trauma: theory and treatment of the lasting effects.* Newbury Park, CA: Sage.

Briere, J. (1992b). Methodological issues in the study of sexual abuse effects. *Journal of Consulting and Clinical Psychology, 60,* 196–203.

Bruce, J., Kroupina, M., Parker, S., & Gunnar, M. R. (2000, July). *The relationships between cortisol, growth retardation, and developmental delay in post-institutionalized children.* Paper presented at the International Conference on Infant Studies, Brighton, UK.

Calverley, R. (1995). *Self in relationship in depressed adolescent girls: Developmental effects of childhood sexual trauma.* Unpublished doctoral dissertation, Harvard Graduate School of Education, Cambridge, MA.

Calverley, R., Fischer, K., & Ayoub, C. (1994). Complex splitting of self-representations in sexually abused adolescent girls. *Development and Psychopathology, 6,* 195–213.

Carrion, V., Weems, C., Eliez, S., Patwardhan, A., Brown, W., Ray, R., et al. (2001). Attenuation of frontal asymmetry in pediatric posttraumatic stress disorder. *Biological Psychiatry, 50*(12), 943–951.

Cicchetti, D. (1991). Fractures in the crystal: Developmental psychopathology and the emergence of self. *Developmental Review, 11,* 271–287.

Cicchetti, D., & Toth, S. (2005). Child maltreatment. *Annual Review of Clinical Psychology, 1,* 409–438.

Courchesne, E. (1991). Neuroanatomic imaging in autism.*Pediatrics, 87*(5), 781–790.

Crittenden, P. (1985). Maltreated infants: Vulnerability and resilience. *Journal of Child Psychology and Psychiatry, 26,* 85–96.

Crittenden, P. M. (1988). Relationships at risk. In J. Belsky & T. Nexworski (Eds.), *Clinical implications of attachment theory* (pp. 136–174). Hillsdale, NJ: Erlbaum.

Cole, M., & Putnam, F. (1992). Effect of incest on self and social functioning: A developmental psychopathology perspective. *Journal of Consulting and Clinical Psychology, 60,* 174–184.

Darwish, D., Esquivel, G., Houtz, J., & Alfonso, V. (2001). Play and social skills in maltreated and nonmaltreated preschoolers during peer interactions. *Child Abuse and Neglect, 25,* 13–31.

DeBellis, M. (2001). Developmental traumatology: The psychobiological development of maltreated children and its implications for research, treatment, and policy. *Development and Psychopathology, 13,* 539–564.

DeBellis, M., Keshavan, M., Clark, D., Casey, B., Giedd, J., Boring, M., et al. (1999). Developmental traumatology. Part II: Brain development. *Biological Psychiatry, 45*(10), 1271–1284.

DeBellis, M., Keshavan, M., Spencer, S., & Hall, J. (2000). N-acetylaspartate concentration in the anterior cingulate of maltreated children and adolescents with PTSD. *American Journal of Psychiatry, 157*(7), 1175–1177.

Diorio, D., Viau, V., & Meaney, M. (1993). The role of the medial prefrontal cortex (cingulate gyrus) in the regulation of hypothalamic–pituitary–adrenal responses to stress. *Journal of Neuroscience, 13*(9), 3839–3847.

Dodge, K. A., Pettit, G. S., Bates, J., & Valente, E. (1995). Social information processing patterns partially mediate the effect of early physical abuse on later conduct problems, *Journal of Abnormal Psychology, 104,* 632–643.

Driessen, M., Herrmann, J., Stahl, K., Zwaan, M., Meier, S., Hill, A., et al. (2000). Magnetic resonance imaging volumes of the hippocampus and the amygdala in women with borderline personality disorder and early traumatization. *Archives of General Psychiatry, 57*(12), 1115–1122.

Dunn, G., Ryan, J., & Dunn, C. (1994). Trauma symptoms in substance abusers with and without histories of childhood abuse. *Journal of Psychoactive Drugs, 26*(4), 357–360.

Egeland, B., & Sroufe, L. (1981). Attachment and early maltreatment. *Child Development, 52,* 44–52.

Eigsti, I., & Cicchetti, D. (2004). The impact of child maltreatment on expressive syntax at 60 months. *Developmental Science, 7,* 88–102.

Ellason, J., Ross, C., Sainton, K., & Mayran, L. (1996). Axis I and II comorbidity and childhood trauma history in chemical dependency. *Bulletin of the Menninger Clinic, 60*(1), 39–51.

Felitti, V., Anda, R., Nordenberg, D., Williamson, D., Spitz, A., Edwards, V., et al. (1998). Relationship of childhood abuse and household dysfunction to many of the leading causes of death in adults. *American Journal of Preventive Medicine, 14,* 245–258.

Fischer, K. (1980). A theory of cognitive development: The control and construction of hierarchies of skills. *Psychological Review, 87,* 477–531.

Fischer, K., & Ayoub, C. (1994). Affective splitting and dissociation in normal and maltreated children: Developmental pathways for self in relationships. In D. Cicchetti & S. L. Toth (Eds.), *Rochester Symposium on Development and Psychopathology: Vol. 5. Disorders and dysfunctions of the self* (pp. 149–222). Rochester, NY: University of Rochester Press.

Fischer, K., Ayoub, C., Singh, I., Noam, G., Maraganore, A., & Raya, P. (1997). Psychopathology as adaptive development along distinctive pathways. *Development and Psychopathology, 9*(4), 729–748.

Fischer, K., & Bidell, T. R. (1998). Dynamic development of psychological structures in action and thought. In R. M. Lerner (Ed.), *Theoretical models of human development* (pp. 467–561). New York: Wiley.

Fischer, K., & Granott, N. (1995). Beyond one dimensional change: Parallel, concurrent, socially distributed processes in learning and development. *Human Development, 38,* 302–314.

Fischer, K., Shaver, P., & Carnochan, P. G. (1990). How emotions develop and how they organize development. *Cognition and Emotion, 4,* 81–127.

Freud, A. (1966). *The ego and the mechanisms of defense.* New York: International Universities Press. (Original work published 1936)

Fuster, J. (1980). *The prefrontal cortex: Anatomy, physiology, and neuropsychology of the frontal lobe.* New York: Raven Press.

Giedd, J., Blumenthal, J., Jeffries, N., Rajapakse, J., Vaituzis, A., Liu, H., et al. (1999). Development of the human corpus callosum during childhood and adolescence: A longitudinal MRI study. *Progress in Neuro-Psychopharmacology and Biological Psychiatry, 23*(4), 571–588.

Gould, E., & Tanapat, P. (1999). Stress and hippocampal neurogenesis. *Biological Psychiatry, 46*(11), 1472–1479.

Greenwald, A. G., Banaji, M. R., Rudman, L., Farnham, S., Nosek, B. A., & Mellott, D. (2002). A unified theory of implicit attitudes, stereotypes, self-esteem, and self-concept. *Psychological Review, 109,* 3–25.

Gunnar, M., & Donzella, B. (2002). Social regulation of the cortisol levels in early human development. *Psychoneuroendocrinology, 27*(1–2), 199–220.

Gunnar, M. R., & Cheatham, C. L. (2003). Brain and behavior interface: Stress and the developing brain. *Infant Mental Health Journal, 24,* 195–211.

Herman, J. (1992). *Trauma and recovery.* New York: Basic Books.

Ito, Y., Teicher, M., Glod, C., & Ackerman, E. (1998). Preliminary evidence for aberrant cortical development in abused children: A quantitative EEG study. *Journal of Neuropsychiatry Clinical Neuroscience, 10,* 298–307.

Ito, Y., Teicher, M., Glod, C., Harper, D., Magnus, E., & Gelbard, H. (1993). Increased prevalence of electrophysiological abnormalities in children with psychological, physical, and sexual abuse. *Journal of Neuropsychiatric Clinical Neuroscience, 5,* 401–408.

Joseph, R. (1999). The neurobiology of traumatic "dissociative" amnesia: Commentary and literature review. *Child Abuse and Neglect, 23*(8), 715–727.

Juraska, J., & Kopcik, J. (1988). Sex and environmental influences on the size and ultrastructure of the rat corpus callosum. *Brain Research, 450*(1–2), 1–8.

Lauder, J. (1983). Hormonal and humoral influences on brain development. *Psychoneuroendocrinology, 8*(2), 121–155.

Lauterbach, E. (1996). Bipolar disorders, dystonia, and compulsion after dysfunction of the cerebellum, dentatorubrothalamic tract, and substantia nigra. *Biological Psychiatry, 40*(8), 726–730.

Macfie, J., Cicchetti, D., & Toth, S. (2001). The development of dissociation in maltreated preschool-aged children. *Development and Psychopathology, 13,* 233–234.

Mostofsky, S., Reiss, A., Lockhart, P., & Denckla, M. (1998). Evaluation of cerebellar size in attention-deficit hyperactivity disorder. *Journal of Child Neurology, 13*(9), 434–439.

Mueller, E., & Silverman, N. (1989). Peer relations in maltreated children. In D. Cicchetti & V. Carlson (Eds.), *Child maltreatment: Theory and research on the causes and consequences of child abuse and neglect* (pp. 529–578). New York: Cambridge University Press.

Newport, D. J., & Nemeroff, C. B. (2000). Neurobiology of posttraumatic stress disorder. *Current Opinion in Neurobiology, 10*(2), 211–218.

Patel, P., Lopez, J., Lyons, D., Burke, S., Wallace, M., & Schatzberg, A. (2000). Glucocorticoid and mineralocorticoid receptor mRNA expression in squirrel monkey brain. *Journal of Psychiatric Research, 34*(6), 383–392.

Pollak, S., Cicchetti, D., & Klorman, R. (1998). Stress, memory, and emotion: Development considerations from the study of child maltreatment. *Development and Psychopathology, 10,* 811–828.

Pollak, S., & Sinha, P. (2002). Effects of early experience on children's recognition of facial displays of emotion. *Developmental Psychology, 38,* 784–791.

Pollak, S., & Tolley-Schell, S. (2003). Selective attention to facial emotion in physically abused children. *Journal of Abnormal Psychology, 112*(3), 323–338.

Porter, C. (2003). *Neurobehavioral sequelae of child sexual abuse.* Unpublished doctoral dissertation, Brigham Young University, Salt Lake City, UT.

Putnam, F. W. (1994). Dissociation and disturbances of self. In D. Cicchetti & S. L. Toth (Eds.), *Rochester Symposium on Development and Psychopathology: Vol. 5. Disorders and dysfunctions of the self* (pp. 251–266). Rochester, NY: University of Rochester Press.

Sapolsky, R., Krey, L., & McEwen, B. (1985). Prolonged glucocorticoid exposure reduces hippocampal neuron number: Implications for aging. *Journal of Neuroscience, 5*(5), 1222–1227.

Sapolsky, R., McEwen, B., & Rainbow, T. (1983). Quantitative autoradiography of [3H]corticosterone receptors in rat brain. *Brain Research, 271,* 331–334.

Sapolsky, R., Uno, H., Rebert, C., & Finch C. (1990). Hippocampal damage associated with prolonged glucocorticoid exposure in primates. *Journal of Neuroscience, 10,* 2897–2902.

Schiffer, F., Teicher, M., & Papanicolaou, A. (1995). Evoked potential evidence for right brain activity during the recall of traumatic memories. *Journal of Neuropsychiatric and Clinical Neuroscience, 7,* 169–175.

Schneider-Rosen, K., Braunwald, K., Carlson, V., & Cicchetti, D. (1985). Current perspectives in attachment theory: Illustration from the study of maltreated infants. In I. Bretherington & E. Waters (Eds.), *Monographs of the Society for Research in Child Development: Growing points of attachment theory and research* (Serial No. 209, pp. 194–210).

Schneider-Rosen, K., & Cicchetti, D. (1984). The relationship between affect and cognition in maltreated infants: Quality of attachment and the development of visual self-recognition. *Child Development, 55,* 648–658.

Seckl, J. (1998). Physiologic programming of the fetus. *Clinical Perionatal, 25*(4), 939–962.

Seckl, J., Cleasby, M., & Nyirenda, M. (2000). Glucocorticoids, 11beta-hydroxysteroid dehydrogenase, and fetal programming. *Kidney International, 57*(4), 1412–1417.

Shields, A., Ryan, R. M., & Cicchetti, D. (1991). Narrative representations of caregivers and emotional dysregulation as predictors of maltreated children's rejection by peers. *Developmental Psychology, 37,* 321–337.

Shipman, K., Zeman, J., Penza, S., & Champion, K. (2000). Emotion management skills in sexually maltreated and nonmaltreated girls: A developmental psychopathology perspective. *Development and Psychopathology, 12,* 47–62.

Stein, M. (1997). Hippocampal volume in women victimized by childhood sexual abuse. *Psychological Medicine, 27*(4), 951–959.

Teicher, M. (2000). Wounds that time won't heal: The neurobiology of child abuse. *Cerebrum, 2*(4), 50–67.

Terr, L. (1991). Childhood traumas: An outline and overview. *American Journal of Psychiatry, 148*(1), 10–19.

Teicher, M., Andersen, S., Dumont, N., Ito, Y., Glod, C., Vaituzis, C., et al. (2000) Childhood neglect attenuates development of the corpus callosum. *Social Neuroscience Abstracts, 26,* 549.

Teicher, M., Andersen, S., Polcari, P., Anderson, C., Navalta, C., & Kim, D. (2003). The neurobiological consequences of early stress and childhood maltreatment. *Neuroscience and Biobehavioral Reviews, 27,* 33–44.

Teicher, M., Glod, C., Surrey, J., & Swett, C. (1993). Early childhood abuse and limbic system ratings in adult psychiatric outpatients. *Journal of Neuropsychiatric Clinical Neuroscience, 5*(3), 301–306.

Teicher, M., Ito, Y., Glod, C., Andersen, S., Dumont, N., & Ackerman, E. (1997). Preliminary evidence for abnormal cortical development in physically and sexually abused children using EEG coherence and MRI. *Annals of the New York Academy of Sciences, 821,* 160–175.

Thatcher, R. (1992). Cyclic cortical reorganization during early childhood. *Brain and Cognition, 20,* 24–50.

U.S. Department of Health and Human Services. (2005). *Child maltreatment 2003.* Washington, DC: U.S. Government Printing Office.

van der Kolk, B., & Fisler, R. (1994). Childhood abuse and neglect and loss of self-regulation. *Bulletin of the Menninger Clinic, 58*(2), 145–168.

Walker, E., Unutzer, J., Rutter, M., Gelfand, A., Saunders, K., VonKorff, M., et al. (1999). Costs of health care use by women HMO members with a history of childhood abuse and neglect. *Archives of General Psychiatry, 56,* 609–613.

Welberg, L., & Seckl, J. (2001). Prenatal stress, glucocorticoids, and the programming of the brain. *Journal of Neuroendocrinology, 13*(2), 113–128.

Westen, D. (1994). The impact of sexual abuse on self structure. In D. Cicchetti & S. L. Toth (Eds.), *Disorders and dysfunctions of the self* (Vol. 5, pp. 223–250). Rochester, NY: University of Rochester Press.

CHAPTER 13

Corticolimbic Circuitry and Psychopathology

DEVELOPMENT OF THE CORTICOLIMBIC SYSTEM

Francine M. Benes

Several brain regions play a role in the integration of affective experience with higher cognitive function. Papez (1937) was the first to draw attention to the fact that links between limbic structures and the neocortex are responsible for the integration of emotion with cognition; he emphasized that the hippocampus, with its extensive limbic connections, and the cingulated cortex, with its elaborate reciprocal interactions with other associative cortical regions, form a central loop of connections. Today, we understand that this so-called "loop of Papez" is only one component in a much more extensive network integrating phylogenetically older and newer portions of the brain. The cortical regions that contribute to this system include not only the hippocampal formation and cingulated cortex, but also the entorhinal region, the prefrontal area, frontal eye field 8, and the inferior parietal lobe (Benes, 1993a); together, these cortical areas subsume, respectively, affective, attentional, motivational, and logical planning components of complex behavioral responses. Although frontal eye field 8 and the inferior parietal lobe do not have direct connections with subcortical limbic structures, they are nevertheless integral to complex behav-

331

iors involving limbic activity, because phylogeneses has established an obligatory (albeit an indirect) role for these regions.

To understand how emotional responses are integrated with thought processes, it is useful to examine the anatomy of the various brain regions that participate in this integration process. Although a discussion of these structures, as they are found in normal adults, can undoubtedly lend some insight into how the brain may achieve a harmonious collaboration between the limbic system and the neocortex, it does not tell us how such a cooperative interplay has been achieved. For this reason, it is useful to examine how such a complex system has been assembled as a result of both phylogenetic and ontogenetic development of the brain. A developmental approach of this type can potentially help us understand not only how the brain has attained its characteristic functions, but also how these functions can be disturbed by perturbations of normal ontogeny.

Yakovlev and Lecours (1967) emphasized that maturation of the human brain follows a sequentially timed process in which phylogenetically older portions of the brain, such as the spinal cord, mature before phylogenetically newer portions, such as the neocortex. Although there are similarities between the evolution of the brain and its early development, there are nevertheless also striking differences. For the purposes of the present discussion, the parallelism identified between phylogenetic evolution and ontogenetic maturation provides a unique opportunity to explore the roots of the emotional and cognitive behaviors found in humans. The discussion that follows begins with a comparison of the hippocampal formation and the neocortex in premammalian species, such as reptiles, with those encountered in mammals, particularly rodents, primates, and humans; however, its main focus is a review of the ontogenetic development of these structures and cortical neurotransmitters in the mammalian brain.

ARCHI- AND ALLOCORTICAL STRUCTURES

The most significant advance in the evolution of the corticolimbic system occurred during the transition from submammalian to mammalian species. In reptiles, the forebrain is composed of a thin cortical mantle surrounding a region called the anterior dorsal ventricular ridge, which invaginates into the lateral ventricle (see Figure 13.1). Although simple in organization, the cortical mantle in reptiles has several different subsidiary areas, including the medial, mediodorsal, dorsal, and lateral regions (Sarnat & Netsky, 1974). Homology of cortical areas found in reptiles with areas found in mammalian brain has been inferred from identified connection patterns with subcortical structures, such as the hypothalamus and the septal region (Bruce & Butler, 1984), as well as with other cortical regions (Ulinski,

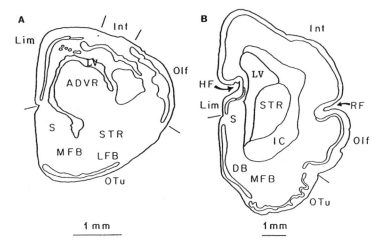

FIGURE 13.1. A comparison of transverse sections through the telecephalon of a reptile (*A*: lizard) and a mammal (*B*: opossum). (*A*) In lizards, the telecephalon has a lateral ventricle surrounded by the pallial region consisting of limbic (Lim; medial and dorsomedial), intermediate (Int; dorsal), and olfactory (Olf; lateral) cortex. In the ventral region, the sepal area (S) is found medially beneath Lim and is dorsal to the medial forebrain bundle (MFB), lateral forebrain bundle (LFB), and olfactory tubercle (OTu). (*B*) In the opossum, the telecephalon has a lateral ventricle (LV) in a position similar to that seen in the lizard. The pallial region also contains three main subdivisions: The limbic cortex (Lim) and hippocampal formation (HF) are found medially; the intermediate cortex (IC) is found dorsally; and the olfactory cortex (OLF) is found laterally, immediately ventral to the rhinal fissure (RF). The RF is not found in the lizard telencephalon. The septal area (S) of the opossum lies ventral to the Lim, and more ventrally, the medial forebrain bundle (MFB) is found. The striatum (STR) in the mammalian telencephalon forms the lateral wall of the ventricle. In lizards (*A*), the striatum is ventrolateral to the anterior dorsal ventricular ridge (ADVR), a component of the cortex that is not found in mammals. The overall appearance of a transverse section through the telecephalon of early mammals, such as marsupials and monotremes, appears similar to that of lizards because there is no corpus callosum, as seen in higher placental mammals. Reproduced with kind permission from Springer Science and Business Media from Ulinski, P. S. (1990). The cerebral cortex of reptiles. In E. G. Jones & A. Peters (Eds.), *Cerebral cortex* (pp. 139–215). New York: Plenum Press.

1990; Ulinski & Peterson, 1981). Its connections with subcortical limbic structures, such as the hypothalamus and septal region, and its extensive intracortical connections have led to the suggestion that the mediodorsal complex is "limbic cortex" (Ulinski, 1990). Additional evidence indicating that the medial–dorsomedial cortex of reptiles is an early homologue of the hippocampal formation comes from the cytology of its neurons and its unique three-layered or trilaminar organization, which is also found in the area dentate and CA subfields of the mammalian hippocampus or archicortex (Ulinski, 1990; see Figure 13.1). Interestingly, neurons in the medial cortex frequently contain zinc (Lopez-Garcia, Martinez-Guijarry, Berbel, & Garcia-Verdugo, 1988; Perez-Clausell, 1988), which is also abundant in the hippocampal formation of the mammalian brain (Haug, 1965; Rosene & Van Hoesen, 1987). Thus, mediotemporal structures in mammals have extensive limbic and intracortical connections that are believed to have first appeared in rudimentary form early in phylogenesis and to have established a foundation for the later appearance of the more intricate corticolimbic system in mammals. In contrast, the dorsal (general) cortex of reptiles may be a precursor of other motor, sensory, and tertiary neocortical regions in the brains of mammalian forms (Bishop, 1959; Herrick, 1933; Orrego, 1961).

THE "LIMBIC LOBE" AND THE EXPANSION OF THE CORTEX

In the course of evolution from reptiles to mammals, there was a transitional form, called *therapsids,* which acquired certain features of mammals (Broom, 1932). Examination of cranial remains of therapsids has revealed evidence consistent with the acquisition of hair, sweat glands, and improved masticatory mechanisms (MacLean, 1985). Broca (1878) noted that in parallel with the first appearance of mammalian features in vertebrates, a *limbic lobe,* consisting of the septal nuclei, amygdala, hippocampus, parahippocampal (entorhinal) cortex, and cingulate gyrus, appeared along the midsagittal plane of virtually all mammalian forms. Interestingly, the elaboration of this so-called *limbic lobe* coincided with the appearance of audition, vocalization, maternal nurturance, and separation calls by the young, suggesting that the integration of visceral responses with cortically mediated behaviors might have facilitated the protection of young offspring (MacLean, 1985). Accordingly, the evolutionary trend toward developing more elaborate behaviors to nurture the young and presumably to perpetuate the species probably involved a corresponding increase in both the amount and complexity of cortical ties with limbic structures. Within the spectrum of mammalian forms, there has been a striking increase in the relative proportion of neocortex. Figure 13.2 shows a comparison of the limbic lobe in rat, cat, and monkey brains (MacLean, 1954).

It is evident from the diagram that there has been a progressive increase in the volume of neocortex surrounding the cingulated and parahippocampal gyri. In primates and humans, this expansion has been accompanied by the most extensive elaboration of connectivity between

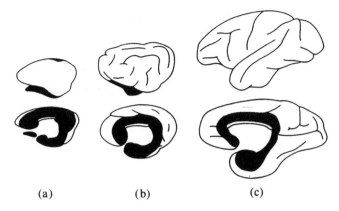

(a)   (b)   (c)

FIGURE 13.2. The "limbic lobe" of the rat (A), cat (B), and monkey (C). According to Broda, the limbic lobe in the human brain consists of several regions, lying along the midsagittal plane, that are similar in subhuman species. It includes the cingulate cortex above, forming a contiguous ring with the parahippocampal gyrus and the hippocampal formation immediately below. Rostral to the hippocampus are the amygdala and, somewhat more medially, the septal nuclei (not shown). As mammalian forms evolved, the general configuration of medial limbic structures was maintained as the neocortex gradually expanded around them. From MacLean, P. D. (1954). Studies on limbic system (visceral brain) and their bearing on psychosomatic problems. In E. R. C. Wittkower (Ed.), *Recent developments in psychosomatic medicine* (pp. 101–125). London: Sir Isaac Pribram and Sons, Ltd. and Philadelphia: J. B. Lippincott Co.

associative cortical regions (e.g., the cingulate region and the hippocampal formation) and the subcortical limbic system (Figure 13.3). The anterior cingulated cortex is involved in the mediation of autonomic and visceral responses (Anand & Dua, 1956; Kaada, 1960; Kaada, Pribram, & Epstein, 1949; Van der Kooy, McGinty, Koda, Gerfen, & Bloom, 1982), making this region a particularly key element in the acquisition of complex emotional behaviors, such as those that are integral to the formation of family units as seen in primates and humans (MacLean, 1985). The visceral and autonomic behaviors elicited by stimulation of the cingulate gyrus are mediated through direct connections of this region with primitive brainstem structures (Figure 13.3), such as the periaqueductal gray (Beckstead, 1979; Domesick, 1969; Hurley, Herbert, Moga, & Saper, 1991; Wyss & Sripanidkulchai, 1984), the nucleus solitarius, and the dorsal motor nucleus of the vagus (Terreberry & Neafsey, 1983, 1987). The spinal cord intermediolateral cell column that gives rise to preganglionic sympathetic fibers also receives direct descending influences from the cingulated gyrus (Hurley et al., 1991). It seems likely that nurturant behaviors would be

The Corticolimbix System

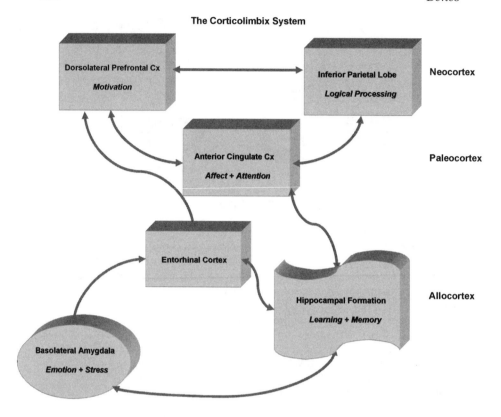

FIGURE 13.3. The corticolimbic system in mammalian brain. An inclusive view of the corticolimbic circuitry of the mammalian brain as consisting of several cortical areas. During the evolution of earliest mammals, the amygdala and hippocampal regions, also called allocortex, developed in relation to basic survival functions but are present only in rudimentary form. As mammals continued to evolve, the paleocortex, including the cingulate gyrus, appeared and attained a remarkable degree of development in rodents. Eventually, in primates and humans, the dorsolateral prefrontal cortex and inferior parietal lobe both became prominent components of the neocortex and helped to mediate executive functions, such as motivation, and intellectual ones, such as logical processing, respectively.

accompanied by emotional responses that include visceral changes. Thus, the complex behaviors embodied in nurturance probably require interplay between cortical and subcortical mechanisms, and the connectivity of the anterior cingulated area is consistent with its proposed role in this function.

The prefrontal area is generally not the first cortical region that comes to mind in relation to the limbic system; however, neuroanatomical investigations have shown that there are extensive reciprocal connections between the dorsolateral prefrontal area and both the cingulated gyrus and the entorhinal cortex (Goldman-Rakic, Selemon, & Schwartz, 1984; Swanson & Kohler, 1986). In this way, the prefrontal area can interface with subcortical limbic structures via these latter two mesocortical regions and the hippocampal formation. Accordingly, the volitional and motivational activity mediated through the prefrontal region can be driven, in part, by limbically derived responses processed through the hippocampal formation and its ties with the amygdala, septal nuclei, and lateral hypothalamus (Figure 13.3), or through the anterior cingulated region and its connections with subcortical regions at various levels of the neuraxis. Another associative cortical region that is particularly well developed in higher mammals is the inferior parietal area, which is believed to play a central role in logical planning (Luria, 1973). Like the prefrontal cortex, this region also has extensive connections with the cingulate cortex, but interacts directly with the hippocampal formation via the presubiculum as well (Seltzer & Van Hoesen, 1979).

The above discussion illustrates that the brain, not having a specific mechanism for deleting phylogenetically older circuits, has integrated some older circuits with newly acquired ones within the corticolimbic system. As a result, there has been a progressive increase in the integration of higher cognitive processes with visceral and instinctual behaviors mediated through subcortical limbic structures. In the human brain, this additive tendency that has occurred during phylogeny has probably been adaptive, because it is doubtful that the human species could have survived without limbic-driven emotions and instincts plus cortically driven logical planning and volition.

THREE- AND SIX-LAYERED CORTEX

To understand how the brain has achieved an exquisite harmony between the cortical and subcortical components of the corticolimbic system, it is useful to examine more closely the cytoarchitectural organization within the cortex of higher mammals and to compare it with that found in reptiles. As noted previously, the cortex of reptiles has a simple three-layered organization (Ulinski, 1977). In the mammalian neocortex, however, the intrinsic organization is much more complex and has been expanded into six layers, which can be distinguished from one another according to the density and size of neurons, as well as their morphological appearance. For example, layer I has sparse numbers of relatively small interneurons, whereas layers II, III, V, and VI contain large numbers of so-called *pyramidal neurons,* which typically project their axons out of the cortex to other distal sites. In contrast, layer IV contains abundant numbers of small inter-neurons, called *granule cells*. With this layer as a reference point, the deeper layers (V and VI) are called *infragranular layers* and the superficial layers (I–III) the *supragranular layers*.

Interestingly, there is a basic dichotomy between infra- and supra-granular layers of the mammalian cortex. Pyramidal neurons in layers V and VI project axons primarily to subcortical structures, whereas those in layers II and III send their axons preferentially to other cortical sites (Jones, 1984). Layer IV receives a rich supply of afferents from the thalamus (White, 1986), whereas layer I has a large number of incoming associated inputs from other cortical regions (Marin-Padilla, 1984). Thus, these latter two receptive layers reflect the subcortical and corticocortical relationship of the other infragranular and supragranular projections layers, respec-tively. In a very general sense, then, the phylogenetic development of the cortex has involved an expansion from three to six layers, and it is of more than passing interest that the three supragranular layers have a more spe-cific role in processing associative activity, with an ever-increasing role in phylogenetically more advanced species such as primates and humans. Interestingly, the thickness of the supragranular layers is proportional to the amount of associative activity that a particular region mediates. For example, the primary visual cortex has a rudimentary amount of the supragranular layers I–III, whereas the tertiary visual association area 19 has a well-developed supragranular zone. Supramodal (tertiary) cortical regions that are purely associative in nature, such as the cingulated cortex, prefrontal areas, and inferior parietal areas, have the most extensive devel-opment of the upper three layers. Overall, the marked expansion of the associative cortex that has occurred in relation to phylogenesis of the brain has involved a dramatic increase in supragranular laminar processing.

ONTOGENESIS OF THE HIPPOCAMPAL REGION

The hippocampal region of the mammalian brain includes the area dentate, the hippocampus proper, the subicular complex, and the entorhinal cortex (Stanfield & Cowan, 1988). Generally speaking, the development of this region involves a carefully timed sequence of events that occurs in virtually all mammalian species, although the period during which the sequential changes occur may be quite different among mammalian forms. For exam-ple, in rats the cells of the region superior (CA1-CA2) are produced within the last half of gestation (Angevine, 1965; Stanfield & Cowan, 1988), whereas in monkeys they are produced during the first half (Rakic &

Nowakowski, 1981). There is also a general tendency for neurons of the hippocampus to be generated internally by mitotic proliferation of precursor elements within a zone closely apposed to the ventricular surface (Angevine, 1965; Rakic & Nowakowski, 1981; Stanfield & Cowan, 1988). When mitoses are complete for a given cell, it begins to migrate upward and eventually assumes its proper position. This *inside-out* progression occurs for the hippocampus proper, the subicular complex, and the entorhinal cortex. For the area dentate, however, the disposition of this subregion within the hippocampal formation is such that the cells migrate in an *outside-in* manner. Thus, the direction of migration is not universal but rather occurs in relation to where the proliferative epithelial zone is found. A second type of developmental gradient occurs along the axis lying between the entorhinal cortex and the area dentata, the *rhinodentate axis* (Stanfield & Cowan, 1988). Specifically, neurons in the entorhinal cortex and area dentata develop earlier, whereas cells in the center of this axis (subicular complex and hippocampus proper) appear later (Rakic & Nowakowski, 1981; Schlessinger, Cowan, & Swanson, 1978).

Developmental changes in the area dentata may continue well into postnatal life. For example, in rats, the numbers of dentate granule cells have been reported to increase during both the juvenile and adult periods (Bayer, Yackel, & Puri, 1982). Some additional evidence has also suggested that the cells arising postnatally may be derived from mitotic neuroblasts (Kaplan & Bell, 1984). These newly generated granule cells of the area dentata may also give rise to axonal projections into subfields CA3 and CA4 of the hippocampus (Stanfield & Trice, 1988). Evidence for postnatal increases of granule cells has not been found in rhesus monkeys, however (Eckenhoff & Rakic, 1988). As yet, no studies have investigated whether similar postnatal changes may occur in the area dentata of the adult human brain, although preliminary evidence suggests that they do not (unpublished data, 1993).

Interestingly, there are some parallels between the ontogenetic development of the hippocampal formation and its evolution in vertebrates. Some investigators believe that the development of the human telecephalon at 8 weeks *in utero* is comparable to that of mature amphibians (Hoffman, 1963), whereas it is thought at 10 weeks to be similar to that of reptiles (Crosby, 1917) and early mammalian forms. In the 8-week-old fetus, at rostral levels of the forebrain, the septal nuclei are immediately ventral to the fornix and medial frontal cortex; at more caudal levels, the fornix is contiguous with the hippocampus (Rakic & Yakovlev, 1968), which also occupies a medial location. Thus, there are similarities in the appearance and relationships of cortical and limbic structures in the forebrains of submammalian and early mammalian species, as well as in the human fetus. The early appearance of limbic cortical structures in the medial forebrain of the human fetus parallels that of phylogenetically earlier forms that lack neocortex; this finding underscores the idea that these regions are developmental precursors to the mesocortical cingulated gyrus, and later, the neocortical prefrontal and inferior parietal lobes (see next section).

ONTOGENESIS OF THE NEOCORTEX

Generally speaking, cortical regions differentiate and mature at varying intervals that reflect phylogeneses. For example, limbically related cortical regions are among the earliest to differentiate. As shown in Table 13.1, by 16–19 weeks of gestational age in humans, the cingulate region is discernible as a gyrus, and at 20–23 weeks the parahippocampal gyrus can be distinguished in the medial temporal area (Gilles, Shankle, & Dooling, 1983). On the other hand, the superior and mediofrontal gyri (prefrontal regions) do not take on a gyral pattern until 24–27 weeks of gestational age, and the angular and supramarginal gyri (inferior parietal area) are not discernible until 28–31 weeks (Gilles et al., 1983).

Within individual cortical regions, ontogenesis follows a carefully timed sequence of events (Poliakov, 1965; Rakic, 1981; Sidman & Rakic, 1973) that also parallels phylogenesis. As in the hippocampal region during ontogeny, all cortical neurons emanate from a region near the ventricular surface. This *marginal zone* appears early and is increasingly displaced outward as precursor cells of the ventricular zone undergo several mitotic divisions and give rise to an intermediate zone between them. According to

TABLE 13.1. Embryonic Development of the Cortical Gyri in Humans

Gestational age (weeks)	Gyri
16–19	Gyrus rectus, insula, cingulate
20–23	Parahippocampal, superior temporal
24–27	Pre- and postrolandic, middle temporal, superior and middle
28–31	Frontal, occipital, cuneus, lingual
32–35	Superior and inferior temporal, medial and lateral orbital, callosomarginal
36–39	Angular, supramarginal, transverse temporal, paracentral, orbital

Note. Data from Gilles, Shankle, and Dooling (1983).

Poliakov (1965), there are five stages of human cortical development. Stage 1 begins at approximately week 7, when postmitotic cells begin to move upward to a position between the intermediate and marginal zones and form an area called the *cortical plate*. In Stage 2, at 10–11 weeks, the cortical plate becomes progressively thicker and more compact; afferent fibers, probably originating in the thalamus, begin to appear in the intermediate zone below the cortical plate. During Stage 3, at 11–13 weeks, the cortical plate has two distinct parts: an inner zone with more mature cells that have an elongated shape and a diffuse distribution and an outer zone with densely packed immature cells. During Stage 4, the ventricular zone becomes less prominent as cells are completing their mitotic division and migrating outward, toward the cortical plate. The longest period is Stage 5, which begins at the 16th fetal week and continues into the early postnatal period. During this stage, postmitotic neuronal cells continue migrating and reach their final destination within the cortical plate.

As neurons enter the cortical plate, those destined for more superficial layer arrive later than those that occupy deeper layers. Accordingly, the cortex, like the hippocampus, shows an *inside-out* progression of development (Rakic, 1974). Studies in humans have shown that by 7 months of gestation, layers V and VI have attained a more advanced degree of development than layers II and III (Marin-Padilla, 1970a). The morphological differentiation of neurons in the various layers mirrors this migratory process, such that large pyramidal neurons with a well-developed dendritic arborization and basket cells (inhibitory interneurons) can be distinguished in deeper layers sooner than in superficial layers (Marin-Padilla, 1970a). By 7.5 months *in utero*, pyramidal neurons in deeper portions of layer III are first beginning to show differentiation of an apical dendrite extending into layer I, whereas in layers V and VI these cells already have elaborate dendritic arborizations. Interestingly, during this same interval, incoming afferent fibers are present in virtually all layers of the cortex. In the months immediately prior to birth, interneurons with a basket cell appearance begin to appear in the deeper portions of layer III, whereas in layers II and outer portions of III they are first beginning to form. By birth, both the second and third laminae contain pyramidal neurons; however, basket cells in layer II are largely absent (Marin-Padilla, 1970b). By 2.5 months postnatally, pyramidal neurons continue to mature, showing a dramatic increase in overall size, in the amount of dendritic branching, and in the numbers of dendritic spines (Michel & Garey, 1984). Interestingly, layers VI and I (the marginal zone) are the first laminae to appear, whereas layers II and III are the last to form and the latest to mature (Marin-Padilla, 1970b).

A COMPARISON OF CORTICAL PHYLOGENY
AND ONTOGENY

It can be seen from the discussion above that there is some tendency for the ontogenesis of the six-layered cortex in mammalian brain to reflect its phylogenetic development. As noted previously, the expansion of the neocortex that has occurred in relation to mammalian evolution has been accompanied by an increase from three to six layers. As shown in Figure 13.4, the supragranular layers are predominantly involved in associative connections and are most extensive in tertiary supramodel regions that have expanded in relative size during evolution. The fact that layers II and III are last to form and mature during mammalian development is in accordance with the idea that similarities between normal ontogenesis and phylogeny can be identified.

Accordingly, the ontogenetic development of layer II may reflect some of the phylogenetic changes that have been traced within this lamina (Sanides, 1969). In certain types of lower mammals, layer II shows an accentuated appearance, resulting from a higher density of neuronal cell bodies; in higher mammals, a lower density of neurons is typically found in this layer (Abbie, 1942). Interestingly, 8-month-old human fetuses also show a similar accentuation of the second lamina, but this disappears during the postnatal period (Sanides, 1969), presumably as increased amounts of neuropil, arising from the elaboration of dendritic branches and synaptic connections, accumulate in layer II of adult primates and humans. Accordingly, it is likely that the high density of neurons in layer II in lower mammals is the result of a much lower quantity of synaptic connections. Thus, both phylogenetic and ontogenetic information concerning laminar organization point to late developmental changes in layer II as a characteristic feature.

Interestingly, in turtles, fibers projecting from the thalamus to the cortex terminate in layer I (Hall & Ebner, 1970); in the mammalian brain, by contrast, these thalamocortical afferents are preponderantly found in layer IV. Thus, in this respect, layer IV of mammals has some homology with layer I in reptiles. The fact that the ontogenetic development of the cortex occurs in an inside-out fashion, with layer IV appearing before layer I and containing a phylogenetically older afferent supply from the thalamus, is consistent with this general idea. It is important to emphasize, however, that neither supragranular nor infragranular layers are exclusively engaged in corticocortical or subcortical processing, respectively. For example, layer I in reptiles receives afferent inputs not only from the thalamus (Hall & Ebner, 1970) but also from other cortical regions, whereas layer I of the cingulated region in mammals also receives afferent fibers from certain

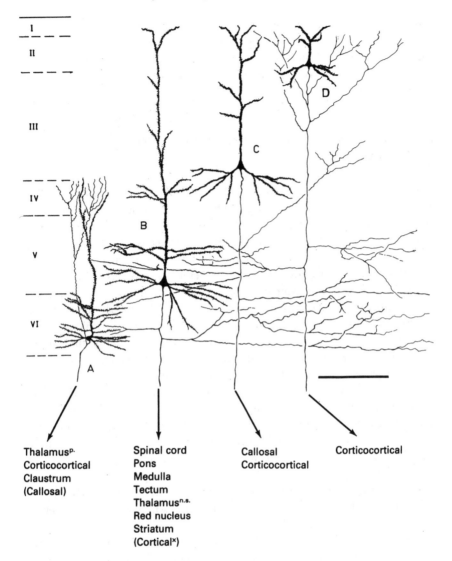

Thalamus[p.]
Corticocortical
Claustrum
(Callosal)

Spinal cord
Pons
Medulla
Tectum
Thalamus[n.s.]
Red nucleus
Striatum
(Cortical[x])

Callosal
Corticocortical

Corticocortical

FIGURE 13.4. A schematic diagram demonstrating the destination of axons of pyramidal neurons in layers II, III, V, and VI of the neocortex. Those in the superficial layers project to other cortical sites, whereas those in deeper laminae project to subcortical regions such as the thalamus, basal ganglia, brainstem, and spinal chord. Reproduced with kind permission from Springer Science and Business Media from Jones, E. G. (1984). Laminar distribution of cortical efferent cells. In A. Peters & E. G. Jones (Eds.), *Cerebral cortex* (pp. 521–548). New York: Plenum Press.

thalamic nuclei (Vogt, Rosene, & Peters, 1981). Thus, it is primarily of heuristic value to emphasize the similarities between phylogeneses and ontogenesis, and in doing so, it is important to avoid the implication that the upper cortical layers were simply added on top of the deeper layers during evolution.

THE DEVELOPMENT OF AFFERENT INPUTS TO THE CORTEX

During normal brain development, the entry of various types of afferent fibers to the cortex also follows a carefully timed sequence. Two principal inputs to the cortex, one arising from the thalamus and one from the contralateral cortex, show such a sequential progression. During prenatal stages in rats, fibers from the thalamus extend toward the cortical mantle and either stop immediately beneath or begin to enter layer IV (Wise & Jones, 1978). In the rat somatosensory cortex, the ingrowth of thalamo-cortical fibers toward specific neuronal elements, particularly those in layer IV, continues after parturition and is not complete until approximately the third postnatal day (Wise & Jones, 1978). In contrast, commissural inputs arising from homologous cortex of the opposite hemisphere begin entering the somatosensory cortex at 5 days postnatally and attain a mature degree of connectivity by day 7 (Wise & Jones, 1978). Thus, pyramidal cell axons grow toward their sites of termination before their dendritic arbors have developed, suggesting that the elaboration of the dendritic tree and the formation of spines on pyramidal neurons may be regulated by extrinsic influences from incoming afferent fibers originating in other cortical areas (Wise, Fleshman, & Jones, 1979).

Interestingly, in primates, the destination toward which commissural afferents travel is determined by the region from which they originate (Goldman-Rakic, 1981). Thus, commissural afferents arising from cortex and surrounding the principal sulcus of the dorsolateral prefrontal area will grow toward the principal sulcus of the opposite hemisphere during the prenatal period (Goldman-Rakic, 1981). If, however, the contralateral cortex to which the fibers would ordinarily project is surgically removed, these commissural afferent fibers deviate from their intended path and course toward a more dorsal location, where they will then enter the cortex to form synaptic connections. Although much of normal brain development is tightly programmed, cortical afferents appear to have considerable flexibility as to where they can terminate, and perturbations of normal developmental sequences can result in the formation of aberrant connections in the cortex of primates (and probably also in humans). Such a process could contribute to the development of psychopathology later in life (Benes, 1993a).

An important developmental change involving projections of the amygdala to the anterior cingulate cortex occurs during the equivalent of adolescence in the rat brain (Plate 13.1). In a recent study using anterograde tracing, a subdivision of the basolateral amygdala showed an increased penetration of labeled fibers in layers II and V of this cortical region (Cunningham, Bhattacharyya, & Benes, 2002). The terminations of these fibers engage in synaptic connections with dendritic spines of pyramidal neurons, but also form nonsynaptic appositions with dendritic shafts of aspiny neurons. The increase of these connections occurs between birth and the beginning of the early adult period. It is well established that the amygdala plays a pivotal role in mediating emotional responses, particularly under conditions of stress (see next section). It seems likely, therefore, that these connections with cingulate neurons may contribute to the integration of affective experiences, with higher cortical functions mediated through the cingulate region.

MYELINATION OF KEY CORTICOLIMBIC PATHWAYS

A broadly accepted marker for the functional maturation of the central nervous system is the acquisition of myelin sheaths around axon shafts. Myelin is the insulating sheath that surrounds axons and enhances conduction velocity; its appearance during development signals the acquisition of functional capabilities for the pathways along which it occurs. It has long been known that various neural pathways myelinate at different stages of development (Flechsig, 1920). There is a general tendency, however, for more cephalad structures to myelinate later than those more caudad, and for subcortical pathways to myelinate before cortical associational paths. For example, the medial longitudinal fasciculus, a pathway that is found along the entire extent of the spinal cord and brainstem, begins myelinating as early as week 20 of the gestational period, whereas the medial lemniscus, a pathway confined to the brainstem, shows similar changes at week 24 (Gilles et al., 1983). Within the cerebral hemispheres, the posterior limb of the internal capsule begins myelinating at week 32, whereas the anterior limb does not show evidence of myelin until week 38. Interestingly, proximal portions of the cingulum bundle do not show evidence of myelin until gestational weeks 38–39 (Gilles et al., 1983), but probably continue myelinating well into the postnatal period (see Figure 13.5). Some paths such as the fornix and mammillothalamic tract, which are not associative in nature, do not begin to myelinate until weeks 44 and 48, respectively. Since the fornix provides an afferent flow from the hippocampal formation to the mammilary body of the posterior hypothalamus, and the mammillo-thalamic tract in turn conveys information to the anterior nucleus of the thalamus, both of these pathways are important components of the loop of Papez and, in a larger sense, the corticolimbic system (see Figure 13.2).

Other cortically based links within this system, however, do not myelinate until well into the postnatal period (Benes, 1989; Benes, Turtle, Khan, & Farol, 1994). For example, the perforant pathway (entorhinal cortex to presubiculum) actively myelinates during postnatal life (see Figure 13.5). After a plateau during the third and fourth decades, myelin increases along the surface of the parahippocampal gyrus during the fifth and sixth decades (Benes, 1989; Benes et al., 1994). As noted in the section on hippo-campal development, the granule cells of the area dentata, to which the perforant pathway axons send a direct projection, may increase in number postnatally in rats. Although similar increases in granule cell numbers have not, as yet, been demonstrated in the human brain, it seems likely that changes in myelination and conduction along the perforant pathway fibers projecting to granule cells in the area dentata do occur. In this setting, other, subtler changes in granule cells at both the cellular and molecular levels could occur, even in the absence of increases in their overall number.

The observation of increasing myelination in the perforant pathway and distal portions of the cingulum bundle, described above, is noteworthy for two reasons. First, it has long been believed that late postnatal changes of this type may occur in the human brain. Yakovlev and Lecours (1967), in noting sequential myelination of the spinal cord, brainstem, and telen-cephalic structures, suggested that the intracortical associational pathways may continue myelinating as late as the fourth decade. Although this paper is often cited as if it had presented empirical evidence for such changes, no data were, in fact, included. The first empirical evidence for such adult developmental changes did not appear until the aforementioned study (Benes, 1989; see Plate 13.1) and its more recent replication and extension (Benes et al., 1994). Second, it is interesting to note that the observation of late myelination of the perforant pathway and distal cingulum bundle pres-ents an unexpected paradox regarding human behavior and development. It has been generally held that late postnatal myelination probably occurs last in the phylogenetically most sophisticated regions of the brain, the associative neocortex, because this would reflect the overall tendency for brain development to parallel phylogeny. It is ironic that this latter idea would have been correct if the associative cortical pathways showing these late postnatal changes were of the neocortical type. Instead, the ones impli-cated in this late myelination are mesocortical transitional types (i.e., the

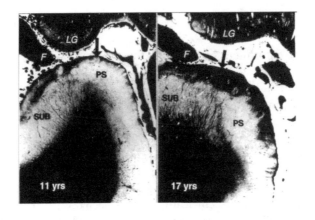

PERFORANT PATHWAY AND DISTAL CINGULUM BUNDLE

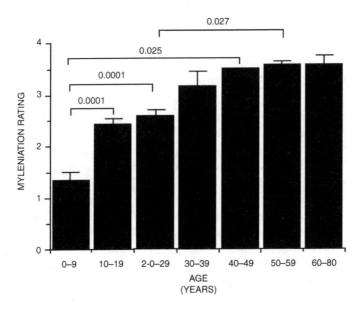

FIGURE 13.5. Postnatal increases of myelination in the hippocampal formation. (*A*) Photomicrographs showing differences in the amount of myelin staining in an 11-year-old (*left*) and a 17-year-old (*right*). (*B*) A set of graphs showing the area of myelin staining in the superior medullary lamina along the surface of the subiculum and presubiculum. Between the first and second decades, there is a doubling in the area of myelin staining ($p = 0.0000005$), then a plateau during the third and fourth decades. Later during the fifth and sixth decades, there is an additional 50% increase in myelin staining. Reproduced with permission from the American Medical Association from Benes, F. M., Turtle, M., Khan, Y., & Farol, P. (1994). Myelination of a key relay zone in the hippocampal formation occurs in the human brain during childhood, adolescence, and adulthood. *Archives of General Psychiatry, 51,* 477–484.

cingulated and entorhinal cortices), and the pathways showing the changes, rather than projecting "upward," send fibers "downward" toward the primitive allocortex of the hippocampal formation. It may be inferred from the known connection patterns of this latter cortical region that increased conduction occurring along the perforant pathway and distal cingulum bundle would probably enhance the flow of activity toward the limbic system. Perhaps it can be concluded from these unexpected findings that late postnatal maturational changes in the human brain, and presumably in human behavior, would involve a tighter modulation of emotional responses in relation to neocortically driven mechanisms. Thus, it would appear from the discussion of the findings illustrated in Plate 13.1 that the advanced phase of human development during adulthood may involve a more effective interplay between cognitive processing and emotional reactivity.

INTEGRATION OF EMOTION

Emotional expression is an attribute that first became apparent in mammals. It is probably mediated in part by primitive relays in the brainstem reticular formation, hypothalamus, amygdala, and septal nuclei. Papez (1937) was the first to postulate that the cingulate gyrus may play a role in the integration of emotional experience with cognition, because it has extensive connections not only with the limbic system but also with other associative cortical regions involved in higher cognitive functions. Consistent with this idea, autonomic responses have been altered by either stimulation or ablation of the anterior cingulate cortex. With electrical stimulation of this region in primates, visceromotor responses—such as eyelid opening, pupillary dilation, respiratory movements, cardiovascular changes, and piloerection (Anand & Dua, 1956; Kaada et al., 1949; Smith, 1945), as well as changes in facial expression (Smith, 1945) and motor arrest (Dunsmore & Lennox, 1950), have been induced. Extensive surgical ablation of the anterior cingulate cortex, in contrast, has resulted in a decrease of emotional responsiveness (Ward, 1948) and even personality changes characterized by either inappropriate purring or growling without provocation in cats (Kennard, 1955). In humans, bilateral infarction of the cingulate gyrus has been associated with increased docility and indifference (Laplane, Degos, Baulac, & Gray, 1981) and an inability to express or experience emotion (Damasio & Van Hoesen, 1983).

The anterior cingulate region has extensive reciprocal connections with several different areas that include the basolateral amygdala, prefrontal region, the presubiculum, and the inferior parietal lobe (Jones & Powell, 1970; Pandya & Kuypers, 1969; Petras, 1971; Seltzer & Pandya,

1978; Seltzer & Van Hoesen, 1979; Van Hoesen, 1982). It is very important to note that the anterior cingulate region also has both afferent and efferent connections with nuclear groups that mediate autonomic functions, such as the periaqueductal gray (Beckstead, 1979; Hurley et al., 1991; Wyss & Sripanidkulchai, 1984), the nucleus solitarius, the dorsal motor nucleus of the vagus (Hurley et al., 1991; Terreberry & Neafsey, 1983; Van der Kooy et al., 1982), and preganglionic sympathetic neurons in the intermediolateral cell column of the thoracic spinal cord (Hurley et al., 1991). Therefore, the anterior cingulate cortex interacts directly with centers that mediate both viscerosensory and visceromotor responses in the periphery, and these connections are believed to be fundamental to its role in integrating emotional responses at the cortical level (Neafsey, Terreberry, Hurley, Ruit, & Frysztak, 1993). Both ablation (Kennard, 1955; Laplane et al., 1981; Ward, 1948) and stimulation (Anand & Dua, 1956; Kaada, 1960) of the anterior cingulate cortex have resulted in autonomic as well as affective changes. In humans with documented seizure activity arising from the cingulate cortex (Devinsky & Luciano, 1993), emotional stimulation is a frequent precipitant of ictal activity (Mazars, 1970), and the majority of such patients exhibit limbically related features such as temper tantrums and fixed psychoses (Mazars, 1970).

The amygdala is a complex corticolimbic region that lies at the temporal pole of the mammalian brain. Considered by some to be an "arbitrarily defined set of cell groups," there are nevertheless subdivisions of this region that can be distinguished by their characteristic architecture, embryogenesis, neurotransmitter profiles, and connectivity and functional roles (Swanson & Petrovich, 1998). The basolateral nuclear complex appears to play a salient role in associative learning and attention (Gallagher & Holland, 1994). This region regulates sensorimotor gating of the acoustic startle response (Wan & Swerdlow, 1997) and contributes to fear conditioning, possibly through a mechanism involving its GABAergic interneurons (Stutzmann & LeDoux, 1999). As discussed above, the postnatal ingrowth of amygdalar fibers into the anterior cingulate cortex, which extends into the early adult period, may play a role in emotional maturation, particularly as it relates to the integration of affect with higher cognitive functions.

LINKAGE OF EMOTION AND ATTENTION

Some researchers believe that the cingulate and parietal cortices may cooperate in the performance of direct attention (Mesulam, 1983). In monkeys (Glees, Cole, Whitty, & Cairns, 1950) and cats (Kennard, 1955), bilateral lesions of the anterior cingulate cortex have been associated with neglect of surrounding objects, including cagemates. In humans with bilateral infarction of the cingulate gyrus, a lack of attentiveness to the surrounding environment has similarly been observed (Laplane et al., 1981), and a cerebral blood flow study reported that human subjects show a marked increase of activity in the anterior part of this region during performance of a Stroop attentional conflict paradigm (Pardo, Pardo, Janer, & Raichle, 1990). The neglect occurring with lesions of the cingulate cortex is thought to involve alterations in the relationship of this area with frontal eye field 8 (Belaydier & Maugierre, 1980), but this may be an indirect effect mediated via the prefrontal and inferior parietal areas. Interestingly, patients with unilateral neglect syndromes associated with lesions of the frontal or parietal regions also show some emotional disturbances, suggesting that there is "a parallelism in the integrity of attention and emotion" (Mesulam & Geschwind, 1978, p. 252).

It is noteworthy that, in monkey posterior parietal cortex, some neurons are activated by hand–eye-coordinated movements, particularly when desirable objects that can satisfy thirst or hunger are employed as targets (Mountcastle, Lynch, Georgopoulos, Sakuta, & Acuna, 1975). Such motivationally driven responses are thought to require both an emotional and an attentional component (Mesulam & Geschwind, 1978). Consistent with this proposal, the inferior parietal region has extensive connections with the anterior cingulate cortex and the presubiculum (Jones & Powell, 1970; Pandya & Kuypers, 1969; Petras, 1971; Seltzer & Pandya, 1978), two important corticolimbic relay areas. Although Luria (1973) emphasized the role of the left (dominant) inferior parietal region in the construction of logical–grammatical relationships, he also noted unilateral neglect syndromes in patients with right-sided posterior parietal lesions. These patients not only neglect extracorporeal space on the left side but also show a peculiar inability to perceive their deficits. It now appears that an anterior attention system mediated by the anterior cingulate area plays a role in semantic processing of words, and the degree of blood flow increases in this region as the number of targets increases (Posner, Peterson, Fox, & Raichle, 1990). In contrast to the contribution of the anterior system to target detection, the posterior attention system is involved in visuospatial shifts of focus (Posner & Peterson, 1990). Both systems seem to be essential to normal attention.

MOTIVATION REQUIRES AFFECT

There is also an important interaction between motivation and affect in humans, as illustrated by a rather distinctive clinical syndrome called *akinetic mutism* that occurs in patients with bilateral occlusion of the anterior cerebral arteries (Barris & Schumann, 1953; Nielsen & Jacobs, 1951) that supply the anterior cingulate cortices and other midsagittal cortical regions. Acute infarctions of this type are associated with an inability to move or speak, as well as considerable negativism. This is quite similar to the catatonic state, wherein muteness, lack of movement, and negativism are also observed. Patients with akinetic mutism who later recover describe a sudden loss of the experience of affect and a concomitant absence of the will to move (Damasio & Van Hoesen, 1983). It seems likely that the extensive reciprocal connectivity between the anterior cingulate region and the prefrontal cortex that plays a direct role in the mediation and volitional drives (Luria, 1973) probably accounts for some of the symptomatology observed in akinetic mutism. Similar defects in motivation and emotional experience are commonly seen in adults with schizophrenia; these defects are thought to arise from a disturbance in connectivity between the dorsolateral prefrontal area and the anterior cingulate cortex (Benes, 1993b).

MATERNAL NURTURANCE, SEPARATION, AND SOCIAL INTERACTIVENESS

In rodents, ablations of the cingulate gyrus are associated with a loss of maternal activities such as nursing, nest building, and retrieval of the young (Slotnick, 1967; Stamm, 1955). It has been suggested that separation calls and play activities—features observed in mammalian offspring—may have emerged in parallel with the development of the cingulate gyrus during the phylogenetic progression of reptiles into mammals (MacLean, 1985). In support of this hypothesis, vocalizations can be elicited by stimulation of the anterior cingulate region in monkeys (Ploog, 1979; Smith, 1945), whereas more extensive ablations that also include the medial subcallosal and preseptal cingulate cortices result in a complete loss of spontaneous isolation calls (MacLean, 1985). In a clinical case report, a child with documented cingulate seizures was noted to run toward her mother during ictal episodes (Geier et al., 1977), an observation suggesting that the cingulate cortex plays a role in human separation behaviors as well (MacLean, 1985). It is not known, however, whether the cingulate gyrus can be implicated in the separation anxiety seen in children.

CINGULATE CORTEX AS KEYSTONE IN CORTICOLIMBIC FUNCTION

Based on the information presented thus far, it can readily be seen that the cingulate region is a central component in a broadly distributed network of cortical and subcortical regions that subsume functions that are altered in disorders of emotion and cognition. In addition to the connections described in the previous sections, and as shown in Figure 13.3, the cingulate cortex is also connected with the dorsolateral prefrontal area, frontal eye field 8, and the inferior parietal lobe. The prefrontal and anterior cingulate cortices receive a rich supply of dopamine afferents from the midbrain ventral tegmental area (Lindvall & Bjorklund, 1984). Some of the areas indicated are phylogenetically newer cortical regions (e.g., the dorsolateral prefrontal and inferior parietal regions) that are most extensively developed in human brain. In contrast, the hippocampal formation is phylogenetically the oldest cortical region and is believed to have first appeared, in a rudimentary form, in reptiles (Ulinski, 1990). The cingulate gyrus is a transitional cortex, or so-called *mesocortex*, that first appeared in early mammals (MacLean, 1990). The anterior portion of this gyrus provides a link between the autonomic centers controlling visceral activity and the neocortical regions, represented in Figure 13.3, that are involved in motivation, attention, and logical processing.

By examining the corticolimbic regions and their interconnections, as illustrated in Figure 13.3, it can be appreciated that defective circuitry in one or several of these areas could give rise to abnormalities in the integration of emotional experience, selective attention, and other neocortically mediated functions such as volition and cognition. Therefore, pathological processes that have an impact on one or several of these corticolimbic regions could give rise to a broad spectrum of symptoms that encompass both the emotional and the cognitive spheres.

IMPLICATIONS FOR THE DEVELOPMENT OF PSYCHOPATHOLOGY

It is well known that various forms of psychopathology show characteristic ages of onset. For example, autism tends to present between 2 and 3 years of age (see also Dawson & Bernier, Chapter 2, and Pelphrey & Carter, Chapter 3, this volume), whereas schizophrenic symptoms begin to appear at approximately 16 years of age, but continue to increase in complexity and intensity for another 5–10 years. It has been suggested that the onset of mental illness in vulnerable individuals may reflect the occurrence of normal developmental changes in the brain. Increases in the maturity of cortical circuitry, including the formation of functional synaptic relationships and the myelination of specific pathways, could serve as "triggers" for the onset of psychopathology (Benes, 1989). Whereas some have emphasized that a defect of synaptic elimination, which normally occurs in the cortex between 5 and 15 years of age, may be the "trigger" in schizophrenia (Feinberg, 1982), others have countered this idea with evidence suggesting that there are major fiber systems growing into the cortex through the period of childhood, adolescence, and even early adulthood (Benes, Vincent, Molloy, & Khan, 1996; Cunningham et al., 2002). In reality, both phenomena may be occurring at the same time: some synapses—presumably ones that are functionally weak—may be retracting as others that have inherently greater strength are undergoing sprouting. Based on what is known about the postnatal development of the medial prefrontal cortex, it seems reasonable to assume that there are complex interactions occurring among various fiber systems, such as those that employ 5-hydroxytryptamine (5-HT) or dopamine as neurotransmitters (Bolte Taylor, Cunningham, & Benes, 1998; Cunningham, Connor, Zhang, & Benes, 2005). The convergence and plasticity of these monoaminergic systems with respect to GABAergic interneurons may provide a neural substrate for the formation of aberrant connection patterns in individuals who carry the susceptibility for various types of psychopathology (Benes, Taylor, & Cunningham, 2000).

CONCLUSIONS

It is evident from the above discussion that the anterior cingulate cortex occupies a unique position in the corticolimbic system of the mammalian brain. Having no homologue in submammalian species and being among the first cortical regions to appear during prenatal development, it is safe to assume that it has an intimate involvement in the mediation of behaviors that are involved in emotional responses to environmental stimuli. Although it is often considered to be *paleocortex,* and therefore primitive in the nature of its functioning, it can also be considered to be *neocortical* in nature, having well-developed supragranular layers. Indeed, it is the upper layers of the cingulate cortex that allow the anterior portion of this region to interact extensively with other neocortical regions and create a network through which limbic-driven emotions can be integrated with higher cognitive functions. It seems reasonable to assume that the associative connections of the anterior cingulate region are most abundant in the human brain among mammalian species because the neocortex is of the greatest size in humans. In terms of cognitive function, this relationship implies that cognitive function in humans may involve the greatest degree of emotional context. On the surface, this view may seem antithetical to conventional perspectives of human cognition that emphasize our ability to think logically and make judgments based on ethical and moral considerations. Although this ability is certainly present, the great paradox and irony inherent in the organization of the human brain is the fact that these "higher" cognitive functions may be driven, not always by the dorsolateral prefrontal cortex, but at least to some degree by the limbic system. What is it that makes us so unique among mammalian species? Is it our massive associational cortices? Or is it the fact that these associations must come to terms with concurrent emotional responses?

This question becomes most critical when we factor in the postnatal development of the human brain during adolescence. The teenage period is a time when active myelination occurs within the limbic lobe (see Figure 13.5) as well as in the prefrontal cortex (Paus et al., 1999). Adolescence is also a period during which major changes in behavior are obviously occurring and these, to a large extent, involve emotional responses to the environment. Indeed, adolescence can be thought of as the period when the greatest degrees of emotional maturation and maternal separation are occurring. Because such changes cannot occur in a neural vacuum, it can be safely assumed that the limbic lobe and its connectivity with many other neocortical areas are changing during this developmental epoch. Accordingly, there must be increased interplay between emotional maturation and cognitive functions. Piaget noted that abstract reasoning develops just prior to the early teen period (Piaget, 1952). The ontogenetic changes occurring during the teen period probably bring the ability to think in the abstract with the ability to experience emotions at the gut level. When these developmental changes proceed in accordance with a carefully timed set of rules that dictates how connections are laid down, then they may "trigger" the ability to think in a goal-directed manner. On the other hand, if these same changes occur in an individual who carries susceptibility genes for a major psychiatric disorder, such as schizophrenia, then they may be a trigger for the appearance of a mental illness phenotype.

Our understanding of the pathophysiology of psychiatric illness will have to take into account a complex interplay between the various risk factors for these illnesses and normal developmental changes in the brain. On the one hand, it is likely that a genetic factor and/or an acquired insult to the brain can alter normal brain development, perhaps focally or in a generalized way. On the other hand, once the brain of an individual who is at risk for a mental illness has been affected by adverse environmental factors, then normal ontogenetic changes may trigger their expression during critical periods of postnatal development. The inherited risk factors for autism are probably different from those for schizophrenia, and the types of environmental factors that influence their expression may also be different. In applying a developmental approach to the study of mental illnesses that present during childhood, adolescence, and adulthood, it will be necessary to define the unique neurobiological consequences of abnormal genes found in relation to each of these illnesses, and to establish an understanding of how the expression of such genes intersects with normal developmental brain changes at critical periods of the life cycle. Overall, it seems reasonable to assume that late maturational changes in the limbic lobe and other regions of the cortex can be related to either normal or abnormal behavioral manifestations.

REFERENCES

Abbie, A. A. (1942). Cortical lamination in a polyprodont marsupial, perameles natusa. *Journal of Comparative Neurology, 76,* 509–536.

Anand, B. K., & Dua, S. (1956). Circulatory and respiratory changes induced by electrical stimulation of the limbic system (visceral brain). *Journal of Neurophysiology, 19,* 393–400.

Angevine, J. B. (1965). Time of neuron origin in the hippocampal region: An autoradiographic study in the mouse. *Experimental Neurology, 13,* 1–70.

Barris, R. W., & Schumann, H. R. (1953). Bilateral anterior cingulate gyrus lesions: Syndrome of the anterior cingulate gyri. *Journal of Neurology, 3,* 44–52.

Bayer, S. A., Yackel, J. W., & Puri, P. S. (1982). Neurons in the dentate gyrus granular layer substantially increase during juvenile and adult life. *Science, 216,* 890–892.

Beckstead, R. M. (1979). An autoradiographic examination of corticocortical and subcortical projections of the mediodorsal projections (prefrontal) cortex in the rat. *Journal of Comparative Neurology, 184,* 46–62.

Belaydier, C., & Maugierre, F. (1980). The duality of the cingulate gyrus in monkey. Neuroanatomical study and functional hypothesis. *Brain, 130,* 525–554.

Benes, F. M. (1989). Myelination of cortical–hippocampal relays during late adolescence. *Schizophrenia Bulletin, 15,* 585–593.

Benes, F. M. (1993a). Neurobiological investigations in cingulate cortex of schizophrenic brain. *Schizophrenia Bulletin, 19,* 537–549.

Benes, F. M. (1993b). Neurobiological investigations in cingulate cortex of schizophrenic brain [Review]. *Schizophrenia Bulletin, 19,* 537–549.

Benes, F. M., Taylor, J. B., & Cunningham, M. C. (2000). Convergence and plasticity of monoaminergic systems in the medial prefrontal cortex during the postnatal period: Implications for the development of psychopathology. *Cerebral Cortex, 10,* 1014–1027.

Benes, F. M., Turtle, M., Khan, Y., & Farol, P. (1994). Myelination of a key relay zone in the hippocampal formation occurs in the human brain during childhood, adolescence, and adulthood. *Archives of General Psychiatry, 51,* 477–484.

Benes, F. M., Vincent, S. L., Molloy, R., & Khan, Y. (1996). Increased interaction of dopamine-immunoreactive varicosities with GABA neurons of rat medial prefrontal cortex occurs during the postweanling period. *Synapse, 23,* 237–245.

Bishop, V. M. (1959). The relation between nerve implications of the afferent innervation of cortex. *Journal of Nervous and Mental Disease, 1281,* 89–114.

Bolte Taylor, J., Cunningham, M. C., & Benes, F. M. (1998). Neonatal raphe lesions increase dopamine fibers in prefrontal cortex of adult rats. *NeuroReport, 9,* 1811–1815.

Broca, P. (1878). Anatomie comparee des circonvolutions cerebrales: Le grand lobe limbique et la scissure limbique dans la serie des manmiferes. *Review of Anthropology, 1,* 385–498.

Broom, R. (1932). *The mammal-like reptiles of South Africa and the origin of mammals.* London: Witherby.

Bruce, L. L., & Butler, A. B. (1984). Telencephalic connections in lizards. *Journal of Comparative Neurology, 229,* 585–601.

Crosby, E. C. (1917). The forebrain of alligator mississippiensis. *Journal of Comparative Neurology, 27,* 325–402.

Cunningham, M. G., Bhattacharyya, S., & Benes, F. M. (2002). Amygdalo–cortical sprouting continues into early adulthood: Implications for the development of normal and abnormal function during adolescence. *Journal of Comparative Neurology, 453,* 116–130.

Cunningham, M. G., Connor, C. M., Zhang, K., & Benes, F. M. (2005). Diminished serotonergic innervation of adult medial prefrontal cortex after 6–OHDA lesions in the newborn rat. *Brain Research: Developmental Brain Research, 157,* 124–131.

Damasio, A. R., & Van Hoesen, G. W. (1983). Emotional disturbances associated with focal lesions of the limbic frontal lobe. In K. M. Heilman & P. Satz (Eds.), *Neuropsychology of human emotion* (pp. 85–110). New York: Guilford Press.

Devinsky, O., & Luciano, D. (1993). The contributions of cingulate cortex to human behavior. In B. A. Vogt & M. Gabriel (Eds.), *Neurobiology of cingulate cortex and limbic thalamus* (pp. 527–556). Boston: Birkhauser.

Domesick, V. B. (1969). Projections from the cingulate cortex in the rat. *Brain Research, 12,* 296–320.

Dunsmore, R. H., & Lennox, M. A. (1950). Stimulation and strychninization of supracallosal anterior cingulate gyrus. *Journal of Neurophysiology, 13,* 207–213.

Eckenhoff, M. F., & Rakic, P. (1988). Nature and fate of proliferative cells in the hippocampal dentate gyrus during the life span of the rhesus monkey. *Journal of Neuroscience, 8,* 2729–2747.

Flechsig, P. (1920). *Anatomie des menschlichen Gehirns und Ruckenmarks auf myelogenetischer.* Leipzig: Gundlange.

Gallagher, M., & Holland, P. C. (1994). The amygdala complex: Multiple roles in associative learning and attention. *Proceedings of the National Academy of Sciences, 91,* 11771–11776.

Geier, S., Bancaud, J., Talairach, J., Bonis, A., Szikla, G., & Enjelvin, M. (1977). The seizures of frontal lobe epilepsy: A study of clinical manifestations. *Neurology, 27,* 951–958.

Gilles, F. H., Shankle, W., & Dooling, E. C. (1983). Myelinated tracts: Growth patterns. In F. H. Gilles, A. Leviton, & E. C. Dooling (Eds.), *The developing human brain: Growth and epidemiologic neuropathology* (pp. 117–183). Boston: Wright-PSG.

Glees, P., Cole, J., Whitty, W. M., & Cairns, H. (1950). The effects of lesions in the cingulate gyrus and adjacent areas in monkeys. *Journal of Neurology and Neurosurgery, 13,* 178–190.

Goldman-Rakic, P. S. (1981). Development and plasticity of primate frontal association cortex. In F. O. Schmitt (Ed.), *The organization of the cerebral cortex* (pp. 69–100). Cambridge, MA: MIT Press.

Goldman-Rakic, P. S., Selemon, L. D., & Schwartz, M. L. (1984). Dual pathways connecting the dorsolateral prefrontal cortex with the hippocampal formation and parahippocampal cortex in the rhesus monkey. *Neuroscience, 12,* 719–743.

Hall, W. C., & Ebner, F. F. (1970). Thalamotelencephalic projections in the turtle (*Pseudemys scripta*). *Journal of Comparative Neurology, 140,* 101–122.

Haug, F. M. (1965). Electron microscopic localization of the zinc in the hippocampal mossy fiber synapses by a modified silver sulfide procedure. *Histochemistry, 8,* 355–368.

Herrick, C. J. (1933). The function of the olfactory parts of the cerebral cortex. *Proceedings of the National Academy of Sciences, 19,* 7–14.

Hoffman, H. H. (1963). The olfactory bulb, accessory olfactory bulb and hemisphere of some anurans. *Journal of Comparative Neurology, 120,* 317–368.

Hurley, K. M., Herbert, H., Moga, M. M., & Saper, C. B. (1991). Efferent projections of the infralimbic cortex of the rat. *Journal of Comparative Neurology, 308,* 249–276.

Jones, E. G. (1984). Laminar distribution of cortical efferent cells. In A. Peters & E. G. Jones (Eds.), *Cerebral cortex* (pp. 521–548). New York: Plenum Press.

Jones, E. G., & Powell, T. P. S. (1970). An anatomical study of converging sensory pathways within the cerebral cortex of the monkey. *Brain, 93,* 793–820.

Kaada, B. R. (1960). Cingulate, posterior orbital, anterior insular and temporal pole cortex. In F. Field (Ed.), *Handbook of physiology* (pp. 1345–1372). Washington, DC: American Physiological Society.

Kaada, B. R., Pribram, K. H., & Epstein, J. A. (1949). Respiratory and vascular responses in monkeys from temporal pole, insula, orbital surface and cingulate gyrus. *Journal of Neurophysiology, 12,* 347–356.

Kaplan, M. S., & Bell, D. H. (1984). Mitotic neuroblasts in the 9-day-old and 1-month-old rodent hippocampus. *Journal of Neuroscience, 4,* 1429–1441.

Kennard, M. A. (1955). The cingulate gyrus in relation to consciousness. *Journal of Nervous and Mental Disease, 121,* 34–39.

Laplane, D., Degos, J. D., Baulac, M., & Gray, F. (1981). Bilateral infraction of the anterior cingulate gyri and of the fornices. *Journal of Neurological Sciences, 51,* 289–300.

Lindvall, O., & Bjorklund, A. (1984). General organization of cortical monoamines. In L. Descarries, T. R. Reader, & H. H. Jasper (Eds.), *Monoamine innervation of cerebral cortex* (pp. 9–40). New York: Liss.

Lopez-Garcia, C., Martinez-Guijarry, F. J., Berbel, P., & Garcia-Verdugo, J. M. (1988). Long-spined polymorphic neurons of the medial cortex of lizards: A Golgi, Timm and electron microscopic study. *Journal of Comparative Neurology, 272,* 409–423.

Luria, A. R. (1973). *The working brain.* New York: Basic Books.

MacLean, P. D. (1954). Studies on limbic system (visceral brain) and their bearing on psychosomatic problems. In E. R. C. Wittkower (Ed.), *Recent developments in psychosomatic medicine* (pp. 101–125). Philadelphia: Lippincott.

MacLean, P. D. (1985). Brain evolution relating to family, play and the separation cell. *Archives of General Psychiatry, 42,* 405–417.

MacLean, P. D. (1990). *The triune brain in evolution: Role in paleocerebral functions.* New York: Plenum Press.

Marin-Padilla, M. (1970a). Prenatal and early postnatal ontogenesis of the human motor cortex: A Golgi study: I. The sequential development of the cortical layers. *Brain Research, 23,* 167–183.

Marin-Padilla, M. (1970b). Prenatal and early postnatal ontogenesis of the human motor cortex: A Golgi study: II. The basket–pyramidal system. *Brain Research, 23,* 185–191.

Marin-Padilla, M. (1984). Neurons of layer: I. A developmental analysis. In A. Peter & E. G. Jones (Eds.), *Cerebral cortex* (pp. 447–478). New York: Plenum Press.

Mazars, G. (1970). Criteria for identifying cingulate epilepsies. *Epilepsia, 11,* 41–47.

Mesulam, M.-M. (1983). The functional anatomy and hemispheric specialization of directed attention: The role of the parietal lobe and its commentary. *Trends in Neuroscience, 6,* 384–387.

Mesulam, M.-M., & Geschwind, N. (1978). On the possible role of neocortex and its limbic connections in the process of attention and schizophrenia: Clinical cases of inattention in man and experimental anatomy in monkey. *Journal of Psychiatric Research, 14,* 249–259.

Michel, A. E., & Garey, L. H. (1984). The development of dendritic spines in the human visual cortex. *Human Neurobiology, 3,* 223–227.

Mountcastle, V. B., Lynch, J. C., Georgopoulos, A., Sakata, H., & Acuna, C. (1975). Posterior parietal association cortex of the monkey: Command functions for operations within extrapersonal space. *Journal of Neurophysiology, 38,* 871–908.

Neafsey, E. J., Terreberry, R. R., Hurley, K. M., Ruit, K. G., & Frysztak, R. J. (1993). Anterior cingulate cortex in rodents: Connections, visceral control functions and implications for emotion. In B. A. Vogt & M. Gabriel (Eds.), *Neurobiology of cingulate cortex and limbic thalamus* (pp. 206–223). Boston: Birkhauser.

Nielsen, J. M., & Jacobs, L. L. (1951). Bilateral lesions of the anterior cingulate gyri: Rreport of a case. *Bulletin of the Los Angeles Neurological Societies, 18,* 231–234.

Orrego, F. (1961). The reptilian forebrain: I. The olfactory pathways and cortical areas in the turtle. *Archives of Italian Biology, 99,* 425–445.

Pandya, D. N., & Kuypers, H. G. J. M. (1969). Cortico–cortical connections in the rhesus monkey. *Brain Research, 13,* 13–36.

Papez, J. W. (1937). A proposed mechanism of emotion. *Archives of Neurology and Pathology, 38,* 725–743.

Pardo, J. V., Pardo, P. J., Janer, K. W., & Raichle, M. E. (1990). The anterior cingulate cortex mediated processing selection in the Stroop attentional conflict paradigm. *Proceedings of the National Academy of Sciences, 87,* 256–259.

Paus, T., Zijdenbos, A., Worsley, K., Collins, D. L., Blumenthal, J., Giedd, J. N., et al. (1999). Structural maturation of neural pathways in children and adolescents: *In vivo* study. *Science, 283,* 1908–1911.

Perez-Clausell, J. (1988). The organization of zinc-containing fields in the brains of the lizard *Podaris hispanica*: A histochemical study. *Journal of Comparative Neurology, 267,* 589–593.

Petras, J. M. (1971). Connections of the parietal lobe. *Journal of Psychiatric Research, 8,* 189–201.

Piaget, J. (1952). *The origins of intelligence in children.* New York: International Universities Press.

Ploog, D. W. (1979). Phonation, emotion, cognition with references to the brain mechanisms involved. In *Brain and Mind Ciba Foundation series* (pp. 79–98). Amsterdam: Exerpta Medica.

Poliakov, G. I. (1965). Development of the cerebral neocortex during the first half of intrauterine life. In S. A. Sarkisov (Ed.), *Development of the child's brain* (pp. 22–52). Leningrad: Medicina.

Posner, M. I., & Peterson, S. E. (1990). The attention system of the human brain. *Annual Review of Neuroscience, 13,* 25–42.

Posner, M. I., Peterson, S. E., Fox, P. T., & Raichle, M. E. (1990). Localization of cognitive operations in the human brain. *Science, 240,* 1627–1631.

Rakic, P. (1974). Neurons in rhesus monkey visual cortex: Systematic relation between time of origin and eventual disposition. *Science, 183,* 425–427.

Rakic, P. (1981). Developmental events leading to laminar and area organization of the neocortex. In F. O. Schmitt (Ed.), *The organization of the cerebral cortex* (pp. 7–28). Cambridge, MA: MIT Press.

Rakic, P., & Nowakowski, R. (1981). The time of origin of neurons in the hippocampal region of the rhesus monkey. *Journal of Comparative Neurology, 196,* 99–128.

Rakic, P., & Yakovlev, P. I. (1968). Development of the corpus callosum and septum cavi in man. *Journal of Comparative Neurology, 132,* 45–72.

Rosene, D. L., & Van Hoesen, G. W. (1987). The hippocompal formation of the primate brain. In A. Peters & E. G. Jones (Eds.), *Cerebral cortex* (pp. 345–456). New York: Plenum Press.

Sanides, F. (1969). Comparative architectonics of the neocortex of mammals and their evolutionary interpretation. In J. M. Petras & C. R. Noback (Eds.), *Comparative and evolutionary aspects of the vertebrate central nervous system* (pp. 404–423). New York: New York Academy of Sciences.

Sarnat, H. B., & Netsky, M. G. (1974). *Evolution of the nervous system.* New York: Oxford University Press.

Schlessinger, A. R., Cowan, W. M., & Swanson, L. W. (1978). The time of origin of neurons in Ammon's horn and the associated retrohippocampal fields. *Anatomy and Embryology, 154,* 153–173.

Seltzer, B., & Pandya, D. N. (1978). Afferent cortical connections and architectonics of the superior temporal sulcus and surrounding cortex in the rhesus monkey. *Brain Research, 149,* 1–24.

Seltzer, B., & Van Hoesen, G. W. (1979). A direct inferior parietal lobule projection to the presubiculum in the rhesus monkey. *Brain Research, 179,* 157–161.

Sidman, R., & Rakic, P. (1973). Neuronal migration with special reference to developing human brain. *Brain Research, 62,* 1–35.

Slotnick, B. M. (1967). Disturbances of maternal behavior in the rat following lesions of the cingulate cortex. *Behavior, 24,* 204–236.

Smith, W. D. (1945). The functional significance of the rostral cingulate cortex as revealed by its responses to electrical excitation. *Journal of Neurophysiology, 8,* 241–255.

Stamm, J. S. (1955). The function of the median cerebral cortex in maternal behavior of rats. *Journal of Comparative Physiology and Psychology, 48,* 347–356.

Stanfield, B. B., & Cowan, W. M. (1988). The development of hippocampal region. In A. Peters & E. G. Jones (Eds.), *Cerebral cortex* (pp. 9–132). New York: Plenum Press.

Stanfield, B. B., & Trice, J. E. (1988). Evidence that granule cells generated in the dentate gyrus of adult rats extend axonal projections. *Experimental Brain Research, 72,* 399–406.

Stutzmann, G. E., & LeDoux, J. E. (1999). GABAergic antagonists block the inhibitory effects of serotonin in the lateral amygdala: A mechanism for modulation of sensory inputs related to fear conditioning. *Journal of Neuroscience, 19,* RC8.

Swanson, L. W., & Kohler, C. (1986). Anatomical evidence for direct projections from the entorhinal area to the rat. *Journal of Neuroscience, 6,* 3010–3023.

Swanson, L. W., & Petrovich, G. D. (1998). What is the amygdala? *Trends in Neurosciences, 21,* 323–331.

Terreberry, R. R., & Neafsey, E. J. (1983). Rat medial frontal cortex: A visceromotor region with a direct projection to the nucleus solitarius. *Brain Research, 278,* 245–249.

Terreberry, R. R., & Neafsey, E. J. (1987). The rat medial frontal cortex projects directly to autonomic regions of the brainstem. *Brain Research Bulletin, 19,* 639–649.

Ulinski, P. S. (1977). Intrinsic organization of snake medial cortex: An electron microscopic and Golgi study. *Journal of Morphology, 152,* 247–280.

Ulinski, P. S. (1990). The cerebral cortex of reptiles. In A. Peters & E. G. Jones (Eds.), *Cerebral cortex* (pp. 139–215). New York: Plenum Press.

Ulinski, P. S., & Peterson, E. (1981). Patterns of olfactory projections in the desert iguana, *Dipsosaurus dorsalis. Journal of Morphology, 168,* 189–228.

Van der Kooy, D., McGinty, J. F., Koda, L. Y., Gerfen, C. R., & Bloom, F. E. (1982). Visceral cortex: Direct connections from prefrontal cortex to the solitary nucleus in the rat. *Neuroscience Letters, 33,* 123–127.

Van Hoesen, G. W. (1982). The parahippocampal gyrus. *Trends in Neurosciences, 5,* 345–350.

Vogt, B. A., Rosene, D. L., & Peters, A. (1981). Synaptic terminations of thalamic and callosal afferents in cingulate cortex of rat. *Journal of Comparative Neurology, 201,* 265–283.

Wan, F. J., & Swerdlow, N. R. (1997). The basolateral amygdala regulates sensorimotor gating of acoustic startle in the rat. *Neuroscience, 76,* 715–724.

Ward, A. A. (1948). The cingular gyrus: Area 24. *Journal of Neurophysiology, 11,* 13–23.

White, E. L. (1986). Termination of thalamic afferents in the cerebral cortex. In E. G. Jones & A. Peters (Eds.), *Cerebral cortex* (pp. 271–289). New York: Plenum Press.

Wise, S. P., Fleshman, J. W., Jr., & Jones, E. G. (1979). Maturation of pyramidal cell form in relation to developing afferent and efferent connections of rat somatic sensory cortex. *Neuroscience, 4,* 1275–1297.

Wise, S. P., & Jones, E. G. (1978). Developmental studies of thalamocortical and commissural connections in the rat somatic sensory cortex. *Journal of Comparative Neurology, 178,* 187–208.

Wyss, J. M., & Sripanidkulchai, K. (1984). The topography of the mesencephalic and pontine projections from the cingulate cortex of the rat. *Brain Research, 293,* 1–15.

Yakovlev, P., & Lecours, A. (1967). The myelinogenetic cycles of regional maturation of the brain. In A. Minkowski (Ed.), *Regional development of the brain early in life* (pp. 3–70). Oxford, UK: Blackwell.

Index

Page numbers followed by *f* indicate figure; *n* indicate note; and *t* indicate table.

The Invisible Bridge